# POPULATION HEALTH and ITS INTEGRATION INTO ADVANCED NURSING PRACTICE

# POPULATION HEALTH and ITS INTEGRATION INTO ADVANCED NURSING PRACTICE

Edited by

## Mary A. Bemker, PhD, PsyS, LADC, LPCC, CCFP, CCTP, CNE, RN

*Associate Professor, School of Nursing, Touro University Nevada*

## Christine Ralyea, DNP, MS-NP, MBA, NE-BC, CNL, OCN, CCRN

*Assistant Vice President Patient Care Services—Carolinas Medical Center
Adjunct Faculty, Queens University Charlotte, NC*

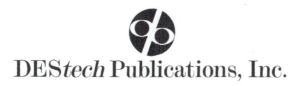

## DEStech Publications, Inc.

**Population Health and Its Integration Into Advanced Nursing Practice**

DEStech Publications, Inc.
439 North Duke Street
Lancaster, Pennsylvania 17602 U.S.A.

Printed in the United States of America
10  9  8  7  6  5  4  3  2

Main entry under title:
    Population Health and Its Integration Into Advanced Nursing Practice

A DEStech Publications book
Bibliography: p.
Includes index p. 517

Library of Congress Catalog Card No. 2018931595
ISBN No. 978-1-60595-392-2

# Table of Contents

CHRISTINE RALYEA, MARY A. BEMKER and
JENNIE PATTISON

## Section III—Tools for Managing Population Health Issues

# Foreword

THIS textbook, *Population Health and Its Integration into Advanced Nursing Practice*, is a welcome and timely addition to the nursing literature. As advanced practice nurses, we have an opportunity for a more significant and far-reaching impact on healthcare by understanding the array of determinants that impact health and by intervening to utilize comprehensive and upstream strategies and solutions. The focus on population health, as offered by this textbook, supports this level of thinking. With a concentration in advanced nursing care, population health strives toward better health outcomes for the group. Population healthcare hinges on the belief that individuals will benefit when the focus is on improving communal healthcare. The contributors to this textbook have provided readers with information on population health, its fit with advanced practice nursing care, obtaining and using data to drive health, specific population foci across the lifespan, illustrative case studies, policy considerations, education, and social media strategies as sources of health advocacy. This is a one of a kind resource that will pave the way for advanced practice nurses and other healthcare providers to see greater possibilities of practice in advancing the health of all.

EDILMA L. YEARWOOD, PhD, PMHCNS-BC, FAAN
Past-President International Society of Psychiatric Nurses
Chair, Department of Professional Nursing Practice
*Georgetown University School of Nursing & Health Studies*

# Preface

**P**OPULATION HEALTH is a topic that is central to healthcare in current times. As the world continues to shrink, care for many becomes prevention- and intervention-focused. It is important to determine how influences within population health impact healthcare for all and how to identify and analyze specific populations. It is also necessary to explain the supports and practices used by advanced practice nurses to enhance population health delivery.

Because of these two distinct needs, the present text is divided into three parts. The first part provides a global review of population health, which includes access to data and application of population health in advanced practice, and then addresses the various roles of the educator, nurse executive, and policy advocate, as these evolve in response to population health and healthcare. The specific variables that healthcare providers need to understand and make an impact in population health (PH) are explained in Chapter 1 and throughout this textbook. In the second part, population health issues that affect vulnerable groups today, such as children, the elderly, the military, substance abusers, the chronically ill, and the obese, are described as major contributing (PH) issues. Disease etiology, cultural influences, and strategies for understanding and addressing such groups are included in this section. The third part takes a deeper look at compassion fatigue and burnout, the use of coaching, social marketing, and other techniques that can foster better care delivery in special populations.

As we begin, it is important we identify what population health is.

Most healthcare leaders agree that population health is directed toward the health outcomes of a specific group of individuals—a subpopulation with specific needs. Defined by Kindig and Stoddart (2003), population health is "the health outcomes of a group of individuals, including distribution of such outcomes within the group" (p. 382). The term may also apply to the total number of residents in a geographic location (Jacobson & Teutsch, 2012; Noble & Casalion, 2013). It can denote classes of individuals with specific health problems and can be defined in terms of health status indicators influenced by a plethora of individual and environmental factors (Dunns & Hayes, 1999).

Population health is addressed best from a holistic perspective, in which it is considered in the context of healthcare in its entirety and for everyone. We are aware that the influence of one aspect of a person's life may impact all others, and the same can apply to groups. Therefore, preventative care for all and care management for those with chronic illnesses are part of this perspective. When both are done, the entire population becomes healthier.

To offer prevention or intervention services, one must understand the factors that influence health. The practitioner must realize both the health dynamics for a given population and the effects of healthcare on everyone within it. Otherwise, practitioners will be left treating symptoms and miss the big picture due to small practices.

Thus, systematic variances in patterns within and between populations need to be investigated, and policies and practices need to address these as a means to improve the overall health and well-being of vulnerable populations (Dunn & Hayes, 1999). Identifying possibilities for interdisciplinary collaboration among nurses, physicians, social workers, the public health system, other healthcare professionals, and supportive economists and demographers can clarify the population health agenda (Noble & Casalino, 2013).

We can no longer work in silos and must collectively put the patient population at the center of our consideration, as we determine how best to address the health dynamic presently confronting our profession. Therefore, this book explores major health concerns from both a theoretical and case-study perspective. Vignettes are interspersed throughout the chapters, so that the reader can consider how specific dynamics come into play within practice. Information is fine on its own; however, it is only through applying knowledge to practice that evidence can make a difference in overall health. Knowing what to do—and when and where to do it—are goals for this text.

Because the healthcare professional is key to the success of population health, support for practitioners is offered. Understanding how to educate and market to populations is critical. Ready access to screens for various conditions, such as substance use disorders and the impact of trauma, is necessary for quality care. Becoming an advocate and having a voice in the scope and role of a practice as it relates to population health are critical to keep all nurses up to speed. Therefore, chapters on these topics, as well as how to use coaching to support health changes, are included.

With many texts on population health available, why should you choose this book? *Population Health and Its Integration into Advanced Nursing Practice* is a textbook that not only looks at the overall dynamics of population health, but also focuses on how this knowledge can be used in practice. To make this easier for readers, a tool kit with key information and resources is provided for each chapter. Discussion questions that focus on application and synthesis are included, which will allow instructors and students to address topics at a graduate level.

Detailed case studies are appended at the end of each chapter. As we are all aware, healthcare is not cut and dried. We nurses cannot claim a given group has issues because of X, and if Y is done, all will be well. Rather, as advanced practitioners and potential policy influencers, we must grasp the complexities of every case we encounter and address such in hypothetical and actual interventions.

For students, applying the information in this volume to real-life situations should support and reinforce their learning and career development. For those already in practice, this text is designed to increase understanding of the highly specific, often economic and cultural, influences on patients and clients in diverse communities. Being able to recognize the social dynamics allows for better comprehension, more effective intervention, and superior outcomes.

## References

Dunns, J., & Hayes, M. (Nov/Dec1999). Toward a lexicon of population health. *Canadian Journal of Public Health Supplement*, S7–10.

Jacobson, D., & Teutsch, S. (2012). An environmental scan of integrated approaches for defining and measuring total population health by the clinical care system, the government public health system, and stakeholder organizations. Washington D.C.: National Quality Forum.

Kindig, D., & Stoddart, G. (2003). What is population health? *American Journal of Public Health, 93*, 3, p. 380–383.

Noble, D., & Casalino, L. (2013). Can accountable care organizations improve population health? *JAMA, 309*(11), 1119–1120.

# Contributing Authors

**Susan R. Allen**, PhD, RN-BC
Assistant Professor
Associate Director of DNP and CNL Programs
Xavier University School of Nursing
Cincinnati, Ohio

**Meliss V. Batchen**, DNS, RN, CFN
LOSS Team Member with St. Tammany Parish Coroner's Office
(STPCO)
Support for Suicide Survivors

**Mary A. Bemker**, PhD, PsyS, LADC, LPCC, CCFP, CCTP, CNE, RN
Associate Professor, School of Nursing
Touro University Nevada

**Mary Biddle**, DNP, RN, CNE, CCFP
Elizabethtown Community and Technical College in
Elizabethtown, Ky

**Kotaya Griffith**, MSN, RN, NP-C, CNL
Carolinas HealthCare System Senior Care, Charlotte NC
Doctoral of Nursing Practice Student at East Carolina University in
(Greenville, NC)

**Carol Ann King**, DNP, MSN, APRN, FNP-BC
Clinical Associate Professor
East Carolina University College of Nursing
Captain, United States Army Reserve/Army Nurse Corp

**Veronica LaPlante Rankin**, MSN, RN-BC, NP-C, CNL, CMSRN
Clinical Nurse Leader Program Coordinator
Affiliation: Carolinas Medical Center, Charlotte North Carolina
Assistant Professor Queens University CNL Program
Doctoral of Nursing Practice Student at East Carolina University in
(Greenville, NC)

**Patrick S. LaRose**, DNP, MSN, RN
Visiting Professor Doctor of Nursing Practice Program
Chamberlain University—College of Nursing

**Mary Lawson Carney**, DNP, RNBC, CCRN, CNE
State Associate Director of Nursing—Indiana
Western Governors University

**Nancyruth Leibold**, EdD, RN, PHN, CNE
Associate Professor in Nursing
Southwest Minnesota State University

**Camille McNicholas**, Phd LLC
Harwinton, Connecticut

**Katharine Murray**, RN, CPHIMS

**Sandra M. Olguin**, DNP, MSN, RN
Assistant Professor
University of Nevada, Reno
Chief Executive Officer
Nevada Nurses Foundation

**Jennie Pattison**, DNP, RN
Associate Dean of Faculty, MSN Specialty Track
Chamberlain University

**Cecilia Ralyea**, BS
Student at Edward Via College of Osteopathic Medicine
(Spartanburg, SC)

**Christine Ralyea**, DNP, MS-NP, MBA, NE-BC, CNL OCN, CCRN
Assistant Vice President Patient Care Services Carolinas HealthCare System
Assistant Professor Queens University CNL Program

**Stephanie J. (Jill) Raps**, Maj USAF DHA SOLUTION DELIV (US)
Chief Stakeholder Engagement Branch

**Laura M. Schwarz**, DNP, RN, CNE
School of Nursing
Minnesota State University Mankato

**Grace Sotomayor**, DNP, MSN, MBA, FACHE, NEA-BC
Chief Nursing Officer- Carolinas Medical Center

# Section 1

# Population Health Overview and Engagement Opportunities for Population Health

## CHAPTER 1

# Population Health Introduction

CHRISTINE RALYEA, DNP, MS-NP, MBA, NE-BC, CNL, OCN, CRRN

## Population Health Overview

**T**HE Institute for Healthcare Improvement (IHI) is a nonprofit organization focused on motivating and building the will for change, partnering with patients and healthcare professionals to test new models of care, and ensuring the broadest adoption of best practices and effective innovations (IHI, 2017a). "It is IHI's belief that new designs must be developed to simultaneously pursue three dimensions, which we call the *Triple Aim*: Improving the patient experience of care (including quality and satisfaction); Improving the health of populations; and Reducing the per capita cost of healthcare" (IHI-Triple Aim, 2017b, para. 1). The Triple Aim incorporates a critical shift in point of view. The concept of treating the health of a population is a systemic approach to identifying and meeting the health needs of a large collective of people.

## Defining Population Health

Population Health is a complex concept and a struggle for many; whether a provider or a consumer, population health can mean many different things. To start, one must understand what a population is or how we define a *population* in healthcare. According to *The Merriam-Webster Dictionary*, a population is "1 a: the whole number of people or inhabitants in a country or region; b : the total of individuals occupying an area or making up a whole; c: the total of particles at a particular energy level—used especially of atoms in a laser; 2: the act or process of populating, 3 a: a body of persons or individuals having a quality or characteristic in common; b (1): the organisms inhabiting a particular locality; (2): a group of interbreeding organisms that represents the level of organization at which speciation begins; and 4: a group of individual persons, objects, or items from which samples are taken for statistical measurement" (Merriam-Webster, 2017). We often think of a population as defined by a group at large. Depending on the patient's or people's view, we can define based on a location, specific characteristics or experiences, or other traits. For example, a nurse practitioner will think of the patients he or she serves in the practice as his/her population. As a provider, he or she will consider the characteristics of the population served to look at assessments, developing treatment plans and plans of care, and ultimately the impact on the health of the population. Note: It is important to understand that throughout this book, the terms patients, clients, and customers are used synonymously and interchangeably.

A population can be a group of people in a community or geographical region. For example, an acute care facility will look at their market share and seek engagement of the providers (e.g., physicians, advanced practice nurses [APNs]) to promote wellness with prevention in clinics and offices. The goal is to reduce progress of precursors for chronic disease, comorbidities, and illnesses. The impact to the acute care facility is a reduction in admissions, length of stay, readmissions, and mortality.

The specialist will view his or her patient population based on a body system or category of diseases he or she treats. The cardiologist will see his or her population through the patients served with such diagnoses as heart failure, acute myocardial infarction, or endocarditis. The cardiologist and cardiac APN can expand care for population health to include multiple preventative programs, such as wellness clinics focusing on weight management, blood pressure control, healthy nutritional intake with cholesterol management, exercise programs with cardio, and more. The specialist will seek to increase preventative measures and compliance for outcome improvements of health and wellness.

Population health is defined with various terms and terminology depending on the setting and groups of patients served. For example, in the acute care setting, the concept of population health can be described as improving the continuum of care with patient (client) medical report sharing and breaking down silos of episodic care to improve the medical management of patients. Improvement of medical management could be measured as less frequent emergency department visits, a reduction in readmissions, an increase of the medial home model, and improved compliance with medical plans of care.

"Probably the most influential contribution to the development of the population health approach is Evans, Barer, and Marmor's *Why Are Some People Healthy and Others Not? The Determinants of Health of Populations*, which grew out of the work of the Population Health Program of the Canadian Institute for Advanced Research" (Kindig & Stoddart, 2003, p. 380). This work strengthens the concept that population health is a focus for larger groups of people (called determinants) concentrating on health (wellness) and preventing disease conditions, and it takes on the new concept of personal ownership in one's (the patient's/client's) health and wellness. APNs must engage patients in active participation and personal ownership of their physical, mental, and psychosocial wellbeing. This includes an understanding of the value of preventive and wellness activities as a driver for population health successes. Simply, the APN who engages her patients within her population she serves to improve compliance with basic principles of weight management, exercise program participation, and dietary controls of fats and sodium, with a net improvement (reduction) in obesity, hypertension, and hyperlipidemia will contribute to the advances in population health.

*Case Vignette*

You are working as a cardiac APN within a large practice, and you want to start a new population health program to invite not only the practice patients, but also the community at large. You speak with the administrative team and share your ideas of twice a week offering a walk in the local park, monthly before the walk leading a meditation exercise with a brief class on stress management and related topics, and twice a year holding a large community screening program for blood pressure, cardiac assessment (monitoring heart sounds), cholesterol testing, health education sessions, and more.

- What would be the information you share with administration to justify and present your case, with the return on investment, to get your project approved?

- What will be the benefits you share for developing such a population health program?

## Food for Thought

As you read this book, we want you to challenge yourself to look beyond your everyday practice and ask, "How can I make a broader difference?" "Can I change, enhance, and improve my practice to make a broader impact focusing on population health?" You want to make an impact that will focus on the Triple Aim in Healthcare, decreasing cost, and improving quality for more people, the greater good, and make a difference. This supports APNs taking the lead in a more proactive manner with a focus on preventative care and improved coordination of care. As an APN, what can be done to engage the patients in their personal ownership for health and wellness? In any practice setting, the APN can make greatest impact in prevention and progression of disease.

## Triple Aim

In the simplest design, Berwick, Nolan, and Whittington (2008) describe the Triple Aim in three components: better health for the population, better care and experience for individuals/patients, and lower cost of healthcare (per capita cost). Figure 1.1 demonstrates the IHI Triple Aim illustration. "The concept is a straightforward way to tackle improvement opportunities for maximum impact: look for opportunities that provide a balance among the health of the populations cared for, the

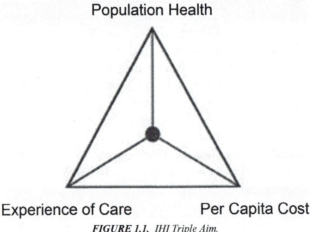

**FIGURE 1.1.** *IHI Triple Aim.*
*Public Domain: www.ihi.org/Engage/Initiatives/TripleAim/pages/default.aspx*

experience of patients or members, and the overall cost of healthcare" (IHI, 2017, para. 2, http://www.ihi.org/engage/initiatives/TripleAim/Pages/default.aspx).

The Triple Aim is not a revelation; we know and understand the cost of healthcare has been on the rise without a net positive impact on quality. Knight (2015) shares maneuvering through a broken system as many countries try to be the best in healthcare. Yet, the data show many deaths per year from hospital acquired conditions, medical errors, and illnesses that are mismanaged. Errors occur not only in acute care, but also in primary care, rehabilitation, and longterm care and in each component across the continuum of care and in every setting. According to Mangat (2015), to make an impact, providers of healthcare must focus on five elements: drive toward cost efficiency, value-based reimbursement, population health management, cost and quality data transparency, and advances in technology.

## Application of Triple Aim in Practice

*Case Vignette*

Do you challenge yourself each day to drive cost efficiency and improve costs and quality? Are you asking about resource allocation and resource use? What is the maximum impact when we prescribe a new medication or a test for a patient? There have been times before noon, I have reflected, and I realize I have seen six patients for whom I prescribed the same treatment plans, and I question why their past treatment plans (medications as an example) were not effective. But I become robotic, chart my notes, and go on to treat the next patients as an advanced care provider. Hence, I start to challenge myself to attempt to understand population health and how I can make a broader impact on the care delivery to/for the patients I serve. The population I treat. Population Health Management is building a culture of wellness and prevention (Mangat, 2015). So, I challenge myself, and I challenge you. How can we embed population health management into our practice each day? Learning about population health, we need to change the focus from the few (approximately 5% of the population) who are sick to the larger portion of the population (20%) who are in good health with chronic illnesses and are likely to become ill later (Hegwer, 2016). As we change this focus, we can transition to health promotion and improve population health. Van Dyke (2016) shared that "population health is creating a sense of urgency . . . timing is vital to consider when rethinking about the pace of transformation" (p. 23). Population health embraces the overall health of larger groups of people, the allocation of resources, targeting maximum impacts, and improving the population's view of health.

According to Berwick *et al.* (2017), "Preconditions for this include the enrollment of an identified population, a commitment to universality for its members, and the existence of an organization (an *integrator*) that accepts responsibility for all three aims for that population. The integrator's role includes at least five components: partnership with individuals and families, redesign of primary care, population health management, financial management, and macro system integration" (p. 759). So back to the question, do we challenge ourselves as advance care practitioners to commit to universality and to accept responsibility for the population we serve? Integrated with accepting the responsibility, are we adding value (quality of care and experience) while reducing cost?

Knight (2015) acknowledges a "systematic approach to care process improvement is necessary to reduce errors and save lives" (p. 4). The future must be grounded in lean process improvements, a changing focus on a value-based versus volume-based structure of fee for service, and improving the transition of care across the continuum. Lean production, also known as the Toyota Production System or justintime production, is an assembly line methodology developed originally for Toyota and the manufacturing of automobiles. Lean production principles are also referred to as lean management or lean thinking. Lean principles of manufacturing have been applied to healthcare and the principles of standardizing workflow processes to reduce the eight wastes in healthcare are essential to reduce errors. The wastes are often remembered using the mnemonic DOWNTIME (**d**efects, **o**verproduction, **w**aiting, **n**ot engaging all, **t**ransportation, **i**nventory, **m**otion, and **e**xtra processing). Improving these processes will enhance the Triple Aim by reducing cost and increasing quality outcomes for populations of people.

*Case Vignette*

Betty Brown, a 40-year-old African American female, has not been to the doctor since she had her fourth child 6 years ago. She is 20 pounds overweight and cannot lose the weight since her last baby. She acknowledges she could lose some weight, but feels comfortable and does not stress about her appearance. Her only complaint is occasional headaches, which she associates with stress at work. Her work has a Live Well program; when Betty went to *check her numbers* to meet a portion of the programs financial reimbursement for teammates, the advanced practice nurse (APN) shared a concern that her blood pressure was elevated 156/90.

You are the APN—what steps will you take with Ms. Brown? How is the treatment of Ms. Brown an application of the principles of Population Health?

## Expanding our Partners

After healthcare focused on the acute episodes of care, rather than developing the health of a population, we created a system in which value was measured by incidents of treatment instead of value reflecting the health of the community served. The cost of healthcare in the United States (U.S.) is disproportionately high. The transition to population health comprises thinking outside the box and expanding our stakeholders and partners to serve a broader community, including the healthy, with preventative measures, screening, and wellness strategies (for example, nutrition and exercise). Additionally, with population health, the goal is to address the bulk of the population who are progressing toward health conditions of chronic illnesses and disease. For example, patients with conditions such as mild hypertension (HTN), *slight* overweight, and lipidemia may state they are in good health, yet they may have silent warning signs for health complications in the future years that will escalate healthcare costs and lead to higher demands of acute care treatment.

Care of complex patients utilizing the principles of the Triple Aim will include affiliating and connecting with a large variety of partners (for example, retail stores and pharmacies, to support access to medications at lower costs, church support groups to enhance compliance to treatment plans). "Not addressing poverty, illiteracy, alcohol, and drug abuse, or even maladaptive cultural beliefs and behaviors that affect healthy behaviors and overall health status will leave the system short of accomplishing all three elements of the triple aim" (Knight, 2015, p.7). For example, engaging the patient in church support groups can help get to the root of many population health issues such as the cultural and socioeconomic barriers to health. These elements are not beyond the scope of an advanced care practitioner; rather they are essential if we are to improve care delivery and quality outcomes.

*Case Vignette*

John Smith, a 54-year-old man, lost his job as manager of a retail store six months ago and has been unable to find another job. He needs to work, because he is supporting two children in college and has a mortgage. He has been suffering from depression and, four months ago, started drinking excessively to cope with everything. He finds himself having beer and cocktails before noon each day and drinking until his head hits the pillow. He no longer has the energy to look for a job or go on interviews, and there is tension at home. He is withdrawn, and the only conversations with his wife and children are with anger, argumentation, and disruption to the household functioning.

- As the APN caring for John, what would your treatment plan be? What community services would you refer him to?

- Are there any measures you could take to impact the broader community related to alcoholism versus caring for one individual, such as John in this case?

**Population Health Management**

The top three investment areas for population health management include the workforce, information technology, and network development (Advisory Board, 2016). Incorporating these three investments can be complex for care management, transition of care, and telehealth pilot programs being developed and implemented. In the past, the focus of healthcare was on acute care, and today we see various roles and opportunities that expand beyond the hospital to provide care, improving access and care delivery. This means that the workforce has different training and insight into expanded roles of value and purpose with a direct impact on population health. For example, in the Charlotte, North Carolina, market, there was a job posting for a Community Outreach Partner, a registered nurse. A potential candidate for this position would be working with schools, churches, nonprofit organizations (such as Classroom Central and Salvation Army), the YMCA, and other organizations to build relationships for health promotion. Looking at the health assessment of the population in the Charlotte area, multiple opportunities exist due to the high percentage of schools with free-lunch and high incidences of diabetes, stroke, and cardiac diseases. The same organization with the Community Outreach position posted has a computer application that is free for anyone to download. It provides health messages and links to clinical experts and access to information related to multiple disease processes and wellness. An individual can be on Medicaid for the children and Welfare, but he or she often has a cell phone. Using a cell phone to send reminders and alerts for health promotion may be the only opportunity to deliver a message to a population prior to seeing them in an acute care setting. When one focuses on population health, innovation and opportunities are welcomed to make a difference.

As advanced care practitioners, we play a vital role in identifying highrisk patients and tracking improvements in care outcomes (Advisory Board, 2016). Healthcare is changing and roles are expanding to include many diverse jobs to build and engage population health principles and roles.

## Framing the Issues

Barr (2015) frames three issues in population health as follows:

"1) Population health management techniques are taking hold in different ways across the country. 2) Technology is playing a big role in population health management, but so is maintaining the human side of the equation. 3) Ignoring population health is probably a mistake" (p.23).

Healthcare systems need to get in the game for population health strategies and implementation investments to be successful. The goal must be to improve the health of the community (population) for as broad as the agency can reach. For example, Trinity Health seeks to reach 20 million people and describes this as a "kid in the candy store" (Barr, 2015, p. 23). An essential element in spread and reach requires a comprehensive technology platform to support coordination and navigation of care. Technology needs to be inclusive of human services, public safety, acute care, rehabilitation, longterm care, office practices, schools, churches, retail businesses, and more. Additionally, technology must be user friendly and without stereotypes, have ease of use, be friendly, and have a meaningful push of data to end users. For example, a friendly reminder could be delivered to take a medication or make an appointment.

## Business Imperatives for Population Health

Six business imperatives for population health management as described by Hegwer (2016) include "physician and clinical integration, contracting strategy, network optimization, operational efficiency, enabling infrastructure, and clinical management" (p. 11). These are slightly different and add the perspective of the value of alignment of goals for improved clinical outcomes. Across the continuum, care must be aligned so all parties accept risk and align with goals. "Creating a high-performance delivery network often requires detailed consumer insight such as knowing how consumers choose their providers and understand which types of consumers prefer specific settings for care" (Hegwer, 2016, p. 14). This changes the focus on consumerism. What do our customers want? How do we deliver upon their needs and not ours? The questions and challenges are as follows: Does this change our practice hours? Does this determine how we care for patients across transitions of care? An example is the geriatric population who wants to see their attending in acute care, when at rehab, and at a skilled nursing facility—how can this new model best be managed? Many questions arise, and we must challenge ourselves to think through the heart, mind, and soul of the clients, community, and population we serve.

Many facets of population health have been identified in the literature. There is no one clear strategy or process for success. Throughout the book, we selected critical concerns related to population health to help the advanced care practitioner shift his or her focus to the broader community, through the eyes of the client/patient, and mobilize change to improve quality while decreasing cost. The shift to population health is a venue for healthcare reform moving from 5% ill to 20% in good health, as described earlier in this chapter.

To start, it is critical that the APN understands how we integrate population health into our practice, thinking outside the box, elevating quality and experience while decreasing cost, and most importantly impacting the broader good of larger groups of people versus the next patient that walks into the office or clinic. This takes understanding the Patient Protection and Affordable Care Act (also referred to as the Affordable Care Act, or ACA) or its replacement, increasing access to care, advancing education for APNs, and getting involved at a local and national level, to close the gaps on health disparity and health literacy. Can we shift our practice to more preventative care? How can we improve compliance with screening for disease or compliance with dietary recommendations to minimize risks from such conditions as obesity and heart disease?

**Advance Practice Nurses Application**

APNs is a broad term that is used throughout the book to reflect generalists and specialists in advanced nursing care delivery who have a minimum of a master's degree and advanced nurse training, including Nurse Practitioners (NPs), Clinical Nurse Specialists (CNSs), Certified Registered Nurse Anesthesiologists (CRNAs), Certified Nurse Midwives (CNMs), and Clinical Nurse Leaders (CNLs). APNs are advanced care providers in all arenas of public health, acute care, long-term care, primary care, and more, who need to know where to find information about their populations. We call this information *big data*. Do you look to the state and community health department(s) for needs assessment and gaps in care, the Center for Disease Control and Prevention (CDC), and many other sources of data to revolutionize your care delivery model and strategy to make a broader impact? "No health system can help an entire population without the right data, and the analytics to derived from the data will identify those in greatest need and suggest strategies" (Knight, 2015, p. 145). Looking at big data, it is important to understand that sources are a collection system to support storage and analysis of data and report data (what, by whom); then the data must be presented in a meaningful way so it applies to populations and the community at large. Knight also suggests reducing data silos and understanding data governance. Do you have an opportunity to share information in a data registry to look at larger sums and collections of data to identify trends and patterns that can improve care delivery? APNs must understand that data are used as a tool to improve outcomes and reduce cost. Data transparency is not new, and as APNs, we will also have our outcomes shared and will be accountable for the care populations receive. The information will be readily available and accessible. The attention and focus are necessary for our success in quality service and cost reductions.

**What is Next in the Book?**

Meaningful data can be used to drive health policy and our work with unique populations. As noted above, population health is defined as "the health outcomes of a group of individuals, including the distribution of such outcomes within the group" (Kindig & Stoddart, 2003). Further, according to the Institute of Healthcare Improvement, population health "is an approach to health that aims to improve the health of an entire human population" (IHI, 2017, para. 1). When we look at groups of individuals, we have selected key population groups that the world has identified as needing focused attention and improvements based on the Triple Aim and opportunities. Several of these populations are the military and care for veterans, pediatrics, geriatrics and the aging, trauma victims, substance abuse, obesity, and those with chronic illness. Remember the win will be when we focus on the large percentage of the population that has a chronic illness, such as hypertension [HTN]; however, currently this group of patients, when asked, will state they are in a *good state of health*. Many patients with HTN say they are asymptomatic for longterm periods, yet the HTN causes systemic ill effects on and throughout the body. Managing the HTN early in the disease management process with frequent blood pressure checks and diet and weight management will offer greater opportunity to reduce chronic disease secondary to HTN. The impact will be greater, and the APN contributes to improving care while lowering cost of care over time.

Additionally, this book will identify valued initiatives the APN can utilize to embrace care for populations, such as health coaching/advisors (leading to behavior modifications). In a study by Hohl *et al.* (2016), health advisors and coaches in the community contributed to compliance of the population in healthier behaviors, improving the outcomes and decreasing disease progression. Ultimately, this demonstrated improved health and reduced cost for healthcare in the community at large.

The use of social media is a way to improve communication about healthcare, options, and preventive care measures. Hence, access to critical data to improve care delivery and compliance in populations can easily be accessed through social media and marketing. This goes beyond WebMd and other sources of medical information that are viewed frequently. There are many applications, games, and other options to support a fun interactive system of information for the APN to strengthen population health.

As APNs focus on providing care with a broader focus on population health, it is critical that they care for themselves, in particular, reducing compassion fatigue and burnout. As APNs, we challenge our effectiveness to make a difference. APNs can drive health policy and advocacy. We must see health policy through the eyes of the receivers of care and from the perceptive of different disciplines (Gatter, 2016). The challenge is developing ways to keep up with policy changes and the shifting data systems. Often nursing education is challenged to include population health in the curriculum, which plays a vital role in the future transitions of care delivery for success. As educators, we are challenged to teach effective communication and outcomes for our behaviors in a variety of practice settings. The APN can work collaboratively with nursing executives to focus on the three dimensions of the Triple Aim. The nurse executive faces the challenges, as care shifts to a varied setting beyond acute care, and must foster innovation and support lean strategies to reduce cost of care. According to Haas, Vlasses, and Havey (2016), population health management lends way to developing new staffing models with a shift to other venues throughout the transitions of care. This requires support for a healthy work environment based on high quality investments in the community. "All of these challenges require highly competent providers willing to change attitudes and culture such as movement towards collaborative practice among the interprofessional team including the patient" (Haas, Vlasses, & Harvey, 2016, p. 126).

These broader aspects will be covered in the book to help the APN make necessary transitions and applications in daily practice, to align with population health and overall improvements in care associated with the Triple Aim. Population Health requires support systems that align providers, communities, incentives, and all aspects of the programs developed. This includes the health services venues, retail market, and the people. Despite the many challenges that lie ahead, the APN can embrace population health and serve as a conduit for success.

**Tool Kit and Resources**

Advisory Board—www.advisoryboard.com

Health Affairs-Population Health—http://healthaffairs.org/blog/2015/04/06/what-are-we-talking-about-when-we-talk-about-population-health/

Institute for Healthcare Improvement—www.ihi.org

Institute for Healthcare Improvement—Triple Aim—www.ihi.org/Engage/Initiatives/TripleAim/pages/default.aspx

Population Health News, a *Health Policy Publishing* publication—(https://www.managedcarestore.com/ypg/hpp.htm), administered by MCOL (http://www.mcol.com/)

1101 Standiford Ave. Suite C-3, Modesto, CA 95350, 209.577.4888—info@populationhealthnews.com

*Discussion Questions*
1. How do you define population health?
2. What are the three elements of the Triple Aim? And how do Advanced Practice Nurses (APNs) play a role in each element?
3. As an APN, what are three measures you can put into practice to advance population health?
4. Who are two stakeholders and community partners that you can include in your practice to improve population health and care outcomes?
5. What is an APN's influence on health determinants focusing on wellness and delaying of chronic illness?

*Case Study*
    As an APN, you are looking for community work. Your son attends a public school that has a high percentage of lowincome people who are eligible for the free lunch program. Last week, you went to the classroom to read to the children and stayed for lunch period. You were concerned about the foods served to the children. As an advocate, you scheduled an appointment to meet with the principal, physical education (PE) teacher, school nurse, and head of the cafeteria food program.

1. Where would you gather information on the free lunch program and the school guidelines for meeting the requirements for federal and state funding?
2. What would be some suggestions you could make to provide healthier foods and portions for the children?
3. Working with the school nurse, are there any additional suggestions you could make for promoting wellness?
4. What suggestions could you make to support the PE teacher and increase the activity level for the school age children?

    Your meeting at your son's school with the team was a success and you were invited to come to school once a week to continue your campaign and efforts for promoting wellness. Many of the teachers wanted you to come to the classroom to speak to the young children.

1. What would your first three lessons be? What materials/curricula would you cover to engage the child's family in wellness?
2. Name one activity you would have the children take home to do as a family to turn in the following week.

3. How would an advocacy program like this improve population health?

4. Identify two other advocacy programs you could lead to support the principles of population health.

## References

Advisory Board (2016). Top three essential population health management investments. Executive Briefing: BJC Accountable Care Organization Case Study. Retrieved from www.advisoryboard.com

Barr, P. (2015). Three practical approaches to population health. *Hospital & Health Networks, 89*(10), 22–27.

Berwick, D. M., Nolan, T. W., & Whittington, J. (2008). *The triple aim: Care, health and cost, 27*(3), 759–769. doi: 10.1377/hlthaff.27.3.759

Gatter, R. (2016). Teaching population health outcomes research, advocacy, and the population health perspective in public health law, *The Journal of Law, Medicine & Ethics, 44*, 41–44. doi: 10.1177/107311051664426

Haas, S., Vlasses, F., & Havey J. (2016). Developing staffing models to support population health management and quality outcomes in ambulatory care settings. *Nursing Economic$, 34*(3), 126–133.

Hegwer, L. R. (2016). Business imperatives for population health management, *Healthcare Executive: The Magazine for Healthcare Leaders, 31*(4), 10–21.

Hohl, S.D., Thompson, B., Krok-Schoen, J. L., Weier, R.C., Martin, M., Bone, L., . . . Paskett, E.D., (2016). Characterizing community health workers on research teams: Results from the Centers for Population Health and Health Disparities. *American Journal of Population Health, 106*(4), 664–670. Retrieved from https://www.ncbi.nlm.nih.gov/pubmed/26794157

IHI (2017). Institute of Healthcare Improvement—Triple Aim, Retrieved from www.ihi.org/Engage/Initiatives/TripleAim/pages/default.aspx

Kindig, D., & Stoddart, G. (2003). What is population health? *American Journal of Public Health, 93*(3), 380–383.

Knight, E. (2015). *The definitive guide to Population health management*. Brentwood, TN: HCPro.

Mangat, M. (2015). Population health management: Building a culture of wellness & prevention. *The Healthcare Executive for Leader Development*, Webinar Series. Retrieved from www.TheHealthcareExecutive.com/webinar.

Merriam-Webster, 2017. Definition of population.

VanDyke, M. (2016). Determining the pace for population health, *Healthcare Executive: The Magazine for Healthcare Leaders. 31*(4), 22–28.

## CHAPTER 2

# Integration of Population Health to Advanced Nursing Care

LAURA M. SCHWARZ, DNP, RN, CNE
NANCYRUTH LEIBOLD, EdD, RN, PHN, CNE

## Integration of Population Health to Advanced Nursing Care

THE advanced practice nurse (APN) is ideally suited to practice population health. There are many ways for APNs to integrate population health into their practices that will be discussed in this chapter. These include changes in advanced nursing practice to accommodate the Patient Protection and Affordable Care Act (also referred to as the Affordable Care Act, or ACA) and steps to accomplish this goal, benefits of APNs including population health in their practices, APNs making global and population health changes through actions on a local level, and transcultural nursing practice.

At the time of the writing of this chapter, the ACA was in place, although slated to be repealed and replaced by current White House administration. It was unclear at the time of the writing of this chapter as to what those changes would be. Therefore, the authors speak to the ACA as it was fully in place at the time of the writing of this chapter, and some parts may remain in place for an indefinite amount of time. The latest revision of the Republican bill created to appeal and replace the ACA is called the American Healthcare Act. The main concern areas expressed at this time by the public and policy makers regarding proposed changes to healthcare coverage include preexisting conditions, cost of premiums, less insurance coverage, and concern about the number of people left without insurance.

Several changes are needed in advanced nursing practice to accommodate the ACA. First, the APN needs to understand the ACA and its implications for healthcare and advanced practice nursing. The first part of this chapter will provide history, background and facts on federal policy guidelines, federal mandates on health insurance coverage, the Health Insurance Marketplace, impacts on Medicare and Medicaid, and how the Affordable Care Act impacts the APN. Other changes/steps needed in Advanced Nursing Practice that serve to accommodate the Affordable Care Act discussed include increasing the number of APNs in the workforce, allowing APNs to practice to their full scope, changes in payment regulations and policies, increased educational levels, increased APN/physician collaboration, and interprofessional education.

## Changes in Advanced Nursing Practice to Accommodate the Patient Protection and Affordable Care Act and Steps to Accomplish this Goal

The APN is ideally suited to practice population health. There are many aspects of population health that APNs can integrate into their practices and venues for which to do so. APNs' educational backgrounds and practice settings make for ideal and indispensable roles in practicing population health for both local and global impact of individuals, families, and society.

## What APNs Need to Know About the ACA: History and Background of the Patient Protection and Affordable Healthcare Act

The first step for APNs to accommodate the ACA is to learn about the history and background of the ACA. President Obama signed *HR 3590: Patient Protection and Affordable Care Act,* also known as the Affordable Care Act (ACA) and "Obamacare," into law in March 2010 after it was signed by Congress. The ACA was originally a healthcare bill created by the Senate. Development of the ACA was designated to move forward comprehensive health insurance reforms over a four-year period and into the future (United States [U.S.] Department of Health and Human Services [HHS], 2015a). The Supreme Court put forth a final decision to uphold the APA on June 28, 2012. A brief history of the implementation of the ACA, as outlined by the HHS (2015a), is provided below.

In 2010, a new Patient's Bill of Rights and cost-free preventative services went into effect. In 2011, those with Medicare began to receive crucial preventative services for free and a 50% reduction on brand name drugs. In 2012, programs such as the Accountable Care Organizations began to assist physicians and healthcare providers to collaborate for better care delivery. On October 1, 2013, open enrollment in the *Health Insurance Marketplace* or HealthCare.gov began. In 2014, the ACA mandated that all Americans are able to have access to affordable health insurance options, tax credits for middle and low-income families to cover a substantial part of coverage costs, and Medicaid was increased to insure a greater number of Americans. Citizens can read more about the year-by-year implementation of changes at http://www.hhs. gov/healthcare/facts-and-features/key-features-of-aca-by-year/index. html#2010. Citizens can read the entire ACA law or specific parts here: http://www.hhs.gov/healthcare/about-the-law/read-the-law/index.html.

**Federal Policy Guidelines**

Key features of the law can be divided into three primary goals, as follows:

1. "Make affordable health insurance available to more people. The law provides consumers with subsidies ('premium tax credits') that lower costs for households with incomes between 100% and 400% of the federal poverty level" (Affordable Care Act, n.d., para 1). A definition of federal poverty level dollar amounts can be found here: https://www.healthcare.gov/glossary/federal-poverty-level-FPL/

2. "Expand the Medicaid program to cover all adults with income below 138% of the federal poverty level" (Affordable Care Act, n.d., para 1). Note that not all states have done so.

3. "Support innovative medical care delivery methods designed to lower the costs of healthcare generally" (Affordable Care Act, n.d., para 1).

The ACA was created to give people back control of their healthcare. This includes a new *Patients' Bill of Rights* that provides Americans with consistent, flexible, and educated choices on their health (U.S. HHS, 2015b). The *Patients' Bill of Rights* was designed to protect the consumer by expanding coverage, containing costs, and increasing access to care. A summary of these changes put forth by the new *Patients' Bill of Rights* is found in Table 2.1.

TABLE 2.1. Summary of Key Features of the Patients' Bill of Rights
(adapted from U.S. HHS, 2015b).

| Coverage |
| --- |
| • Bans health insurance plans from denying limits or benefits to any child under age 19 who has a pre-existing condition. |
| • Allows young adults under the age of 26 to be covered by parent's health plan. This even includes persons under the age of 26 who are married, not living with their parents, attending school, not financially dependent on their parents, and or eligible to enroll in their employer's plan. |
| • Bans insurers from canceling someone's insurance because they made an honest mistake or omitted information that had little relationship to their health. |
| • Guarantees people the right to appeal insurer's denial of payment. |
| Costs |
| • Bans lifetime and annual limits on most benefits for all new healthcare plans. Previously, many plans had lifetime and annual caps. Note: This does not include annual limits for grandfathered plans. |
| • Requires insurance companies to justify all unreasonable premium increases. |
| • Requires healthcare providers spend premium dollars primarily on healthcare and not on administrative costs. |
| Care |
| • Stipulates preventative care has no cost to the consumer, including no copayment. |
| • Allows people to choose the primary care provider they want from their plan's network. |
| • Allows people to get emergency care at a hospital outside of their plan's network. |

## Federal Mandates on Healthcare Insurance Coverage

The Kaiser Family Foundation (2013) provides an excellent summary of the ACA requirements, including health insurance coverage requirements. The overall approach to the ACA is that it requires most U.S. citizens and legal residents to have qualifying health insurance. The law mandates state-based healthcare Exchanges for individuals to purchase health insurance and Exchanges for small businesses to purchase coverage. Employers (except small businesses) are required to pay penalties for employees who receive tax credits for health coverage obtained through an Exchange. It enforces new rules on health insurance plans in the Exchanges and those in the individual and small group markets. The law also expanded Medicaid to 133% of the federal poverty level.

The law mandates individuals who do not have coverage must pay whichever is greater: a tax penalty of $695/year up to a cap of $2,085 per family, or 2.5% of household income. The penalty was phased in as follows: $95 or 1.0% of taxable income in 2014, $325 or 2.0% of taxable income in 2015, and $695 or 2.5% of taxable income in 2016. After 2016, the penalty was set to be increased annually by the cost-of-living adjustment. There are several exemptions that are granted, such as financial hardship, religious objections, and income below guidelines (Kaiser Family Foundation, 2013). The law also fines employers that do not offer health insurance, have 50 or more full-time employees, "and have at least one full-time employee who receives a premium tax credit (Kaiser Family Foundation, 2013, para. 4). Employers with more than 200 employees are required by the ACA to have health insurance plans that they offer and to which they automatically enroll employees. Employees may decline the coverage (Kaiser Family Foundation, 2013).

## Health Insurance Marketplace

The Health Insurance Marketplace is also known as the Health Insurance Exchange and is located at www.HealthCare.gov. The Marketplace is important for the APN to understand so that he or she can teach and assist patients with navigation through this website. The Marketplace is a federally facilitated website at which individuals and families who do not have healthcare insurance, such as from an employer, spouse, or partner, can find information about health insurance options and purchase healthcare insurance. The website also has information about eligibility for assistance with paying premiums and reducing out-of-pocket costs. The open enrollment period for the next year begins November 1 and ends on January 31, but people must enroll by December 15 to have coverage begin on January 1 of the following year.

Besides the Health Insurance Marketplace and HealthCare.gov, some states have a state-based Marketplace. Whether an individual or family will use HealthCare.gov or a state-based Marketplace depends on the state in which they live. Those who visit HealthCare.gov are asked to provide their ZIP code. If the person or family lives in a stateserved Marketplace area, they will be redirected to the state-based Marketplace that serves them. Training for people who use the Health Insurance Marketplace, including consumers, those who assist consumers, and small employers, can be accessed conveniently from a link at the bottom of the HealthCare.gov website or at https://marketplace.cms. gov/technical-assistance-resources/training-materials/training.html.

## The Affordable Care Act Impacts on Medicare and Medicaid

Because the APN will likely care for those who are qualified and/or insured under Medicare and/or Medicaid, it is paramount for the APN to understand the impacts of the ACA on these two insurance entities. The ACA mandated Medicaid be expanded to all non-Medicare qualified persons who are under the age of 65. This includes "(children, pregnant women, parents, and adults without dependent children) with incomes up to 133% FPL based on modified adjusted gross income (as under current law undocumented immigrants are not eligible for Medicaid)" (Kaiser Family Foundation, 2013, para. 6). The Supreme Court upheld the ACA expansion of Medicaid, but limited the power of the HHS to enforce it, leaving the decision on whether to expand Medicaid up to the individual states (Kaiser Family Foundation, 2013).

Since the Affordable Care Act was enacted in March 2010, The Centers for Medicare & Medicaid Services (CMS) has worked together with states "to determine essential implementation priorities and provide the guidance needed to prepare for the significant changes to Medicaid and the Children's Health Insurance Program (CHIP). Specifically, CMS has provided a variety of guidance and federal support for states to develop new or upgrade existing *eligibility systems*" (Medicaid.gov, n.d.). Specific provisions for Medicare and Medicaid can be found at https://www.medicaid.gov/affordable-care-act/index.html.

## The Advanced Practice Nurse and the Affordable Healthcare Act

It is necessary for the APNs to understand how the ACA impacts them and their practices. The ACA has a non-discrimination provision that includes nurse practitioners and recognition of their practice as follows:

"... as primary care providers and leaders in public and home care medical home pilots and demonstrations, funding for nurse managed clinics; funding for graduate nurse education and post graduate experience demonstrations, inclusion in primary care Medicare payment increases, and inclusion in ACOs (Accountable Care Organizations)." (American Association of Nurse Practitioners, n.d., para. 2).

The bill language contains an abundance of provider-neutral language that will assist with the use of nurse practitioners in many different settings. The ACA's broad determination of roles and scope for the APN has potential implications for an increase in the APN workforce, opportunities, and scope of practice and a learning curve for healthcare navigation (American Association of Nurse Practitioners, n.d.).

## Increase Supply of Advanced Practice Nurses in Primary Care

The supply of APNs needs to grow in order to accommodate the ACA. Although it is expected that under the ACA, 32 million more people will have access to primary care, the number of primary care physicians is decreasing as fewer residents choose to enter internal and family medicine areas. The ACA requires greater numbers of primary care providers (Lathrop & Hodnicki, 2014). However, it is unlikely that there will be enough physicians to cover this increase in need for primary care (Poghosyan, Lucero, Rauch, & Berkowitz, 2012). APNs have formal preparation that makes them uniquely suited primary care providers (Hain & Fleck, 2014; Lathrop & Hodnicki, 2014). Over 58 million Americans live in primary care Health Professional Shortage Areas (HPSAs) and almost half the states have at least a 20% HPSAs (Van Vleet & Paradise, 2015). Almost 90% of all nurse practitioners are prepared in primary care (American Association of Nurse Practitioners, 2014). A strong nurse practitioner workforce can help meet the growing need for primary care providers (Poghosyan *et al.*, 2012; Van Vleet & Paradise, 2015). The Institute of Medicine (IOM) (2011) further recommends increasing the number of nurse practitioners in primary care.

## Practice to the Full Extent of Education and Training

There are challenges to meeting the need of the ACA and increased need for primary care providers. Perhaps the greatest challenge, and a change that needs to occur to accommodate both the ACA and APNs' service in primary care is to allow APNs to practice to the full extent of their education and training. Increasing APN scope of practice may help increase the supply of APNs (Poghosyan *et al.*, 2012). Various bodies and authors have argued for policy makers to enact policies to lift practice restrictions and allow APNs to effectively utilize them by allowing them to practice to their full scope. The National Council of State Boards of Nursing (NCSBN, 2008) recommends that nurse practitioners practice to the full extent of their scope and endorses the American Association of Colleges of Nursing (AACN) advanced practice registered nurse (APRN) *Consensus Model* to promote uniformity in the APRN role across all 50 states. The IOM (2011) key message

#1 is "*Nurses should practice to the full extent of their education and training*" and the IOM recommendation #1 is "Remove scope of practice barriers provides further endorsement." At issue, and a barrier, is that although nurse practitioners have a common educational and training background directed by a common accreditation body and national certification, scope of practice laws lack consistency from state to state (Poghosyan *et al.*, 2012); in many states, there are legislative and regulatory barriers that prevent nurse practitioners from practicing to their full potential (Van Vleet & Paradise, 2015).

Nurse practitioner practice is in fact regulated by a range of agencies varying from state to state, including state boards of nursing and/or medicine, pharmacy, and others and, with this, a varying scope of practice. Some states allow nurse practitioners to practice independently, whereas others require oversight by a physician (Poghosyan *et al.*, 2012). Poghosyan *et al.* (2012) argue that it is important that policy be enacted to establish regulations for a consistent scope of practice across all states to help clarify the professional identity of nurse practitioners. Lastly, allowing APNs to practice fully saves money. The RAND Corporation, for example (Eibner, Hussey, Ridgely & McGlynn, 2009), determined that 4.2 to 8.4 billion dollars could be saved in the state of Massachusetts with full scope of practice. The IOM (2011) report states ". . . what nurse practitioners are able to do once they graduate varies widely for reasons that are not related to their ability, education or safety concerns, but to the political decisions of the state in which they work" (p. 5). The IOM (2011) has asked that the Federal Trade Commission and Department of Justice review state regulations "to identify those that have anticompetitive effects without contributing to the health and safety of the public" (p. 10). Further, the IOM has deemed that states with regulations that are overly restricted should be urged to change them to allow APNs to provide care to the full extent of their education and training.

**Changes in Payment Regulations and Policies for APN Practice**

Payment regulations provide a barrier to growing the APN workforce and scope of practice; therefore, policy makers should help work toward their removal. Medicare, Medicaid, and private/commercial payers, for example, have complex systems to pay providers, and these vary significantly between how APNs and physicians in primary care are reimbursed and in the percent of reimbursement (Chapman, Wides,

& Spetz, 2010; Hain & Fleck, 2014; Van Vleet & Paradise, 2015). One in four health maintenance organizations do not recognize nurse practitioners as primary care providers. Poghosyan *et al.* (2012) describe that billing discrepancies lead to discouragement of nurse practitioners being billed independently and, hence, hidden under physician practice. This in turn does not allow for APN care to be tracked and evaluated, limits the consumer from seeing quality care indicators of the APN who provided the care, and does not provide incentives to hire and keep APNs as autonomous care providers. Chapman *et al.* (2010) explain that nurse practitioners have lower wages and reimbursement in comparison to physicians, which makes it hard for nurse practitioners to sustain practicing in primary care. It is clear that the policies regulating pay for APNs need to be changed to be commensurate with that of physicians.

## Increased Levels of Nursing Education

The ACA creates a greater need for APNs; however, there are not enough APN programs to accommodate that need. Although the ACA launched increased loan forgiveness programs and a demonstration grant for nurse practitioner residency in federally qualified centers, it did not increase funding for education of nurse practitioners (Poghosyan *et al.* 2012). The IOM (2011) key message #2 is *"Nurses should achieve higher levels of education and training through an improved education system that promotes seamless academic progression"* and the IOM recommendation #5 is *"Double the number of nurses with a doctorate degree by 2020"* to provide further credence for advancing education of APNs.

Although a doctorate is not currently required for APN practice, the Doctor of Nursing Practice (DNP) education should be encouraged because it provides graduates with more advanced knowledge in nursing inquiry and quality improvement (Hain & Fleck, 2014). The DNP is the most fitting degree for the APN, and advancing to the DNP is congruent with the IOM recommendation of higher levels of education and training. The DNP is a terminal degree and is practice-focused rather than research focused, such as the PhD (American Association of Colleges of Nursing, 2006). A DNP education consists of two components, as follows: (1) Eight essentials that are foundational outcome competencies necessary for all DNP graduates regardless of specialty or practice focus (see Table 2.2) and (2) "Specialty competencies/content prepare

*TABLE 2.2. The Essentials of Doctoral Education
for Advanced Nursing Practice.*

| |
|---|
| I. Scientific Underpinnings for Practice |
| II. Organizational and Systems Leadership for Quality Improvement and Systems Thinking |
| III. Clinical Scholarship and Analytical Methods for Evidence-Based Practice |
| IV. Information Systems/Technology and Patient Care Technology for the Improvement and Transformation of Healthcare |
| V. Healthcare Policy for Advocacy in Healthcare |
| VI. Interprofessional Collaboration for Improving Patient and Population Health Outcomes |
| VII. *Essential*: Clinical Prevention and Population Health for Improving the Nation's Health |
| VIII. *Essential*: Advance Nursing Practice |

*Source*: American Association of Colleges of Nursing, 2006.

the DNP graduate for those practice and didactic learning experiences for a particular specialty. Competencies, content, and practical experiences needed for specific roles in specialty areas are delineated by national specialty nursing organizations" (American Association of Colleges of Nursing, 2006, p. 8). The entire AACN document including each essential in detail can be found at the following website: http://www.aacn.nche.edu/publications/position/DNPEssentials.pdf.

In their article, *The Affordable Care Act: Primary Care and the Doctor of Nursing Practice* Nurse, Lathrop and Hodnicki (2014) discuss how the changes from the Affordable Care Act, such as a preventative model, emphasis on primary care, funds for community health initiatives, and quality care, created a need for well-prepared healthcare providers. Lathrop and Hodnicki (2014) maintain that APNs who hold a DNP are wellsuited to meet this need through their "leadership in community health centers, serving on interdisciplinary teams, and advocating for and directing future policy initiatives" (p. 1). Statistics indicate that the need for primary care DNP-prepared APNs will grow with the ACA; however, scope of practice and reimbursement rules and regulations are a barrier. Lending further support to the need to increase scope of practice and the need for reimbursement commensurate with that of physicians, as discussed earlier in this chapter, Lathrop and Hodnicki (2014) wrap up their article by citing the professional and legal barriers that must be dissolved in order for the DNP nurse to provide care to the full extent of their preparation.

## Increased APN/Physician Collaboration to Promote National Health Goals

IOM (2011) key message #3 states that *"nurses should be full partners, with physicians and other health professionals, in redesigning healthcare in the United States."* Under key message #3, the IOM (2011, p. 230) further states the following:

> Nurses should have a voice in health policy decision making and be engaged in implementation efforts related to healthcare reform. Nurses should also serve actively on advisory committees, commissions, and boards where policy decisions are made to advance health systems to improve patient care.

Newhouse *et al.* (2011) conducted a systematic review of the literature that revealed outcomes of patients cared for "by nurse practitioners and certified nurse midwives in collaboration with physicians were similar and in some ways, better than care provided by physicians alone" (p. 230). This finding serves to underscore IOM key message #3. Some professional organizations maintain that physicians have a longer and more rigorous preparation than nurse practitioners and, therefore, nurse practitioners cannot provide safe care on the same level as physicians (Hain & Fleck, 2014). According to Newhouse *et al.* (2011), study results demonstrate that APNs provide safe, effective, and quality care and that APN-Physician collaborative delivery models be moved forward by health professionals in the United States to promote joint health goals. Hain and Fleck (2014) maintain that several other researchers have found the same and that the traditional hierarchical model contributes to ineffective teamwork, promotes physician dominance, and further endorses the collaborative model.

Nurse practitioners should be active members and/or leaders in interprofessional teams. Nurse practitioner-physician collaboration is essential to healthcare transformation. Nurse practitioner students can assist others in understanding the significance of Care vs. Cure (Hain & Fleck, 2014). IOM recommendation #2, which states to *"expand opportunities for nurses to lead and diffuse collaborative improvement efforts,"* emphasizes the importance of APN collaboration with physicians and others. Lastly, it is important to note that *Interprofessional Collaboration for Improving Patient and Population Health Outcomes* is also a Doctoral Education for Advanced Nursing Practice Essential (Essential VI, American Association of Colleges of Nursing, 2006).

## Interprofessional Education

The importance of interprofessional education (IPE) should also be recognized, because it serves to increase physician knowledge of the nurse practitioner role (Hain & Fleck, 2014). IPE may also improve patient outcomes, an important factor for care of individuals, families, and populations. In a systematic review, Reeves, Perrier, Goldman, Freeth, and Zwarenstein (2013) found that IPE compared to no education had positive outcomes with increased patient satisfaction, improved health outcomes in persons with certain types of chronic diseases, and fewer medical errors. Although these results need careful consideration because of the small sample sizes and lack of generalizability, the findings help underscore the value of IPE and the need for further research in this area.

## Benefits of APNs Including Population Health in Their Practices

Population health is an important focus of the ACA, and with it comes improved safety, outcomes, and health. The ACA supports several issues of concern to advanced practice nursing. The ACA helps create more value with its significant contribution to primary care. It promotes leadership opportunities for nurse practitioners. such as the appropriation of up to $50 million dollars toward NurseManaged Health Centers or Clinics (Poghosyan *et al.*, 2012; Van Vleet & Paradise, 2015). ANPs help fill the gaps in urban and rural areas, because a far greater percentage of nurse practitioners work in these areas than do physicians. Further, they serve a wider range of community settings and a high percentage of patients from vulnerable populations, including the uninsured (Buerhaus, DesRoches, Dittus, & Donelan, 2015).

## Making a Difference through Nurse-Managed Health Centers

Nurse-managed health centers (NMHCs) are one way for APNs to make a difference. The NMHC is an effective model for providing safety-net healthcare to underserved populations, a great proportion of whom suffer health disparities (Esperalt, Hanson-Turton, Richardson, & Debisette, 2012; Waite, Nardi, & Killian, 2014). "NMHCs are based on a philosophy of commitment and care, particularly for the most vulnerable residents and communities" (Esperalt *et al.*, 2012,

p. 24). This philosophy is congruent with nursing's beliefs in social justice and cultural competence and provides an ideal opportunity for the APN to make a difference in the health and welfare of the nation's population. NHMCs provide holistic care, health promotion, disease prevention, and wellness, as well as a full spectrum of primary care to low income, minority, vulnerable, and underserved populations. These centers are often owned and operated by or affiliated with schools of nursing. The APN is the primary provider of healthcare in the NMHC (Esperalt *et al.*, 2012; Waite *et al.*, 2014). NMHCs create opportunities for APNs to lead these centers and underscore values of nursing, including patient-centered care, comprehensive primary care, and preventative services to underserved and vulnerable populations (Poghosyan *et al.*, 2012).

## Leadership Opportunities for the DNP-Prepared APN to Utilize DNP Education

The DNP-educated APN has significant educational preparation suited to leadership and other opportunities to population health. Although not yet required, it is the best degree for the APN. Population health is a central value and congruent with the practice of nursing. Three of the eight AACN (2006) DNP Essentials have population health as a central focus. *Essential V: Healthcare Policy for Advocacy in Healthcare* states "the DNP graduate is able to design, implement and advocate for healthcare policy that addresses issues of social justice and equity of healthcare" (2006, p. 13). These are leadership functions that are uniquely suited to APNs. *Essential IV: Interprofessional Collaboration for Improving Patient and Population Outcomes* is directly related to population health and advocates for not only working as part of an interprofessional team, but serving as the team leader as appropriate. The APN serving as leader promotes operating to the full educational scope and serves to elevate the APN role and its credibility.

*Essential VII: Clinical Prevention and Population Health for Improving the Nation's Health* also speaks directly to population health. This essential describes how health activities toward clinical prevention and population health is essential to the health of the nation's population. Again, a major focus is leadership: "DNP graduates engage in leadership to integrate and institutionalize evidence-based clinical prevention and population health services for individuals, aggregates, and populations" (2006, p. 15).

### APNs Making Global and Population Health Changes Through Actions on a Local Level

The IOM (2011) places nurses on the front line of leading change and advancing health. The IOM "committee envisions a future system that makes quality care accessible to the diverse populations of the United States, internationally promotes wellness and disease prevention, reliably improves health outcomes, and provides compassionate care across the lifespan" (p. 2). This vision is an ideal opportunity for APNs to make an impact in global and population health. The Consensus Model for APRN Regulation (American Association of Colleges of Nursing, 2008) in fact suggests a new APRN role with a population foci that may develop over time. Education and action on a local level can promote population and global health.

### Definitions of Global Health and Global Nursing

The Sigma Theta Tau International (STTI) *Global Advisory Panel on the Future of Nursing* (GAP-FON) studied literature from articles published between 2005 and 2015 to develop consensus definitions of global health and global nursing (Wilson *et al.*, 2016). The proposed definition of global health according to GAP-FON (p. 1530) is as follows:

"An area for practice, study and research that places a priority on improving health, achieving equity in health for all people and ensuring health-promoting and sustainable sociocultural, political and economic systems . . . and it emphasizes transnational health issues, determinants and solutions; involves many disciplines within and beyond the health sciences and promotes interdependence and interdisciplinary collaboration; and is a synthesis of population-based prevention with individual holistic care."

Further, GAP-FON suggests a definition for global nursing as "the use of evidence-based nursing process to promote sustainable planetary health and equity for all people. Global nursing considers social determinants of health, includes individual and population-level care, research, education, leadership, advocacy and policy initiatives" (p. 1530). These definitions make apparent the relationship between individual, population, and global care and can be used to guide the APN in global health and global nursing.

## Including Population and Global Health Content in Nursing Education

Nurses for the most part have been educated in caring for the individual and most nurses entering APN programs have a background of practice in facilities that focus primarily on the individual (Hatcher, 2015). Hatcher advocates for a paradigm shift in APN education from focus on the individual to a blend in individual and population health and promotion of a better grasp of the social determinants of health in all courses, including clinical and didactic. When possible, education programs should promote goal health clinical experiences. The Consensus Model for APRN Regulation (American Association of Colleges of Nursing, 2008, p.11) states that the APRN education must have the following related to population and global health:

- Additional content, specific to the role and population, in these three APRN core areas should be integrated throughout the other role and population didactic and clinical courses;
- Prepare the graduate to assume responsibility and accountability for health promotion and/or maintenance as well as the assessment, diagnosis, and management of patient problems, which includes the use and prescription of pharmacologic and non-pharmacologic interventions; and
- Ensure clinical and didactic coursework is comprehensive and sufficient to prepare the graduate to practice in the APRN role and population focus.

### *Glocal*: Think Global-Act Local

Organizations such as The Nightingale Initiative for Global Health (NIGH) endorse glocalization: thinking global by acting locally. NIGH "challenges nurses everywhere to think and act both locally and globally, to raise their voices about the contribution of nursing, and to become authentic advocates, particularly in addressing" (Beck, Dossey & Rushton, 2013, p. 366). Further illustrating the Glocal concept is an analysis whereby an extensive review of the literature revealed "several nursing authors argue that nurses globally are increasingly sharing concerns expressed by nurses at a local level" (Grootjans & Newman 2013, p. 78). Healthy People 2020, the Global Health Initiative, and STTI Global Health all support the notion of thinking globally to act locally.

The Healthy People 2020 topical goal for global health is to *"Improve public health and strengthen U.S. national security through global disease detection, response, prevention, and control strategies"* (Office of Disease Prevention and Health Promotion, 2016). The healthy people goal for global health states that "Rapid identification and control of emerging infectious diseases helps: promote health abroad, prevent the international spread of disease and protect the health of the U.S. population" (Office of Disease Prevention and Health Promotion, 2016, para. 1). The APN is at the front lines of caring for patients in primary care, public health, and other settings and, thus, plays a very important part in rapid identification and control of emerging infectious diseases locally to think globally. Improved global health helps the United States in several ways. Global health can impact the United States both directly and indirectly, including spread of diseases, food-borne illnesses, and contaminated products such as pharmaceuticals. The United States can learn from other countries who have better outcomes and can use comparisons to recognize ways to improve its own country's health (Office of Disease Prevention and Health Promotion, 2016).

**STTI Involvement in Glocal Health**

In July 2012, the United Nations (U.N.) Economic and Social Council (ECOSOC) granted special consultative status to the Honor Society of Nursing, STTI, based on expertise in the field of nursing and global health. This U.N. designation recognizes the STTI commitment to the charter of the UN, which seeks to achieve international cooperation toward solving humanitarian issues (Sigma Theta Tau International Honor Society of Nursing, 2016, para. 1). STTI developed 17 sustainable development goals (SDGs) and a website with several ideas for how nurses can act locally to make a difference globally: http://www.nursingsociety.org/connect-engage/our-global-impact. These ideas include using your passion and talent to get involved with a local organization, such as volunteering for an organization like the YMCA. Another idea is using chapter resources to make a difference, for example, STTI chapters at the local level raising funds for communities in need around the globe and global projects, such as community drives to have soap, pencils, paper, crayons, etc., supplies to send with missionaries who were going to help an underdeveloped community.

## IHI Open School Change Agent Network (I-CAN)

The Institute for Healthcare Improvement Open School Change Agent Network (I-CAN) "offers leadership and community organizing training to equip students, residents, faculty, and health professionals with the skills they need to lead a health improvement project in their local setting" (Institute for Healthcare Improvement, 2016a, para. 1). "The I-CAN course, Leadership and Organizing to Improve Population Health, provides tools in improvement science, leadership, and community organizing to help you create change in real-world projects" (Institute for Healthcare Improvement, 2016b, para. 2). The I-CAN website—http://www.ihi.org/education/IHIOpenSchool/ICAN/Pages/Projects.aspx—offers ideas on how professionals can get involved in projects in their own community. Ideas for activities in four areas—access to care, health behaviors, social determinants of health, and clinical care—are given at this website: http://www.ihi.org/education/IHIOpenSchool/ICAN/Pages/Topic-Activity-Pages.aspx.

### Global Strategic Directions for Strengthening Nursing and Midwifery

This publication by the World Health Organization (WHO, 2016) provides rich information on ways in which nursing and midwifery professionals can change the way healthcare is organized and provided. "The strategic directions for nursing and midwifery provide policymakers, practitioners and other stakeholders at every level of the healthcare system with a flexible framework for broad-based, collaborative action to enhance capacity for nursing and midwifery" (World Health Organization, 2016, p. 5). The report may be found at the following website: http://www.who.int/hrh/nursing_midwifery/global-strategic-midwifery2016-2020.pdf.

### Transcultural Nursing Practice

The APN must include transcultural nursing as an integral part of practice. Transcultural nursing practice starts with culturally competent care. This part of Chapter 2 will provide information on transcultural nursing, cultural competence, culturally and linguistically appropriate care, and health disparities. An overview of cultural nursing assessment and care is provided. In order to understand the meaning of transcultural practice, some definitions are in order. Although there is not one agreed upon definition for the terms for cultural competence (Shen, 2015), we do have some starting points. *Transcultural Nursing* (TCN) is a theory-based humanistic discipline, designed to serve individuals, organizations, communities, and societies. Human care/caring is defined within the context of culture (Transcultural Nursing Society, 2016). One definition of *culturally competent nursing care* that is well endorsed by the literature and nursing practice is by Madeline Leininger. Leininger (in Shen, 2015 describes it as follows:

> The explicit use of culturally based care and health knowledge that is used in sensitive, creative, and meaningful ways to fit the general lifeways and needs of individuals or groups for beneficial and meaningful health and well-being or to face illness, disabilities or death.

A comprehensive listing of definitions for cultural competence can be found in a literature review by Shen (2015. The Transcultural Nursing Society (2016) argues that culturally competent care can occur only when culture care values are known and serve as the foundation for meaningful care.

APNs are not only ideally situated in their practice settings to provide culturally competent care, but also are well equipped to do so. In fact, authors of a multisite study (Matteliano & Street, 2012) found that nurse practitioners stood out above other professionals in the level of comprehensiveness of their approaches to cultural competence, both with patients and in healthcare teams. "NPs established culturally sensitive partnerships with patients, encouraged self-advocacy, addressed contextual considerations and adjusted practices to meet the patient needs" (Matteliano & Street, 2012, p. 425). Related to cultural competence, nurses in general embrace a holistic approach in their care of patients, but this was especially endorsed by nurse practitioners (Matteliano & Street, 2012).

## Health Disparities, Healthcare Disparities and Health Equity

The APN needs to understand the meanings of health disparities, healthcare disparities and health equity, and their relationship to transcultural nursing practice. Health disparities, healthcare disparities, and health equity are intertwined. *Health disparities* is defined by (U.S. Department of Health and Human Services, 2008) as follows:

> A particular type of health difference that is closely linked with social, economic,

and/or environmental disadvantage. Health disparities adversely affect groups of people who have systematically experienced greater obstacles to health based on their racial or ethnic group; religion; socio-economic status; gender; age; mental health; cognitive, sensory, or physical disability; sexual orientation or gender identity; geographic location; or other characteristics historically linked to discrimination or exclusion (U.S. Department of Health and Human Services, 2008, p. 28).

Healthcare disparities are: "Differences in the receipt of, experiences with, and quality of healthcare that are not due to access-related factors or clinical needs, preferences, or appropriateness of intervention" (Health Care Disparities, n.d.). *Health equity* is defined as follows:

"the attainment of the highest level of health for all people. Achieving health equity requires valuing everyone equally, with focused and ongoing societal efforts to address avoidable inequalities, historical and contemporary injustices, and the elimination of health and healthcare disparities" (Health Equity n.d.).

### Culturally Competent Transcultural Nursing Practice

The HHS Office of Minority Health (OMH) offers an outstanding free online elearning program *What is Culturally Competent Nursing Care: A Cornerstone of Caring?* The program is based on the National Standards for Culturally and Linguistically Appropriate Services (CLAS), which are discussed next in more detail. Nurses and social workers can earn nine continuing education credits for completing the program, which is divided into three manageable courses that may be completed at the learner's own rate. The program may be found online at the following location: https://ccnm.thinkculturalhealth.hhs.gov/

### National Standards for Culturally and Linguistically Appropriate Services (CLAS)

The National Standards for CLAS in Health and Healthcare (The National CLAS Standards) are also important for the APN to know and understand. The APN can take a leadership role in implementation in practice settings. The National CLAS Standards "aim to improve healthcare quality and advance health equity by establishing a framework for organizations to serve the nation's increasingly diverse communities" (U.S. Department of Health and Human Services, 2016, para. 1). The CLAS Standards are 15 action steps that are divided under four headings. The first standard will "provide effective, equitable, under-standable and respectful quality care and services that are responsive to diverse cultural health beliefs and practices, preferred languages, health literacy and other communication needs," (para. 3) and is, by itself, under the heading *principle standard*. Standards 2 to 4 fall under the heading *governance, leadership, and workforce*, Standards 5 to 8 are grouped under the heading *communication and language assistance*, and Standards 9 to 15 are grouped under the heading *engagement, continuous improvement, and accountability*. You can view all 15 standards at the following website: https://ccnm.thinkculturalhealth. hhs.gov/PDFs/EnhancedNationalCLASStandards.pdf.

### Connection Between CLAS and Health Equity

It is paramount for the APN to realize the connection between CLAS and health equity. The HHS describes this connection as follows:

> Though health inequities are directly related to the existence of historical and current discrimination and social injustice, one of the most modifiable factors is the lack of culturally and linguistically appropriate services, broadly defined as care and services that are respectful of and responsive to the cultural and linguistic needs of all individuals. Health inequities result in disparities that directly affect the quality of life for all individuals. Health disparities adversely affect neighborhoods, communities, and the broader society, thus making the issue not only an individual concern but also a public health concern (U.S. Department of Health and Human Services, 2016).

### Providing Culturally Competent Nursing Assessment and Care

The Giger and Davidhizar (2002) Transcultural Assessment Model provides a model and theoretical foundation for culturally competent nursing care and an excellent foundation for assessing a family's culture, including one's own. The model includes "(1) transcultural nursing and culturally diverse nursing, (2) culturally competent care, (3) culturally unique individuals, (4) culturally sensitive environments, and (5) health and health status based on culturally specific illness and wellness behaviors" (Giger, 2017, p. 5). The Transcultural Assessment Model incorporates six connected cultural phenomena related to the culturally unique individual: communication, space, social organization, time, environmental control, and biological variation. "This nursing assessment and intervention model helps raise nurses' awareness of the differences between people from different cultural backgrounds and consider each

TABLE 2.3. *The Giger and Davidhizar Transcultural Assessment Model. Adapted from U.S. Department of Health and Human Services (HHS, n.d.).*

| Phenomena | Description | Examples |
|---|---|---|
| Communication | • Language spoken<br>• Voice quality<br>• Pronunciation | • Use of silence<br>• Use of nonverbal communication |
| Space | • Degree of comfort observed (conversation)<br>• Proximity to others | • Body movement<br>• Perception of space |
| Social organization | • Culture<br>• Race<br>• Ethnicity<br>• Family role function | • Work<br>• Leisure<br>• Church<br>• Friends |
| Time | • Use of time<br>• Measures<br>• Definition | • Social time<br>• Work time<br>• Time orientation (future, present, or past) |
| Environmental control | • Cultural health practices<br>• Values<br>• Definitions of health and illness | |
| Biological variation | • Body structure<br>• Skin color<br>• Hair color<br>• Other physical dimensions | • Biochemical and genetic factors<br>• Susceptibility to illness and disease<br>• Psychological characteristics and coping and social support |

individual's unique cultural identity" (U.S. Department of Health and Human Services, n.d., para. 1). The Tool kit, by Think Cultural Health (U.S. Department of Health and Human Services, n.d.), has an excellent overview of the tool and is depicted in Table 2.3.

## Cultural Awareness

The first step to cultural competency and improving cultural understanding is discovering one's own cultural identity. Cultural awareness is "the ability to understand one's own culture and perspective alongside the stereotypes and misconceptions associated with other unknown or less known cultures and statuses" (Matteliano & Street, 2012, p. 426). A care provider's sensitivity improves as the provider realizes how his or her own values and beliefs influence interactions with patients (Matteliano & Street, 2012).

## Culturagram

The *Culturagram* is another tool that may be used to assess a family's culture. It was developed by Elaine Congress in 1994 and revised in 2000. Originally developed for use by social workers, the culturagram has since been used by many other professions. The culturagram assesses the 10 areas below (Congress, 2005, p. 252):

- Reasons for relocation
- Legal status
- Time in community
- Language spoken at home and in the community
- Health beliefs
- Crisis events
- Holidays and special events
- Contact with cultural and religious institutions
- Values about education and work
- Values about family–structure, power, myths, and rules

A list of individual family members is placed in a box at the center of the Culturagram, and the 10 areas assessed are placed in boxes surrounding the family box, with spokes stemming from the family box to each of the 10 other boxes. The Culturagram diagram and an example Culturagram may be found in a journal article written by Congress (2005).

## Conclusion

The Population Health Advanced Practice Nurse, who is well versed in healthcare policy (such as the ACA, Global, and Glocal Population Health) and transcultural nursing practice, is best suited to interact as a strong leader in the interprofessional team. A sound understanding of payment policies in the workplace lay the foundation for application of responsible economic practices. Familiarity with the ACA allows APNs to explain it to others in the community and interprofessional team. APNs can lead the way to diminishing healthcare disparities by being aware of their own culture, understanding the 15 CLAS action steps, understanding cultural assessment, and utilizing resources.

## Tool Kit and Resources

Further Resources on the ACA include the following websites:

**Healthcare.gov**, the official site of the *Health Insurance Marketplace*, at which families and individuals can find information about health insurance options and purchase healthcare insurance. The website also has information about eligibility for assistance with paying premiums and reducing out-of-pocket costs. http://www.Healthcare.gov

**CMS Site—Health Insurance Marketplace**: A federal government website managed by the Centers for Medicare & Medicaid Services for healthcare providers as a central location for updated resources to assist families and individuals with application, enrollment, and coverage. http://marketplace.cms.gov

**Information About ACA for Consumers** from the American Association of Nurse Practitioners, which includes information on the Health Insurance Marketplace that is helpful to the Advanced Practice Nurse in assisting patients with navigation and enrollment: https://www.aanp.org/legislation-regulation/federal-legislation/affordable-care-act-aca/19-legislation-regulation/federal-legislation/1335-affordable-care-act-aca-2

**A Complete Summary of the Affordable Healthcare Act** from the Kaiser Family Foundation: http://kff.org/health-reform/fact-sheet/summary-of-the-affordable-care-act/

**Medicaid and ACA**: https://www.medicaid.gov/affordablecareact/affordable-care-act.html

**Medicare and ACA**: https://www.medicare.gov/about-us/affordable-care-act/affordable-care-act.html

**A Primer on Medicare: Key Facts About the Medicare Program and the People it Covers** from the Kaiser Family Foundation. http://files.kff.org/attachment/report-a-primer-on-medicare-key-facts-about-the-medicare-program-and-the-people-it-covers

### Tool Kit of Resources for Transcultural Nursing

| Source | URL |
| --- | --- |
| National Standards for Culturally and Linguistically Appropriate Services (CLAS) in Health and Healthcare-Website | https://www.thinkculturalhealth.hhs.gov/clas |
| CLAS Standards-PDF | https://ccnm.thinkculturalhealth.hhs.gov/PDFs/EnhancedNationalCLASStandards.pdf |
| Think Cultural Health: Culturally Competent Nursing Care-Online Learning Module | https://www.thinkculturalhealth.hhs.gov/GUIs/GUI_TCHRegister.asp?mode=new&site=3 |
| Caring Across Cultures-PDF | https://www.roswellpark.org/sites/default/files/node-files/page/nid940-21946-caring-across-cultures-web.pdf |
| Transcultural Nursing Society-Membership, Journal, Certification, Foundation Conferences, Scholars, Theories | http://www.tcns.org/ |
| End of Life Care Tutorial | http://edoc.ucdavis.edu/doctoring/media/Tutorials/Culture/4Cs/index.html |
| Theories/Textbooks | http://www.tcns.org/Theories.html |

*Assignments*

---

**The Importance of Self Awareness—
Your Cultural Identity Assignment**

For this exercise, use the Giger and Davidhizer model to assess the six cultural phenomena for yourself.

---

*Cultural Assessment Interview Assignment*

Choose a family from a different cultural or ethnic background than your own. Ask the family if they would like to be interviewed and inform them that they are under no obligation to do so, that the interview is completely voluntary. Explain to the family that the purpose of the assignment is to learn about the culture of a family from a diverse population. Use the Giger and Davidhizar Transcultural Assessment Model and Culturagram to formulate questions and observations for the family you will interview. During the interview, choose and implement an evidence-based "family level" culturally appropriate nursing action you will implement during the interview to assist a family member, or members, or the entire family, based on your assessment. Write a paper based on your findings. Include an introduction of the family, narrative of the interview/assessment, the Culturagram, the nursing action including why you chose it and results, rationale for the nursing action (peer-reviewed literature), your thoughts on experience of doing the assessment, and a reflection of what you have learned about analyzing and responding to marginalized populations.

## Discussion Questions

1. What are the primary goals and features of the ACA?
2. What is needed in order to facilitate advanced practice nurses' role in healthcare in order to realize their role in the ACA?
3. Explain at least three benefits that advanced practice nurses realize by including population health in their practice.
4. What is one specific way you can make a global and population health impact through your actions in your own local community?
5. Explain what constitutes health disparities and healthcare disparities and how these disparities impact health equity.

## Case Study 1
*Assisting Patients/Families with Navigating ACA to Acquire Healthcare Insurance.*

You are the advanced practice nurse caring for a family who consists of a single mother Tanya and two children Serena and Kip, ages three and five. Tanya is employed 30 hours per week making $10/hour plus tips at a local restaurant. She does not receive insurance from her employer, nor does she receive child support or insurance for her children from the father who is out of the picture. At present, the family has no health insurance coverage. How might you assist Tanya in navigating the ACA to acquire health coverage in your state? Does Tanya qualify for Medicaid in your state? Explain.

## Case Study 2

*The Uninsured Amish Couple*

You are working as a primary care provider in a rural outreach clinic in an area with a large Amish population. Samuel and Anna, a married couple ages 26 and 22, respectively, bring their 2-year-old daughter Samantha to your clinic for an earache. You notice in the intake paperwork that the couple is uninsured. The couple states they do not wish to be insured and that their community will provide for them. Is this couple exempt from being required to purchase medical insurance for the family under the Affordable Care Act? Why or why not? If not, what if any paperwork needs to be filed? How will your clinic handle payment?

## Case Study 3

*Medicare and the Insurance Exchange*

You are visiting a 72-year-old patient named Amir in his home. Amir is insured through Medicare. Amir is concerned about the costs of medications and asks if it would be better for him to drop Medicare and get insurance through the Exchange. What questions may you ask and what response would you provide Amir?

## Case Study 4

*Cobra versus the Insurance Exchange*

Juan is a 42-year-old patient you are seeing at your local primary care clinic. Juan has a question on dropping COBRA. He asks, "My COBRA is too expensive; can I drop it and enroll in the Marketplace instead"? What explanation will you provide Juan? What assistance can you provide Juan in navigating the Marketplace?

## Case Study 5

*Pregnant College Student Insured by Parents*

You are working in a local clinic in a college town. A 24-year old college student, Courtney, is seeing you for prenatal care. Courtney is currently covered on her parent's insurance. She asks you what her insurance options are after the baby is born. What response will you provide Courtney?

## Case Study 6

*Cultural and Religious Beliefs in Death and Dying*

Choose a religion other than your own. It is best to select one you are not very familiar with.

You are working as a Hospice Nurse with a patient named George and his family. George and his family practice the religion you choose above. How will you assess the cultural needs of George and his family related to their religious beliefs, death, and dying?

## References

Affordable Care Act. (n.d.). In Healthcare.Gov Glossary. Retrieved from https://www.healthcare.gov/glossary/affordable-care-act/

American Association of Colleges of Nursing. (2006). *Essentials of doctoral education for advanced practice nursing.* Retrieved from www.aacn.nche.edu/publications/position/DNPEssentials.pdf

American Association of Colleges of Nursing. (2008). *The consensus model for APRN regulation: Licensure, accreditation, certification & education.* Retrieved from http://www.aacn.nche.edu/education-resources/APRNReport.pdf

American Association of Nurse Practitioners. (2014). *NP fact sheet.* Retrieved from http://www.aanp.org/all-about-nps/np-fact-sheet

American Association of Nurse Practitioners (n.d.). General information about ACA. Retrieved from https://www.aanp.org/legislation-regulation/federal-legislation/affordable-care-act-aca/19-legislation-regulation/federal-legislation/1336-aca-general-information

Beck, D. M., Dossey, B. M., & Rushton, C. H. (2013) Building the nightingale initiative for global health—NIGH—Can we engage and empower the public voices of nurses worldwide? *Nursing Science Quarterly 26*(4), 366–371. doi:10.1177/0894318413500403

Buerhaus, P. I., DesRoches, C. M., Dittus, R., & Donelan, K. (2015). Practice characteristics of primary care nurse practitioners and physicians. *Nursing Outlook, 63*(2), 144–153. doi: 10.1016/j.outlook.2014.08.008

Chapman, S. A., Wides, C. D., & Spetz, J. (2010). Payment regulations for advanced practice nurses: Implications for primary care. *Policy, Politics, & Nursing Practice, 11*(2), 89–98.

Congress, E. P. (2005). Cultural and ethical issues in working with culturally diverse patients and their families. *Social Work in Health Care. 39*(34), 249–262. doi:10.1300/J010v39n03_03

Eibner, C., Hussey, P. M., Ridgely, M. S., & McGlynn, E. A. (2009). *Controlling health care spending in Massachusetts: An analysis of options.* Santa Monica, CA: RAND Corporation. Retrieved from https://www.rand.org/pubs/technical_reports/TR733.html.

Esperalt, M. C., Hanson-Turton, T., Richardson, M., & Debisette, A. T. (2012). Nurse-managed health enters: Safety-net care through advanced nursing practice. *Journal of the American Academy of Nurse Practitioners, 24*, 24–31. doi:10.1111/j.1745-7599.2011.00677.x

Giger, J. N. (2017). *Transcultural nursing: Assessment and intervention* (7th ed.). St. Louis, MS: Elsevier.

Giger, J., & Davidhizar, R. (2002). The Giger and Davidhizar transcultural assessment model. *Journal of Transcultural Nursing, 13*(3), 185–188. doi:10.1177/10459602013003004

Grootjans, J., & Newman S. (2013). The relevance of globalization to nursing: A concept analysis. *International Nursing Review 60*(1),78–85. doi:10.1111/j.1466-7657.2012.01022.x

Hain, D., Fleck, L. (2014). Barriers to Nurse Practitioner practice that impact healthcare redesign. *OJIN: The Online Journal of Issues in Nursing,19*(2), 5. doi: 10.3912/OJIN.Vol19No02Man02

Hatcher, B. J. (2015). Toward a paradigm shift in advanced practice nursing education: From an individual to a blended population/individual perspective. *Quality in Primary Care, 23*(3), 179–180.

Health Care Disparities. (n.d.). In *Think Cultural Health Glossary*. U.S. Department of Health and Human Services. Retrieved from https://ccnm.thinkculturalhealth.hhs.gov/Content/Toolkit/Glossary/Glossary1.asp

HealthCare.gov. (n.d.). *Affordable Care Act (ACA)*. Retrieved from https://www.healthcare.gov/glossary/affordable-care-act/

Health Equity. (n.d.). In *Think Cultural Health Glossary*. U.S. Department of Health and Human Services. Retrieved from https://ccnm.thinkculturalhealth.hhs.gov/Content/Toolkit/Glossary/Glossary1.asp

Institute for Healthcare Improvement. (2016a). Open-School: I-CAN frequently asked questions (FAQ). Retrieved from http://www.ihi.org/education/IHIOpenSchool/ICAN/Pages/FAQ.aspx

Institute for Healthcare Improvement. (2016b). Open-School: Take action with I-CAN learning activities. Retrieved from http://www.ihi.org/education/IHIOpenSchool/ICAN/Pages/FAQ.aspx

Institute of Medicine (2011). The future of nursing: Leading change, advancing health. Retrieved from https://www.ncbi.nlm.nih.gov/books/NBK209880/

Kaiser Family Foundation. (2013). Summary of the Affordable Care Act. Retrieved from http://kff.org/health-reform/fact-sheet/summary-of-the-affordable-care-act/

Lathrop, B., & Hodnicki, D. R. (2014). The Affordable Care Act: Primary care and the doctor of nursing practice nurse. *Online Journal of Issues in Nursing, 19*(2), 2. doi:10.3912/OJIN.Vol198No02PPT02

Matteliano, M. A., & Street, D. (2012). Nurse practitioners' contributions to cultural competence in primary care settings. *Journal of The American Academy of Nurse Practitioners, 24*(7), 425–435. doi:10.1111/j.1745-7599.2012.00701.x

Medicaid.gov. (n.d.). *Affordable Care Act*. Retrieved from https://www.medicaid.gov/affordable-care-act/index.html

National Council of State Boards of Nursing. (2008). *Consensus model for APRN regulation: Licensure, accreditation, certification & education*. Retrieved from https://www.ncsbn.org/2276.htm

Newhouse, R. P., Stanik-Hutt, J., White, K. M., Johantgen, M., Bass, E. B., Zangaro, G., Weiner, J. P. (2011). Advanced practice nurse outcomes 1990-2008: A systematic review. *Nursing Economic$, 29*(5), 230-251. doi:10.1234/1234567

Office of Disease Prevention and Health Promotion. (2016). Global health. In *Healthy People 2020*. Retrieved from https://www.healthypeople.gov/2020/topics-objectives/topic/global-health

Poghosyan, L., Lucero, R. Rauch, L. & Berkowitz, B. (2012). Nurse practitioner workforce: A substantial supply of primary care providers. *Nursing Economic$, 30*(5), 268–274.

Reeves, S., Perrier, L., Goldman, J., Freeth, D., & Zwarenstein, M. (2013). Interprofessional education: Effects on professional practice and healthcare outcomes (update). *Cochrane Database of Systematic Reviews, 3*. doi: 10.1002/14651858.CD002213.pub3

Shen, Z. (2015). Cultural competence models and cultural competence assessment instruments in nursing: A literature review. *Journal of Transcultural Nursing, 26*(3), 308-321. doi:10.1177/1043659614524790

Sigma Theta Tau International Honor Society of Nursing. (2016). United Nations: Sustainable development goals. Retrieved from http://www.nursingsociety.org/connect-engage/our-global-impact/stti-and-the-united-nations.

Transcultural Nursing Society. (2016). *Philosophy and values*. Retrieved from http://www.tcns.org/

U.S. Department of Health and Human Services. (2008). The Secretary's Advisory Committee on National Health Promotion and Disease Prevention Objectives for 2020. Phase I report: Recommendations for the framework and format of Healthy People 2020. Section IV: Advisory Committee findings and recommendations. Retrieved from http://www.healthypeople.gov/sites/default/files/PhaseI_0.pdf.

U.S. Department of Health and Human Services. (2015a). Key features of the Affordable Care Act. Retrieved from http://www.hhs.gov/healthcare/facts-and-features/key-features-of-aca/index.html

U.S. Department of Health and Human Services. (2015b). *About the law*. Retrieved from http://www.hhs.gov/healthcare/about-the-Blaw/index.html

U.S. Department of Health and Human Services. (2016). National CLAS Standards. In *Cultural Competency*. Retrieved from https://www.thinkculturalhealth.hhs.gov/clas

U.S. Department of Health and Human Services. (n.d.). Giger and Davidhizar transcultural assessment model. In *Think Cultural Health*. Retrieved from https://ccnm.thinkculturalhealth.hhs.gov/Content/Toolkit/ResourceLibrary/Course1/ResourceLibrary3.asp

Van Vleet, A., & Paradise, J. (2015). Tapping nurse practitioners to meet rising need for primary care. *Kaiser Family Foundation*. Retrieved from http://kff.org/medicaid/issue-brief/tapping-nurse-practitioners-to-meet-rising-demand-for-primary-care/

Waite, R., Nardi, D., & Killian, P. (2014). Context, health, and cultural competence: Nurse managed health care centers serving the community. *Journal of Cultural Diversity, 20*(4), 190–194.

Wilson, L., Mendes, I. A. C., Klopper H., Catrambone, C., Al-Maaita, H. R., Norton M. E., & Hill, D. (2016). 'Global health' and 'global nursing': Proposed definitions from The Global Advisory Panel on the Future of Nursing. *Journal of Advanced Nursing 72*(7), 1529–1540. doi: 10.1111/jan.12973.

World Health Organization. (2016). *Global strategic directions for strengthening nursing and midwifery 2016–2020.* Retrieved from http://www.who.int/hrh/nursing_midwifery/global-strategic-midwifery2016-2020.pdf

## CHAPTER 3

# Population Health and Data Analysis

STEPHANIE J. (JILL) RAPS, Maj USAF DHA Solution Deliv (US)
KATHARINE W. MURRAY, RN, CPHIMS

## Population Health and Data Analysis

T HE continuing need to proactively prepare to address emerging public health problems and emergency responsiveness, and to be accountable to the public, has intensified national and global efforts to collect data and information from multiple sources. Data analysis has reshaped the practice of public health by streamlining public health surveillance, disease and injury investigation and control, decision making, quality assurance, and policy development (https://www.ncbi. nlm.nih.gov/pmc/articles/PMC4371418/). Health departments are collecting and analyzing data on a scale that was inconceivable, even five years ago (Brixey, Brixey, Saba & McCormick, 2011). To be able to manage this overwhelming surge of data and information, the public health field has tapped into information technology (IT).

Current Centers for Disease Control and Prevention (CDC) Public Health Service initiatives (Table 3.1) require effective data collection and information from multiple sources. Information systems have become widely adapted to fit the special needs within public health. Recognizing the importance of connections among electronic health systems and public health information systems has helped establish data and information exchange standards to support system interoperability (Brixey *et al.*, 2011). This chapter provides a brief overview of the evolution of electronic health records, clinical informatics, big data in healthcare, and how data helps drive population health and introduces concepts of how

49

*TABLE 3.1. CDC Public Health Service Initiatives.*
*https://www.cdc.gov/stltpublichealth/publichealthservices/*
*essentialhealthservices.html*

| |
|---|
| 1. Monitor health status to identify and solve community health problems. |
| 2. Diagnose and investigate health problems and health hazards in the community. |
| 3. Inform, educate, and empower people about health issues. |
| 4. Mobilize community partnerships and action to identify and solve health problems. |
| 5. Develop policies and plans that support individual and community health efforts. |
| 6. Enforce laws and regulations that protect health and ensure safety. |
| 7. Link people to needed personal health services and assure the provision of health care when otherwise unavailable. |
| 8. Assure competent public and personal healthcare workforce. |
| 9. Evaluate effectiveness, accessibility, and quality of personal and population-based health service. |
| 10. Research for new insights and innovative solutions to health problems. |

to obtain and apply population health data. The chapter also includes historical examples and several case studies to illustrate these concepts.

## The Evolution of Clinical Informatics and Big Data in Healthcare

*Electronic Health Records*

Early design and development of computer-based patient records (CPRs), now called electronic health records (EHRs), began back in the late 1960s when multiple, small scale efforts began appearing throughout the United States (U.S.). These efforts started a new health IT era that changed the way healthcare providers recorded and shared data. These early efforts were largely driven by the U.S. Centers for Medicare & Medicaid Services (CMS) requirements to direct the adoption of electronic financial systems to improve the accuracy of billing, timely payment for services, and tracking and to reduce fraud.

However, even with these early efforts, prior to 2009, the majority of healthcare documentation was still captured on paper and stored in silos. Sharing health information was largely reliant upon hand carrying records, mailing, or the use of unsecured fax machines, presenting numerous challenges in an ever-increasing digital world. During the 1980s and 1990s, there came an explosion in computer technology development, resulting in the IT industry delivering larger and larger amounts of computing power and bandwidth and larger storage capacity, at lower costs. The advent of personal computers in the 1980s brought health IT to the patient bedside for the first time and the concept of a world-wide internet was being realized. Today, IT continues to mature and evolve at breakneck speed, producing more sophisticated hardware and software solutions.

In 1997, an Institute of Medicine (IOM) Committee report defined the CPR as an "electronic patient record (i.e., a repository of healthcare information about a single patient) that resides in a system specifically to support users through the availability of complete an accurate data, alerts, reminders, clinical decision support systems, links to medical knowledge, and other aids" (Dick, Steen & Detmer, 1997, p. 1). The report further identified 12 specific attributes (listed below) that a robust CPR must possess. This was the first time (on a large scale) that the CPR was viewed as a routinely used healthcare tool, not just a digitized representation of the paper record.

1. The CPR contains a problem list that clearly delineates the patient's clinical problems and the current status of each (e.g., the primary illness is worsening, stable, or improving).

2. The CPR encourages and supports the systematic measurement and recording of the patient's health status and functional level to promote more precise and routine assessment of the outcomes of patient care.

3. The CPR states the logical basis for all diagnoses or conclusions as a means of documenting the clinical rationale for decisions about the management of the patient's care. (This documentation should enhance use of a scientific approach in clinical practice and assist the evolution of a firmer foundation for clinical knowledge.)

4. The CPR can be linked with other clinical records of a patient—from various settings and time periods—to provide a longitudinal (i.e., lifelong) record of events that may have influenced a person's health.

5. The CPR system addresses patient data confidentiality comprehensively—in particular, ensuring that the CPR is accessible only to authorized individuals. (Although absolute confidentiality cannot be guaranteed in any system, every possible practical and cost-effective measure should be taken to secure CPRs and CPR systems from unauthorized access or abuse.)

6. The CPR is accessible for use in a timely way at any and all times

by authorized individuals involved in direct patient care. Simultaneous and remote access to the CPR is possible.

7. The CPR system allows selective retrieval and formatting of information by users. It can present custom-tailored "views" of the same information.

8. The CPR system can be linked to both local and remote knowledge, literature, bibliographic, or administrative databases and systems (including those containing clinical practice guidelines or clinical decision support capabilities) so that such information is readily available to assist practitioners in decision making.

9. The CPR can assist and, in some instances, guide the process of clinical problem solving by providing clinicians with decision analysis tools, clinical reminders, prognostic risk assessment, and other clinical aids.

10. The CPR supports structured data collection and stores information using a defined vocabulary. It adequately supports direct data entry by practitioners.

11. The CPR can help individual practitioners and healthcare provider institutions manage and evaluate the quality and costs of care.

12. The CPR is sufficiently flexible and expandable to support not only today's basic information needs but also the evolving needs of each clinical specialty and subspecialty (Dick, Steen & Detmer, 1997).

Fast forward to today, and the goals for an EHR remains principally the same, as follows:

- To systematically eliminate the logistical problems created by paper records, thereby making clinical data readily available electronically to authorized users (healthcare providers, claims adjudicators, case managers, and researchers), wherever the user (or record) physically resides

- To support healthcare providers with clinical documentation workflow, error checking, and decision support to ultimately improve patient safety and outcomes, decrease duplication of tests, decrease costs, and improve patient satisfaction

- To make healthcare data accessible to support clinical, epidemiological (surveillance and prevention), and outcomes research.

EHRs are designed to digitally capture detailed accounts of a patient's health information, generated by multiple healthcare providers, in a variety of scenarios (e.g., patient reported health data, walk-in clinics, healthcare provider offices, emergency rooms, and hospital encounters) throughout the patient's lifetime. An EHR typically contains vast amounts of information, such as demographic and contact information, vital signs, allergies, current and past medications, immunizations, radiology text reports, laboratory results, procedures, hospitalizations, and family and social history.

As adoption of the EHR grows and the amount of data captured and stored in EHRs increases, the secured sharing of electronic data between organizations becomes important. For example, since 2001, the Department of Defense (DoD) and Department of Veterans Affairs (VA) securely share a significant amount of health information electronically, continue to support interagency health data sharing activities, and continue to deliver IT solutions that significantly improve the secure sharing of appropriate electronic health information for their shared patient population. These initiatives enhance healthcare delivery to beneficiaries and improve the continuity of care for those who have served our country. Additionally, advances in the eHealth Exchange and Health Information Exchange (HIE) initiatives in the past 10 years continue to support interagency and multiagency health data sharing between federal and private sector partners (eHealth Exchange, 2017).

*Security Concerns*

The federal government enacted the Health Insurance Portability and Accountability Act of 1996 (HIPAA) Privacy Rule to ensure patients have rights over their health information, no matter what form it is in (paper or digital). The government also created the HIPAA Security Rule to require specific protections to safeguard electronic health information. Protective measures that can be built in to EHR systems should include the following:

- Access control tools like passwords and PIN numbers, to help limit access to personal and health information to authorized individuals.
- Encrypting stored health information such that it cannot be read or understood except by those using a system that can decrypt it with a key.
- An audit trail feature, which records who accessed health information, what changes were made, and when.

Finally, the law requires covered entities (e.g., clinics, hospitals, and other healthcare providers) to notify patients of a potential "breach." A breach of personally identifiable information (PII) or protected health information (PHI) occurs when information is lost, disclosed to, accessed by, or potentially exposed to unauthorized individuals or compromised in a way in which the subjects of the information are negatively affected. These requirements help patients know if something has gone wrong with the protection of their information and helps keep healthcare providers accountable for the protection of PII/PHI.

### The HITECH ACT—Spurring EHR Adoption

Initiatives such as CMS' *meaningful use* (https://www.healthit.gov/policy-researchers-implementers/meaningful-use-regulations) are good examples of EHRs beign used to support quality health care for all. The regulations are accelerating the adoption of EHRs and, as a result, the volume and detail of patient information is growing rapidly. The surge in the creation and broadening use of EHRs was driven in part by a $30 billion federal government stimulus package, provided by the Health Information Technology for Economic and Clinical Health (*HITECH*) Act in 2009. The Act was designed specifically to provide incentives to adopt EHRs and encourage the sharing of patient information by healthcare providers everywhere in an attempt to lower costs, speed diagnosis, and improve patient outcomes.

Since the passage of the HITECH Act, the healthcare industry has undergone rapid changes in technology. The adoption of EHRs among healthcare providers has been one of the most transformative changes to occur, and fluctuations in both the market and in EHR systems show no signs of slowing down. In 2008, only 17% of physicians and 9% of hospitals had at least a basic EHR (i.e., electronic order entry and results reporting, clinical note documentation, and consolidated medication, allergy, and problem lists). By 2015, 96% of hospitals and 78% of physician offices were using certified EHRs (Report to Congress, 2016). As a result, today the majority of the U.S. population has at least part of their healthcare record accessible electronically.

### Health IT Trends

A number of industries, including healthcare, are making the move to EHR software applications and analytic tools in the cloud. *Cloud-based EHRs* offer attractive benefits, particularly to smaller and mid-sized medical groups and smaller hospitals, because there are little upfront financial investments needed for infrastructure and sustainment. By reducing the significant startup costs of a typical workstation and server solution, more healthcare providers are likely to turn to a cloud-based EHR alternative that is flexible, scalable, and cost-effective. The ability to access an EHR from outside the office/hospital through a mobile device is also supported by a cloud solution. Remote EHR access not only has the potential to increase productivity among healthcare providers, but also it can also improve continuity of care and have a positive impact on patient outcomes.

The healthcare industry, perhaps more than any other industry, is on the brink of a major transformation through the use of *advanced analytics and big data technologies*. Providers continue to employ meaningful big data analytics strategies to convert EHR information into actionable insights. EHRs have been transformative in the healthcare industry, enabling faster patient information access, improved workflow, reduced costs, and information sharing across organizations. The ability to combine and analyze a variety of structured and unstructured data across multiple data sources aids in the accuracy of diagnosing patient conditions, matching treatments with outcomes, and predicting patients at risk for disease or readmission. Predictive modeling and machine learning on large sample sizes, with more patient data, can uncover nuances and patterns that couldn't be previously observed. Additional trends include increased usage of and support for telehealth and improved patient portals to increase the patient's involvement in his or her health and wellness plan.

## The Role of the Clinical Informaticist

As the health technology landscape has changed over the past 30 years, so has the job and responsibilities of the clinician. Federal mandates are pushing healthcare providers to embrace health IT solutions and transition to EHRs. Clinicians with an interest in health technology have opportunities worth pursuing in the rapidly evolving role of the *clinical informaticist*. Clinical informatics as a specialty is relatively new, so the job description may differ, depending on the location and nature of the healthcare facility and work being done. Clinical informatics, also known as healthcare or medical informatics, is defined as the interdisciplinary study of the design, development, adoption and application of IT-based innovations in healthcare services delivery (HIMSS, 2016). The field typically includes the following:

- Methods to electronically collect, store, and analyze healthcare data
- Analysis of information needs and cognitive processes and optimal ways to meet those needs
- Methods to support clinical decisions, including summarization, visualization, provision of evidence, and active decision support
- Optimizing the flow of information and coordinating it with care providers' and patients' workflows to maximize patient safety and care quality
- Methods and policies for information infrastructure, including privacy and security

The American Medical Informatics Association (AMIA) considers the term "informatics," when used within a healthcare delivery scenario, to be essentially the same regardless of the health professional group involved (i.e., dentist, pharmacist, physician, nurse, or other health professional). The AMIA Board of Directors approved the Core Content for the Sub-Specialty in Clinical Informatics in November 2008. The core content defines the boundaries of the discipline and informs the recommended clinical informatics program requirements. The core content includes four major categories: fundamentals, clinical decision making and care process improvement, health information systems, and leadership and management of change (Gardiner, Overhage, Steen, Munger, Holmes, Williamson, & Detmer, 2009).

Nursing informatics (NI) is a sub-specialty that integrates nursing science with multiple information management and analytical sciences to identify, define, manage, and communicate data, information, knowledge, and wisdom in nursing practice. NI supports nurses, consumers, patients, the healthcare team, and other stakeholders in their decision-making in all roles and settings to achieve desired outcomes. This support is accomplished through the use of information structures, information processes, and IT (ANA, 2015). Nursing informatics professionals also simplify documentation of patient care and enter patient notes using computers, mobile devices, and voice recognition software. Nursing Informatics professionals aim to improve the accuracy of patient data and enable critical data analysis to improve efficiency of overall patient care.

Clinical informatics is a rapidly expanding career field. According to the AMIA, around 70,000 specialists in this field will be needed within the next few years because of the impact that federal laws have had on the healthcare system—specifically, the mandate for EHRs. Seeing the need for education in this discipline, many colleges and universities now offer graduate level health informatics degree and certificate programs via distance learning or in traditional on-campus settings. For nurses seeking a different career path or wanting to specialize and have an interest in the field of IT, clinical informatics is a career path to consider.

The field of clinical informatics is on the cusp of its most exciting period to date, entering a new era in which technology is starting to handle "Big Data," bringing about unlimited potential for information growth and secondary usage. Data mining and Big Data analytics are helping to realize the goals of diagnosing, treating, helping, and healing patients in need of healthcare, with the end goal of this domain being improved health outcomes or the quality of care that healthcare can provide to patients.

*What is "Big Data?"*

The amount of data produced and captured within the healthcare landscape has grown to such an extent that analysis of this data grants potentially limitless possibilities for advanced levels of study to be done and knowledge to be gained. However, there are a number of issues that arise when dealing with these vast quantities of data, especially how to analyze this data in a reliable manner. A basic goal of clinical informatics is to take in real world medical data from all levels to help advance the understanding of medicine and medical practice. The ultimate objective of any big data analytics project should be to generate some sort of value for the organization doing the analysis. Otherwise, they are just performing some technological task for technology's sake.

The term "Big Data" is somewhat vague with definitions that are not universally agreed upon. Big data, as defined by Gartner, Inc., (Sicular, 2013) includes high-volume, high-velocity, and/or high-variety information assets that demand cost-effective, innovative forms of information processing which enable enhanced insight, decision making, and process automation. It is becoming generally accepted that there are specific attributes that define big data. In most big data circles, these are called the five Vs: volume, variety, velocity, veracity, and value. These data sets are so complex that traditional data processing application software is inadequate to deal with them in order to derive intelligence for effective decisions.

• Volume refers to the sheer size or amount of data

- Variety describes whether the data is structured, semi-structured, or unstructured
- Velocity is the frequency of incoming data that needs to be processed
- Veracity measures to genuineness or trustworthiness of the data
- Value evaluates how good the quality of the data is in reference to the intended results

Today, health data repositories exhibit all of these qualities. *Big volume* in health data comes from the vast amount of electronic data captured and stored. *Big variety* in health data pertains to datasets with a large amount of varying types of independent attributes (structured data elements like laboratory values and unstructured data like scanned clinical notes) and datasets that are gathered from many sources. *Big velocity* in health data occurs when new data is coming in at high speeds, which can be seen when trying to monitor real-time events, such as monitoring a patient's current condition through medical devices during a critical hospital stay. *High veracity* of health data, as in any profession using analytics, is of concern when working with possibly noisy, incomplete, or erroneous data (as could be captured from faulty clinical sensors or self-reported patient information). The *high value* of health data is seen all throughout clinical analytics, because the primary goal is to improve clinical care and outcomes.

The value of big data in healthcare today is largely limited to research, because analyzing and studying big data requires a very specialized skill set. Big data has the potential to impact multiple areas across the continuum of healthcare, such as improving clinical, financial, and operational decision making; reducing the cost of healthcare; and providing greater savings under federal and pay-for-performance incentive programs. Cost pressure in the U.S. healthcare system in not new—healthcare expenses have continued to rapidly increase over the last two decades. In 2015, U.S. healthcare spending increased 5.8% to reach $3.2 trillion, or $9,990 per person.

The coverage expansion that began in 2014 as a result of the Patient Protection and Affordable Care Act (also referred to as the Affordable Care Act, or ACA) continued to have an impact on the growth of healthcare spending in 2015. Additionally, faster growth in total healthcare spending in 2015 was driven by stronger growth in spending for private health insurance, hospital care, physician and clinical services, and the continued strong growth in Medicaid and retail prescription drug spending. Finally, the overall share of the U.S. economy devoted to healthcare spending was 17.8% in 2015, up from 17.4% in 2014 (CMS, 2015). Healthcare decision makers have the opportunity to enhance clinical outcomes by unlocking these data to generate actionable intelligence. Some analysts have proposed that the value derived from big data could potentially be worth $300 to $450 billion per year to the U.S. healthcare industry.

Big data gets its name for a reason; the information sets are vast and complex. Big data, and the use of business intelligence, genomics, and analytics, have the potential to decode the intricacies of a multitude of medical diagnoses, for example, cancer and dementia. *Analytics* is the discovery, interpretation, and communication of meaningful patterns in data. Digital *analytics* is a set of business and technical activities that *define*, create, collect, verify or transform digital data into reporting or research results. Federal plans such as the Precision Medicine Initiative and Cancer Moonshot are huge strides in a direction to realize great benefits of big data in healthcare.

### Case Study 1—National Cancer Institute, Cancer Moon Shot: Building an IT Structure

*National Cancer Center. (n.d.)*

An essential component for optimizing the impact of an expanded early cancer detection capability is the establishment of an IT infrastructure that will assemble quantitative image data, molecular analysis results, genomic data, and patient history into a widely-accessible and analyzable database. The importance of this IT infrastructure has been conclusively demonstrated by the impact of the International Early Lung Cancer Program (I-ELCAP) database of more than 75,000 participants from 72 institutions, which represents a paradigm for future research collaborations. The database consists of baseline and follow-up metadata (e.g., pertinent medical information, smoking history, and quality of life measures), diagnostic reports (e.g., CT examination reports), diagnostic images (e.g., CT, MRI, PET), treatment information if performed (e.g., surgical, radiotherapy, and chemotherapy procedures and results), and long-term follow-up of screenings and diagnoses. All data are entered into the I-ELCAP Management System, a web-based database that also provides for patient management and follow-up reports. This database has enabled seminal research on early lung cancer detection and treatment and has provided key information for the development of national guidelines for efficient implementation of

CT screening for lung cancer, which is now covered by the CMS for high-risk smokers. Data in the I-ELCAP database has been used in over 300 publications. The I-ELCAP Data Repository collects the patient metadata and images in a distributed system that provides participating institutions with a web-based interface to enter patient data and manage the follow-up of their participants/patients according to a common protocol. The system is hosted in a "private cloud" in a U.S. datacenter, with backup systems in place at a separate location in the United States. Each datacenter has multiple power and Internet connections to provide redundancy. The security and privacy of patient data are ensured by using industry standard encryption technologies to protect the data between all the I-ELCAP institution and servers. The clinical metadata can be directly entered into the system from any Internet connected computer, and images are transferred automatically from each institution's scanner or PACS (Picture Archiving and Communication System) to the I-ELCAP repository. In addition to data collection, the I-ELCAP Management System provides for download of all data in a format that can be parsed by any statistical package and, thus, enables data analysis for research, patient follow-up, and quality image and data monitoring, both on an institutional level and a national/global level. The I-ELCAP Data Repository has collected the metadata and images for over 75,000 patients, totaling approximately 40 TB of data. The average file size for an individual patient is less than one gigabyte. If all new patients diagnosed with cancer in the United States (1.6 million per year) were included in a similar national database, the total storage required per year would be approximately one petabyte. This amount of data is easily handled by existing commercial cloud storage facilities. For comparison, approximately seven petabytes of photos are uploaded to Facebook accounts and six petabytes of videos are uploaded to You-Tube every month.

## How Does Data Drive Population Health?

Data and information are the foundation of public health (Saba & McCormick, 2011). As discussed in the previous section, electronic health information and big data have become widely available and massive amounts of data are produced each day that provide opportunities to understand social interactions, environmental, and social determinants of health and their impact on individuals (Tomines, Readhead, Readhead & Teutsch, 2013).

Despite the abundant sources of public health data and information, the sources lack standardization in organization, nomenclature, and electronic transmission (Brixey *et al.*, 2011). The powerful analytic tools utilized in commercial marketing and other fields are not commonly present in public health departments. It is important to understand the limitations of healthcare data resources when searching for and collecting reliable data. Public health systems are commonly defined as "all public, private, and voluntary entities that contribute to the delivery of essential public health services within a jurisdiction" (p. 12). The public health system includes public health agencies at state and local levels, healthcare providers, public safety agencies, human service and charity organizations, education and youth development organizations, recreation and artsrelated organizations, economic and philanthropic organizations, environmental agencies and organizations.

The Public Health Nursing field strives to provide continuous surveillance and assessment of the multiple determinates of health with the intent to promote health and wellness; prevent disease, disability and premature death; and improve neighborhood quality of life. These population health priorities are addressed through identification, implementation, and evaluation of universal and targeted evidence-based programs and services that provide primary, secondary, and tertiary preventive interventions (Brixey *et al.*, 2011). Public health or population health management improves healthcare outcomes while containing costs. Many of the IT initiatives currently underway are related to population health in one way or another: "electronic health records, meaningful use, interoperability, accountable care organizations, disease state management, payforperformance and patient-centered medical home" all have elements that relate to managing patients in groups. IT and data are often the starting point for managing population health issues, whereas point of care data drive informed decision making. How one idenitifes within a population may vary, but in terms of health individuals are often identified by diseases, such as diabetes, asthma, COPD, heart disease and cancer (http://www.healthcareitnews.com/news/data-key-population-health-management ).

Public health authorities are required to drill down for individual data and risk factors in order to diagnose, investigate, and control disease and health hazards in the community, including disease that "originates with social-, environmental-, occupational- and communicable-disease exposures." The community relies on public health to control exposure across jurisdictions and sectors, which may involve closing a school or business, isolating infectious individuals, or limiting exposures to health hazards. For example, a clinician or laboratory reports a case of active tuberculosis to the local health department. In response, public health staff performs chart reviews and patient interviews to identify exposed community members and immediately ensure appropriate precautions. For the next year, they ensure that all affected patients receive appropriate care and case management. They may provide direct clinical services, expert consultation for drug-resistant and other challenging cases, or oversight of private sector care, to ensure an appropriate treatment regimen and patient adherence. This process is resource intensive and time-consuming for both the public health department and clinicians, which can lead to a suboptimal response and public health control measures. Access to EHR data can improve the efficiency of both the investigation and quality assurance process, because health department staff no longer need to travel to multiple sites, manually abstract data from multiple electronic medical records (EMRs), or reenter abstracted data into an electronic public health information system. EHR data may offer more longitudinal, complete, and accurate information than a onetime interview with a patient. Data obtained from a personal health record (PHR) may be different in content or time frame and may also include information on patients who have not had a clinical visit (http://www.healthcareitnews.com/news/data-key-population-health-management).

The mission of the public health field is to promote the health of the population rather than to treat individuals. Public health professionals collect and utilize data to monitor the occurrence of health events, conditions, and deaths on health and ideally identity preventive measures to treat populations. The following provides an example of using data and predictive analytics to drive population health:

*Data and Predictive Analysis—Example 1*

From clean water supplies to the polio vaccine, the most effective public health interventions are typically preventative policies that help stop a crisis before it starts. But predicting the next public health crisis has historically been a challenge, and even interventions like chlorinating water or distributing a vaccine are in many ways reactive. However, with predictive analytics, it is possible to pilot new ways to predict public health challenges and intervene before they begin. Currently, predictive analytics are used to leverage seemingly unrelated data to predict trends in data like "who is most susceptible to birth complications" or "chronic diseases or where and when a virulent outbreak is most likely to occur." With this information, public health officials should be able to respond before an issue manifests itself and provide the right prenatal treatments to mitigate birth complications, identify those most likely to be exposed to lead, and/or finding food establishments most at risk for violations. Most importantly predictive analytics helps information and data to become actionable.

Predictive models may help determine the allocation of resources and prioritize home inspections in high lead poisoning risk areas (an active approach), instead of waiting for reports of children's elevated blood lead levels to trigger an inspection (the current passive approach). An active predictive approach shortens the amount of time and money spent in mitigation by concentrating efforts on those homes that have the greatest risk of causing lead poisoning in children. Incorporating predictive models into the electronic medical record interface will serve to alert healthcare providers of lead poisoning risk levels to their pediatric and pregnant patient populations so that preventive approaches and reminders for ordering blood lead level laboratory tests or contacting patients lost to follow-up visits can be done. There is a great opportunity in public health to use analytics to promote data-driven policies. As public health professionals, it will be vital to use data better, share these data with the public and our partners, and then leverage those data to create better policies, systems, and environmental changes (https://hbr.org/2014/09/how-cities-are-using-analytics-to-improve-public-health).

## How Do We Obtain and Apply the Data?

The previous section highlighted the importance of understanding how data drive population health and the limitations of healthcare data resources. This section focuses on effective strategies to obtain and apply data and provides numerous sources for reliable public health data and information. Data collection and sharing in public health occur at three levels: local, state/territorial, and federal. Programs at each level have similar organization and management structures. Since most funding is based on programmatic need, many information systems have been built to support specific programs, thereby creating "silo"-like systems. To be productive, the program-oriented funding streams and information systems need to flow together (Brixey *et al.*, 2011). Efforts are underway to assist healthcare providers in overcoming barriers to data collection and sharing through the implementation of regional, state/territorial, and local HIEs. This comprehensive, rather than disease-specific, approach to data collection and sharing is the foundation of public health information sharing and informatics.

Unlike incentives in the clinical care system, scant funding is available to public health departments to develop the necessary information infrastructure and workforce capacity to capitalize on EHRs, personal health records, or Big Data. Current EHR systems are primarily built to serve clinical systems and practice rather than being structured for public health use. In addition, there are policy issues concerning how broadly the data can be used by public health officials. Because these issues are resolved and workable solutions emerge, they should yield a more efficient and effective public health system (https://www.ncbi. nlm.nih.gov/pmc/articles/PMC4371418/). Finding data sources and effectively using statistics are of vital importance as national, state, and local public health departments are called upon to respond quickly to ever and more pressing emergencies. To make informed decisions and policies, public health practitioners require timely, quality information (Saba & McCormick, 2011).

The CDC, the Council of State and Territorial Epidemiologists (CSTE), and the National Notifiable Diseases Surveillance System (NNDSS) are the most reliable resources to obtain public health data. The CDC's primary role includes detecting and responding to new and emerging health threats; tackling the biggest health problems causing death and disability for Americans; putting science and advanced technology into action to prevent disease; promoting healthy and safe behaviors, communities, and environment; developing leaders and training the public health workforce, including disease detectives; and taking the health pulse of our nation (CDC, 2014). NNDSS is a nationwide collaboration that enables all levels of public health—local, state, territorial, federal, and international—to share notifiable disease-related health information. Public health uses this information to monitor, control, and prevent the occurrence and spread of statereportable and nationally notifiable infectious and noninfectious diseases and conditions. NNDSS is a multifaceted program that includes the surveillance system for collection, analysis, and sharing of health data. It also includes policies, laws, electronic messaging standards, people, partners, information systems, processes, and resources at the local, state, territorial, and national levels (CDC, 2015). The CSTE works to advance public health policy and epidemiologic capacity by promoting effective use of epidemiologic data to guide public health practice and improve health; supporting effective public health surveillance and epidemiologic practice through training, capacity development, and peer consultation; developing standards for practice; and advocating for resources and scientifically based policy (http://www.cste.org/?page=About_CSTE). Below is a description of how these organizations support public health surveillance in jurisdictions:

*Data and Predictive Analysis—Example 2*

Notifiable disease surveillance begins at the level of local, state, and territorial public health departments (also known as jurisdictions). Jurisdictional laws and regulations mandate reporting of cases of specified infectious and noninfectious conditions to health departments. Health Departments work with healthcare providers, laboratories, hospitals, and other partners to obtain the information needed to monitor, control, and prevent the occurrence and spread of these health conditions. In addition, health departments notify the CDC about the occurrence of certain conditions.

The CDC Division of Health Informatics and Surveillance (DHIS) supports NNDSS by receiving, securing, processing, provisioning, and releasing nationally notifiable infectious diseases data to disease-specific CDC programs. The DHIS also supports local, state, and territorial public health departments in collecting, managing, and analyzing their data and in submitting case notification data to the CDC for NNDSS. The DHIS provides this support through funding, HIE standards and frameworks, electronic health information systems, and technical support. Together, the DHIS and CDC programs prepare annual summaries of infectious and noninfectious diseases and conditions, which are published in the *Morbidity and Mortality Weekly Report.*

These programs collaborate with the Council of State and Territorial Epidemiologists (CSTE) to determine which conditions reported to local, state, and territorial public health departments are nationally notifiable. The CDC programs, in collaboration with subject matter experts in the CSTE and in health departments, determine what data elements are included in national notifications. Health departments participating in NNDSS voluntarily submit infectious disease data to the DHIS and also submit some data directly to CDC programs.

With the evolution of technology and data and exchange standards, the CDC now has the opportunity to strengthen and modernize the infrastructure supporting NNDSS. As part of the CDC Surveillance

Strategy, the NNDSS Modernization Initiative (NMI) is underway to enhance the system's ability to provide more comprehensive, timely, and higher quality data for public health decision making. Through this multiyear initiative, the CDC seeks to increase the robustness of the NNDSS technological infrastructure so that it is based on interoperable, standardized data and exchange mechanisms (CDC, n.d.).

The Partners in Information Access for Public Health Workforce website (https://phpartners.org/health_stats.html) is another resource that provides a collection of links to data on the health of a population. The website is a collaboration of U.S. government agencies, public health organizations, and health sciences libraries. The resources are from health data news, county and local health data, state health data, individual state and metropolitan data, national health data, global health data, statistical reports, demographic data, geographic information systems (GIS), training and education, health information technology and standards, tools for data collection and planning.

There are various ways to apply data in the public health field. Having a basic understanding of informatics and data analytics will provide insights and opportunities to improve each of the ongoing elements of any public health surveillance system. The following examples, quoted directly from the CDC, highlight how clinical informatics and data can be applied in the public health field:

- *Planning and system design*—Identifying information and sources that best address a surveillance goal; identifying who will access information, by what methods and under what conditions; and improving analysis or action by improving the surveillance system interaction with other information systems.
- *Data collection*—Identifying potential bias associated with different collection methods (e.g., telephone use or cultural attitudes toward technology); identifying appropriate use of structured data compared with free text, most useful vocabulary, and data standards; and recommending technologies (e.g., global positioning systems and radiofrequency identification) to support easier, faster, and higher-quality data entry in the field.
- *Data management and collation*—Identifying ways to share data across different computing/technology platforms; linking new data with data from legacy systems; and identifying and remedying data-quality problems while ensuring data privacy and security.

- *Analysis*—Identifying appropriate statistical and visualization applications; generating algorithms to alert users to aberrations in health events; and leveraging high-performance computational resources for large data sets or complex analyses.
- *Interpretation*—Determining usefulness of comparing information from one surveillance program with other data sets (related by time, place, person, or condition) for new perspectives and combining data of other sources and quality to provide a context for interpretation.
- *Dissemination*—Recommending appropriate displays of information for users and the best methods to reach the intended audience; facilitating information finding; and identifying benefits for data providers.
- *Application to public health programs*—Assessing the utility of having surveillance data directly flow into information systems that support public health interventions and information elements or standards that facilitate this linkage of surveillance to action and improving access to and use of information produced by a surveillance system for workers in the field and health-care providers (https://www.cdc.gov/mmwr/preview/mmwrhtml/su6103a5.htm).

## Case Study 2—Millennium Cohort Study 2013—A DoD Research Project (DoD, 2013)

"The Millennium Cohort Study" is a project recommended by the U.S. Congress in 1999 and sponsored by the DoD. The study is being conducted by the Naval Health Research Center in San Diego, California. (DMDC Reference #: 000019. RCS #: DD-HA(AR)2106. OMB approval #: 0720-0029.) The Millennium Cohort Study is an ongoing longitudinal cohort study designed to evaluate long-term health effects of military service, including deployment related issues and illnesses. It is the largest population-based prospective health project in U.S. military history, currently collecting data on over 200,000 enrolled participants. Investigators that conduct The Millennium Cohort Study include uniformed and nonuniformed scientists from the Army, Navy, Air Force, VA, and academic institutions. Ultimately, the greatest benefits of this study will not be known for many years. Multiple, targeted research projects within The Millennium Cohort Study have been conducted since 2013, resulting in improved surveillance and treatment of active duty and separated service members. One example is included below.

## Sleep and Health Resilience Metrics in a Large Military Cohort Study (DoD, 2013)

Longitudinal analyses were conducted from 2001 to 2008 using subjective data collected from The Millennium Cohort Study questionnaires and objective data from military records that included demographics, military health, and deployment information (Seelig, Jacobson, Donoho, Trone, Crum-Cianflone & Balkin, 2016). Subjective sleep duration and insomnia symptoms were collected on the study questionnaire. Resilience metrics included lost work days, self-rated health, deployment, frequency, and duration of healthcare utilization, and early discharge from the military. Generalized estimating equations and survival analyses were adjusted for demographic, military, behavioral, and health covariates in all models.

*Results*: The presence of insomnia symptoms was significantly associated with lower self-rated *health*, more lost work days, lower odds of deployment, higher odds of early discharge from *military* service early, and more *health*care utilization. Those self-reporting less than 6 hours (short sleepers) or longer than 8 hours (long sleepers) of *sleep* per night had similar findings, except for the deployment outcome in which those with the shortest *sleep* were more likely to deploy.

## Conclusions

Poor sleep is a detriment to service members' health and readiness. Leadership should redouble efforts to emphasize the importance of healthy sleep among military service members, and future research should focus on the efficacy of interventions to promote healthy sleep and resilience in this population.

## Chapter Summary

As public health, clinical care, information science, computer science, and IT continue to come together, the field of public health and informatics will continue to expand to support the public health functions of assessment, policy development, and assurance to promote a healthy nation (Brixey *et al.*, 2011). Federal, state, and local public health leaders need to continue the commitment to public health informatics and the development of a sustainable centralized HIE. Just as electronic health information will transform the day-today practice of medicine, it

will also transform the practice of public health (https://www.ncbi.nlm.
nih.gov/pmc/articles/PMC4371418/).

## Tool Kit and Resources

Centers for Disease Control and Prevention (CDC). (2017). National
health initiatives, strategies & action plans. CDC. Retrieved from
https://www.cdc.gov/stltpublichealth/strategy/index.html

Health IT Regulations. (2016). Meaningful use regulations. Retrieved
from https://www.healthit.gov/policy-researchers-implementers/
meaningful-use-regulations

HIMSS (2016). Fundamental Issues. Retrieved from http://www.himss.
org/clinical-informatics/medical-informatics

Institute of Medicine (U.S.) The computer-based patient record: An essential technology for healthcare revised edition. Revised Edition.
Washington D.C.: National Academy Press.

International Medical Infrmatics Association (IMIA) Retrieved from
http://www.imia.org/

National Cancer Center. (n.d.). Cancer moonshot: Building an IT structure. Retrieved from https://www.cancer.gov/research/key-initia-
tives/moonshot-cancer-initiative

National Database of Nursing Quality Indicators. American Nurses As-
sociaiton. Retrieved from http://www.nursingquality.org/

TIGER Initiative (Technology Informatics Guiding Education Reform)
– includes best practices and technological capabilities within nursing. Retireved from: http://www.tigersummit.com

U.S. Department of Health & Human Services. The Office of the National Coordinator for Health Information Technology. Retrieved
from http://healthit.hhs.gov/portal/server.pt

*Discussion Questions*
1. What role has the adoption of electronic health record (EHR)
   systems played in enabling enhanced population health and data
   analytics?

2. Discuss two major health IT trends and the impact on population
   health and data analytics.

3. Identify specific skills that have evolved the role of the Clinical

and Nurse Informaticist and why that role is important in population health efforts.

4. What is "Big Data?" Why is it important? What are some concerns? How does data drive population health? Give examples.

5. What role has the adoption of electronic health record (EHR) systems played in enabling enhanced population health and data analytics?

6. Discuss two major health IT trends and the impact on population health and data analytics.

7. Identify specific skills that have evolved the role of the Clinical and Nurse Informaticist and why that role is important in population health efforts.

8. What is "Big Data?" Why is it important? What are some concerns? How does data drive population health? Give examples.

*Definitions*

**Analytics**—is the discovery, interpretation, and communication of meaningful patterns in data. Digital *analytics* is a set of business and technical activities that *define*, create, collect, verify or transform digital data into reporting or research results.

**Big Data**—Extremely large data sets that may be analyzed computationally to reveal patterns, trends, and associations, especially relating to human behavior and interactions.

**Cloud-Based Computing**—A model for enabling ubiquitous, convenient, on-demand network access to a shared pool of configurable *computing* resources (e.g., networks, servers, storage, applications, and services) that can be rapidly provisioned and released with minimal management effort or service provider interaction.

**Cohort Study**—A cohort study follows a distinct group of people over an extended period of time.

**Decision Support System**—A computerized information system used to support decision making in an organization or a business.

**Electronic Health Record**—An electronic version of a patient's medical history that is maintained by the provider over time and may include all of the key administrative clinical data relevant to that person's care under a particular provider, including demographics, progress notes, problems, medications, etc.

**Informatics (Clinical)**—The interdisciplinary study of the design, development, adoption, and application of IT-based innovations in healthcare services delivery, management, and planning.

**Information Management**—The collection and *management* of *information* from one or more sources and the distribution of that *information* to one or more audiences.

**Information Technology**—The study or use of systems (especially computers and telecommunications) for storing, retrieving, and sending information.

**Interoperability**—The ability of different information technology systems and software applications to communicate and exchange data and to use the information that has been exchanged.

**Morbidity**—The incidence or prevalence of a disease or of all diseases.

**Mortality**—Relative incidence of death within a particular group categorized according to age or some other factor, such as occupation.

**Surveillance**—The ongoing systematic collection and analysis of data and the provision of information which leads to action being taken to prevent and control a disease, usually one of an infectious nature.

## References

American Nurses Association (ANA), (2015). Nursing informatics: Scope and standards of practice (2nd ed.) Atlanta, GA: Nursebooks.org.

Andrews, J. (2012). Data is key to population health management. Healthcare IT News. Retrieved from http://www.healthcareitnews.com/news/data-key-population-health-management

Brixey, J. J., Brixey, J.E., Saba, V.K., & McCormick, K. (2015). Essentials of nursing informatics (6th ed.). New York: McGraw-Hill Education.

Centers for Disease Control and Prevention (CDC). (2011). Core function of public health and how they relate to the 10 essential services. Retrieved from https://www.cdc.gov/nceh/ehs/ephli/core_ess.htm

Centers for Disease Control and Prevention (CDC). (n.d.). NNDS Modernization Initiative. Retrieved from https://www.cdc.gov/nmi/documents/nmi.pdf

Centers for Disease Control and Prevention (CDC). (2014). Mission, role and pledge. Retrieved From https://www.cdc.gov/about/organization/mission.htm

Centers for Disease Control and Prevention (CDC). (2015). National notifiable disease

Centers for Disease Control and Prevention (CDC). (2017). National health initiatives, strategies & action plans. CDC. Retrieved from https://www.cdc.gov/stltpublichealth/strategy/index.html

Choucair, B., Bhatt, J., & Mansour, R. (2014). How cities are using analytics to improve public health. Harvard Business Review. Retrieved from https://hbr.org/2014/09/how-cities-are-using-analytics-to-improve-public-health.

CMS (n.d.). National Health Expenditures 2015 highlights. Retrieved from https://www.cms.gov/Research-Statistics-Data-and-Systems/Statistics-Trends-and-Reports/NationalHealthExpendData/downloads/highlights.pdf

Council of State and Territorial Epidemiologists. (CSTE). (n.d.). About CSTE. Retrieved from http://www.cste.org/?page=About_CSTE.

Department of Defense (DoD).( 2013). Millennium cohort study. Retrieved from https://www.millenniumcohort.org/about

Dick, R., Steen, E., Detmer, D. (1997). Institute of Medicine (US) Committee on Improving the Patient Record; The Computer-Based Patient Record: An Essential Technology for Health Care. Washington (DC): National Academies Press (US); 1997.

eHealth Exchange. (2017). What is eHealth Exchange? The Sequoia Project. Retrieved from http://sequoiaproject.org/ehealth-exchange/

Education. Surveillance system (NNDSS). Retrieved from https://wwwn.cdc.gov/nndss/

Gardiner, R., Overhage, J.M., Steen, E.B., Munger, B., Holmes, J., Williamson, J., & Detmer, D. (2009). Core content for the subspecialty of clinical informatics. *Journal of the American Medical Informatics Association, 16*(2), 153–157.

Health IT Regulations. (2016). Meaningful use regulations. Retrieved from https://www.healthit.gov/policy-researchers-implementers/meaningful-use-regulations

HIMSS (2016). Fundamental Issues. Retrieved from http://www.himss.org/clinical-informatics/medical-informatics

Institute of Medicine (U.S.) The computer-based patient record: An essential technology for healthcare revised edition. Revised Edition. Washington D.C.: National Academy Press.

National Cancer Center. (n.d.). Cancer moonshot: Building an IT structure. Retrieved from https://www.cancer.gov/research/key-initiatives/moonshot-cancer-initiative

Savel, T., & Foldy, S. (2012) The role of public health informatics in enhancing public health Surveillance. *Morbidity and Mortality Weekly Report. 61*(03), 20-24. Retrieved from https://www.cdc.gov/mmwr/preview/mmwrhtml/su6103a5.htm

Seelig, A., Jacobson, I., Donoho, C., Trone, D., Crum-Cianflone, N., & Balkin, T. (2016). Sleep and health resilience metrics in a large military cohort. *Sleep, 39*(5),1111-20.

Sicular, S. (2013, March27). Gartner's big data definition consists of three parts, not to be confused with three "V"s. Forbes Retrieved from https://www.forbes.com/sites/gartnergroup/2013/03/27/gartners-big-data-definition-consists-of-three-parts-not-to-be-confused-with-three-vs/#17bb8c142f68

Report to Congress (2016). Report to Congress on Health IT Progress, Office of the National Coordinator for Health Information Technology (ONC), Office of the Secretary, United States Department of Health and Human Services.

The Medicare and Medicaid EHR Incentive Programs provide financial incentives for the "meaningful use" of certified EHR technology. Retrieved from https://www.healthit.gov/policy-researchers-implementers/meaningful-use-regulations

The Office of the National Coordinator for Health Information Technology. (2016). 2016 report to congress on health IT progress. U.S. Department of Health and Human Services. Retrieved from https://www.healthit.gov/sites/default/files/2016_report_to_congress_on_healthit_progress.pdf

Tomines, A., Readhead, H., Readhead, A., Teutsch, S. (2013). Applications of electronic health information in public health: Uses, opportunities & barriers. *EgEMS*, *1*(2), 1019.

## CHAPTER 4

# Population Health: Making a Difference in Policy

PATRICK S. LaROSE, DNP, MSN, RN

## Population Health: Making a Difference in Policy

**P**OPULATION HEALTH is a broad and often challenging concept to understand, especially for nurses who want to engage in some level of political advocacy. Let's take a moment to explore what population health is and how we can better narrow our focus to address healthcare priorities that impact populations and health determinants within the local community. Kindig and Stoddart (2003) first brought order to the definition of population health in 2003 by saying population health is "the health outcomes of a group of individuals, including the distribution of such outcomes within the group" (p. 382) and continued to further the definition by adding "the field of population health includes health outcomes, patterns of health determinants, and policies and interventions that link these two" (p. 380). In summary, population health can be considered the health goals for a specific community of people in which the development of healthcare policy is aligned to achieve the health goals for the community. For practical purposes, the community or population represents the patient.

Nurses have customarily worked with specific populations of people to address healthcare issues within communities, hospitals, and other types of healthcare organizations (American Association of Colleges of Nursing, 2008). Within this context, the word population simply means the group that has been targeted for care, services, or research on a "population." If we narrow our view and define a population of people with congestive heart failure (CHF) within our community, for example, we are indeed looking at the health and well-being of a specific population. Looking at this issue from a more global view, we can address CHF issues on a national level and link the goals and objectives of Healthy People 2020 (U.S. Department of Health and Human Services, 2010). Our view on population health and the outcome of health determinants becomes something that is more familiar to us and more understandable in terms of our professional approach to care for a group of people. The overall idea of population health is not much different than the definition of public health. According to the American Public Health Association (2017) "public health promotes and protects the health of people and the communities where they live, learn, work and play" (para. 1).

Health policy development is predicated on the overall goals and objectives of the population and should align with initiatives that are based nationally for wellness and illness prevention. The Healthy People 2020 (U.S. Department of Health and Human Services, 2010) campaign serves as an excellent framework for wellness promotion and provides examples of population health initiatives. These initiatives have had a positive impact on the health and well-being of communities across the United States (U.S.) for many years. The framework of population health provides a perspective on ways the advanced practice nurse (APN) can participate in population or public health policy to drive better health outcomes. This goal is achieved by becoming more politically aware and having a working knowledge of how healthcare policies are developed. Understanding the formal definition of policy makes operationalizing the term a bit easier. Mason, Gardner, Outlaw, and O'Grady (2016, p. 3) defines policy as "the deliberate course of action chosen by an individual or group to deal with a problem." Arguably, this would mean healthcare policy is about solving a healthcare problem within a community or larger population to improve the health determinants. The role of the healthcare policy advocate is one in which the APN brings his or her education, knowledge, experience, and passion to support policy that drives positive change for a specific population.

Including a chapter relating to political advocacy within a population health textbook speaks to the important roles APNs play in terms of advocating for their patients and communities as a whole. APNs have a long-standing history of providing advocacy for patients within the hospital, physician's office, and in community care. As respected members of the healthcare community, APNs are well-situated to provide advocacy on healthcare policy that provides benefit to the community. Evans (2013) asserts that nurse practitioners have a clear opportunity to influence local policy development that can impact health determinates within a specific population. Moreover, APNs can assemble a body of empirical evidence and utilize this evidence to bring about change in care standards. APNs have been using evidence for years and understand the importance of evidence as the underpinning for practice. However, APNs need to become more familiar with the issues impacting the health and well-being of their community. This awareness often helps to drive the development of policies that are important to the community and improve the standards of care overall. The importance of the APN's role in political advocacy cannot be understated and is an integral part of advanced practice (Evans, 2013). Nurses with advanced education have a moral and ethical obligation to be part of the national healthcare conversation as it relates to the development, approval, implementation, and evaluation of healthcare policy. Sadly, many nurses and APNs do not see themselves as an active part of the national or community healthcare conversation. There are many reasons for this limited engagement, but the most important aspect is the overall lack of education on political advocacy.

Nurses typically are not engaged in political advocacy, which may be due to a lack a general understanding of the legislative process (Byrd *et al.*, 2012). Although APNs possess many of the elementary skills necessary to be successful with political advocacy, there are a number of reasons why nurses are simply not involved. Kostas-Polston, Thanavaro, Arvidson, & Taub (2015) suggest that APNs are too busy and, in some cases, do not possess the political competency to be engaged. Congruent with this line of thinking, Gleeson, Hemingway, and Rosser (2015, p. 40), assert that "policy-practice gap exists where advanced practice nurses have too many barriers for engagement such as limited time and limited awareness of policy issues to become more involved." Des Jardin (2001) suggests fear and apathy may be another cause of limited or no engagement in policy development. Regardless of the reason, it is apparent from empirical studies that APNs must become more involved in the legislative process as a means for their voices to be heard and to help improve the health and well-being of groups within the community and nation. Kostas-Polston *et al.* (2015, pg. 12) says, "The NP's [Nurse Practitioner's] voice is necessary in the dialog to transform our country's health-care system, secure the NPs role in healthcare delivery, and to have an influence on determinants of health."

Kostas-Polston *et al.* (2015, pg. 12) say "the difficult and challenging work of the nurse practitioner political advocate is to educate and demonstrate to powerful policymakers that supporting and advancing policies that promote better health and healthcare is in the best interest of the larger community." Driving a healthcare policy that shapes healthcare systems requires political savvy and competency. Political competency means the APNs possess an understanding of the legislative process, identify how to assess healthcare policy needs within their communities (policy identification), can formulate healthcare policy that may be used to advance a political platform (policy formulation), collaborate and align with lobbying groups (coalitions) or other stakeholders to ensure healthcare policy success (approval and advancement of healthcare policy), and can evaluate the effectiveness of healthcare policy in existence (Gleeson *et al.*, 2015). However, if APNs lack political competence, as is suggested by Kostas-Polston *et al.* (2015) and do not understand or feel comfortable with political activism, more focus needs to be placed on helping APNs acquire these skills. Once APNs feel compelled and prepared to enter the political arena, they can become more engaged in the advancement of healthcare policies that provide a positive impact on their communities through well-designed healthcare initiatives that address the health determinates of the population as a whole.

To develop some level of political competence, nurses need to be exposed to the practical application of healthcare policy development to better understand the overall process. As nurses develop more experience and gain a better sense of confidence in their abilities to be active and valuable members of the political (or legislative) processes, more of them may become involved.

Formal educational preparation for APNs is defined by the American Association of Colleges of Nursing (AACN) through both *The Essentials of Doctoral Education for Advance Practice Nursing* (2006a) and *The Essentials of Masters Education for Advance Practice Nursing* (2006b). Health policy and advocacy is central to the education of nurses in advance practice and should reflect pedagogy and learning experiences that directly provide the student with practical application of concepts to help acquire political astuteness and competency. According to the AACN (2006a, 2006b), APNs engage on political activism to improve the health and well-being of communities, advance the profession of nursing, and collaborate with stakeholders to provide advocacy for populations. Effective preparation and practical experiences in political advocacy drives the acquisition of these skills and the knowledge to enhance political competency and increased awareness of the important role nurses play in social change and healthcare policy development (Gleeson *et al.*, 2015).

## Political Advocacy

The role of the nurse political advocate may appear to be limited; however, nursing as a profession has a rich history of nurses stepping outside of the normal work environment to promote and advocate for healthcare policy to improve the health and well-being of their patients. Prominent nurses, such as Florence Nightingale, Sophia Palmer, and Dr. Mary Elizabeth Carnegie, worked within policy and politics to advance the cause for care, civil rights, and improvements to nursing education (Mason *et al.*, 2016). Modern day nurses are actively engaged in healthcare policy advocacy on local and national levels. Now is the time to encourage APNs to become politically involved and assume roles of leadership in the political advancement of causes that are important for populations and the discipline of nursing. This process can begin at the grass roots or clinical level (Evans, 2013). Becoming involved with a practice council or agreeing to lead a committee on evidence-based policy changes is an excellent way for nurses to start.

Other avenues for involvement include joining a professional association and working with the legislative or healthcare policy committee. National organizations such as the American Nurses Association (ANA) and The American Association of Nurse Practitioners (AANP) have legislative arms within the organizations that are focused on advancing healthcare policy for many different issues that impact communities, the nation, and the profession of nursing. For example, the ANA has student slots on committees that can promote committee participation and networking for students. This experience can also drive the development of confidence and competence in the nurse and promote additional engagement in the future (Fackler, Chambers, & Bourbonniere, 2015).

### Case Vignette

Mary is an advanced practice registered nurse (APRN) working in a small rural clinic in Western North Carolina. Over the course of the last year, Mary has witnessed a dramatic increase in mumps and measles outbreaks in children from the community. A majority of these children are just entering school. Mary is growing curious about the vaccination history of these children and begins to research the medical records. She discovers the vaccination rate of children in her practice is much lower than she anticipated. She decides to send a survey to the parents of the children in her practice to determine the parents' overall understanding of the importance of vaccinations. Much to her surprise, even parents that have vaccinated their children are uninformed about the importance of vaccinations. She knows providing education to parents is a central element to ensuring a healthier community and addresses her concerns with the local school board. The school board agrees with Mary and, because of her advocacy, enacts a policy that requires parents to attend a one-hour education on vaccinations for new students entering kindergarten.

Mary developed an awareness of a healthcare policy issue. As you reflect on this case vignette, determine how Mary became aware of this healthcare policy issue. What beginning steps did Mary take to determine the root cause of the issue? As an APRN, Mary understood the problem to be larger than her practice and determined a lack of education as a primary issue. Why did Mary feel compelled to meet with the school board about this issue? Did the action of the school board, by requiring mandatory education for all parents enrolling students in kindergarten, go far enough to help resolve the educational deficit with parents? What additional work can Mary advocate for in relationship to educating parents?

**Nurses in Political Roles**

APNs have been largely underrepresented in healthcare politics for many years. The reasons for the under-representation relate to many factors, such as a lack of formal preparation in political advocacy and lack of direct access to be part of policy change (Molina-Mula & De Pedro-Gómez, 2013). APNs are on the front lines of care and are often the first healthcare professionals to become exposed to a healthcare policy issue that needs to be addressed locally, within the nurses' community, state, or even nationally. As such, APNs can leverage their education, experience, and knowledge to effect change that can provide positive outcomes for the population served. However, when the profession of nursing fails to interact as a political advocate for healthcare policies, which are important on the national stage, the nation loses the valuable and important perspective nurses bring to the conversation. Moreover, APNs can bring clarity to their roles, both with advance practice and in primary care. As APNs become more visible in the national healthcare conversation, this lends to the development of practice credibility, which can often foster public confidence (Weston, 2010).

Nurses have a moral and ethical obligation to develop political competency and engagement to address pressing healthcare issues within the community and population. An excellent example of nurses working to advance the cause of public health policies is the National Nurse Movement. The National Nurse Act (NNA), originated by Ms. Terri Mills, RN, MS, CNE, calls for the appointment of a Chief Nursing Officer to work alongside of the Surgeon General to address pressing public and population health issues within the United States (National Nurse Act, 2017). Ms. Mills and a number of nurse volunteers have tirelessly worked to gain legislative approval on the NNA for over eight years and continue to build support and coalitions to help move this house bill into law.

The Robert Wood Johnson Foundation, in partnership with the American Association of Retired Persons (AARP), helped to fund the development of the Nurses on Board Coalition (Nurses on Board Coalition, 2017). This coalition was founded to address the Institute of Medicine's (IOM's) call to action, which encourages more nurses to play greater roles on boards and with commissions in which nurses can demonstrate their knowledge and problem-solving abilities (IOM, 2010). The overarching goal of this coalition is to encourage nurses to serve on boards, commissions, and other important decision-making bodies to effect change within their communities, focusing on achieving 10,000 nurse placements on boards by the year 2020 (Nurses on Board Coalition, 2017). This goal may seem challenging, but coalitions like this and others represent a perfect platform for nurses to be recognized for the contribution they can offer as healthcare leaders.

Although organizations like Nurses on Board Coalition focus on creating awareness for nurses to become politically engaged, there are a number of nurses who serve their communities as policymakers. According to the ANA (American Nurses Association, 2017), there are currently five nurses who serve the people in Congress as of the writing of this chapter. Each of these nurses holds prominent positions within Congress and can effect real changes to the political landscape through the advancement of healthcare policies that meet the needs of their individual constituent communities and the nation as a whole. There are currently no nurses serving as Senators in the 115th Congress (Manning, 2017). In comparison, however, in the 115th Congress, there are a total of 14 physicians elected into office, with three physicians elected as Senators and eleven elected into the house (Manning, 2017). The

Congressional Research Office publishes the profile of Congress after each election to identify professional (occupational) demographics of elected members. The occupational summary page highlights political leaders, physicians, educators, and business professionals. Most notably missing are nurses, and this is because the number of nurses elected into office are still very low.

Although this chapter is not focused on how to get elected to office, it is focused on the important role nurses and APNs play in advancing the political cause for their respective communities and populations of service. APNs stand at the forefront of healthcare today in our nation. There is no other profession as well suited as nurses to address the pressing needs of the population. APNs understand the complexities of care, the needs within their own communities, and the importance of being a voice for effective healthcare policy development. APNs not only understand the complexities of the needs within their own communities, but also, as political advocates, they can stand up for the profession and scope of practice changes and can advocate for the increasing role of APNs within the community (Weston, 2010). If APNs, as the leaders of our own destinies, remain quiet and silent, others will make policy for us and will dictate the role that APNs play in important issues such as national healthcare reform, the role of nurses in advance practice, scope of practice, and patient safety. APNs simply must become more familiar and aware of political opportunities for healthcare policy engagement and take the bold steps needed to advance causes that are important.

*Case Vignette*

Cory is an APN working in a busy urgent care clinic, in a state that restricts Cory's ability to prescribe narcotics. He must have the supervising physician see the patient and prescribe the narcotics as a part of the treatment plan for the patient. This frustrates Cory and the physician, impacts the efficiency of the practice, and delays the patient's discharge from the clinic. Cory wants to change these practice restrictions and increase the scope of practice for the APN in his state.

Political awareness often comes to the APN when he or she is part of an ineffective healthcare policy that can delay care to patients. Cory is frustrated with the practice restrictions with his state. What can Cory do initially to become more involved with scope of practice issues for the APN in his state? Cory has made the decision to use evidence to assemble a policy platform to help the state reform scope of practice issues. To whom should Cory address this policy platform in relationship to promoting this positive change for nurse practitioners? How would you advise Cory in regards to joining grass roots efforts to change practice? Is there a particular nursing organization that would help Cory advance his policy platform?

## Developing Political Confidence and Clout

APNs provide advocacy (e.g., securing approval for a medically needed procedure from the insurance company or providing orders for home healthcare to improve recovery or patient safety) for their patients on a number of different levels. Whatever the issue, research over the years on the role of the APN is very clear about the very important role these nurses play in advancing quality healthcare to patients. Developing confidence in taking the advocacy role outside of the nurse-patient relationship may be a little easier than APNs realize. According to Brokaw (2016), nurses already possess many skills in advocacy that will serve them well as they look to focus on healthcare policy changes to address community need. Brokaw (2016) says, "When nurses influence the politics that improve the delivery of healthcare, they are ultimately advocating for their patients" (para. 1). Other research that supports this argument reveals that nurses already possess many of the skills and attributes to transition into the role of political advocate. Although it may appear overwhelming initially, refining the skill to develop political awareness and competency requires some additional learning, but is manageable for the APN looking to play a larger role in defining effective healthcare policies for the community.

## Getting Started—Nurse Political Awareness

Beginning to develop awareness of the healthcare policy needs within a community can be a challenging task initially. However, if the APN has a passion about an issue, it appears from the research that he or she is more likely to become involved in some form of political activism. In a study conducted by Kung and Lugo (2015), 884 APNs participated in a survey concerning practice barriers and political engagement. According to the authors, 23% of the respondents were likely to participate in political action if the issue was related to practice barriers. This seems to confirm the notion that passion plays a role in political awareness and involvement. Another interesting aspect relates to policy awareness when APNs are forced to work with policies they view to be ineffective.

As awareness develops concerning the ineffective nature of the policy, nurses appear to be more engaged in working collaboratively to revise the policy to bring about new policy that is effective. Weston (2010) asserts that nurses have been working to improve healthcare policies at the organizational level for many years. Translating these skills into political competency simply requires a plan for this growth.

Public and population health policies can impact an individual the same as hospital policy may impact a nurse's practice. The only difference is that the reach of public health policies is much broader and can have a direct impact on the healthcare system as a whole. Developing political awareness requires APNs to pay attention to policies that not only affect them, but also have the ability to impact a community or populations. Mason *et al.* (2016) addresses the significant impact policies can have by identifying the spheres of political influence (p. 7). The spheres of political influence include the workplace, community, government, and professional organizations (Mason *et al.*, 2016). Central to this is the idea that each sphere overlaps, providing commonality at which the impact of a new healthcare policy can be felt. This model makes perfect sense if you consider enacting of the Patient Protection and Affordable Care Act (also referred to as the Affordable Care Act, or ACA). The ACA was enacted into law by the government (government sphere). Many different stakeholders addressed the positive and negative aspects of the proposed law prior to being enacted through their professional organizations (associations and interest groups). The impact of ACA was felt across both the workplace and community. As nurses develop a sense of understanding of how laws are made and the impact a healthcare law can have in the workplace and within the community, this understanding can be translated into action.

### Case Vignette

Tifani Jefferson, RN, has a passion regarding noise pollution in her community. With a major airport 10 minutes from the community's downtown, numerous plants and a motor speedway all within 20 miles of the city, both urban and suburban residents are impacted by loud sounds. Nurse Jefferson has spoken before the City Council and State Legislation. By demonstrating the community backing and using her expertise as a nurse, she was able to demonstrate some solid alternatives to minimize the impact of noise on her community (e.g., received a grant for improved insulation window replacement near the airport).

What problem are you passionate about? What are key points you can pull together about this problem, and what can you do to get support for this concern? What legislation might you support, and if so how would you advocate for such?

## Taking the First Steps

Political engagement and involvement by nurses in the development of new healthcare policies can be rather intimidating and is often cited as the primary reason why nurses do not get involved with political advocacy (Gleeson *et al.*, 2015). However, for APNs to become more engaged in defining policies for the community and promoting political advocacy, there needs to be a starting point. A number of research articles and opinion pieces call for nurses to develop a strategic plan to promote political competence (Kostas-Polston *et al.*, 2015). The development of a strategic plan for political competence should focus on supporting skills and knowledge that need to be developed to promote competence and life-long learning. One of the key elements to gaining political confidence is for the APN to take inventory of the skill set that he or she already possesses and construct a plan of learning that will help to support this new-found competence. Nurses are all too familiar with the word competence and understand the importance of knowing how to do something because this often impacts the quality of care that is delivered to patients. Within the framework of this understanding, nurses need to become familiar with the political climate of the community. This is accomplished by getting to know the issues that are important in the community and identifying important policymakers and elected officials. Becoming more aware of the political landscape promotes additional knowledge and confidence (Kostas-Polston *et al.*, 2015). APNs provide clinical leadership every day and understand the healthcare system. As political confidence increases, APNs can self-regulate their knowledge to learn what they do not know in preparation for accomplishing the first steps in their strategic plan—getting to know policymakers. According to Fackler *et al.* (2015), "Nurses believe power develops from the acquisition of knowledge, experience, and self-confidence" (p. 267).

Self-confidence grows as the APN become more familiar with the political landscape and develops relationships with policymakers. Getting to know policymakers is one of the most important initial steps the APN can take as a part of the political competence plan. Staying local and developing relationships with local politicians, such as the Mayor, members of the county commission, elected school board officials, and other local policymakers, is one of the best ways to start. APNs must also understand that they are healthcare experts. The knowledge and frontline experience nurses possess can be translated into a skill set that may be extremely helpful to a policymaker. According to Gallup, in 2016, the profession of nursing once again ranked as the most trusted profession and has maintained this designation for the last 15 years. This makes nurses uniquely qualified and credible when speaking about healthcare issues to a policymaker, and this level of credibility also makes arranging for a meeting with a policymaker a little easier.

APNs that do not possess political competency may find meeting with a policymaker a bit overwhelming. If this is the case, the next practical step within the competency plan is to join a national organization that is focused on grass root efforts to lobby for healthcare policy changes. Involvement with a national organization will expose the APN to political tactics and strategies as a means of helping to advance a political platform.

APNs involved with a professional nursing organization; where the focus is on legislative activities, have the opportunity to develop negotiation skills, work within coalitions, and define policy recommendations important to causes supported by the organization. Eventually, the APN will develop the confidence to meet one to one with a policymaker to share his or her thoughts and interest on issues that are important. In the first quarter edition of *Georgia Nursing* (Morales, 2017), the author of this opinion piece encourages nurses to find their passions and voices. She further encourages nurses to get involved with their respective professional organizations to increase the voice of nurses and start a national conversation on healthcare. It makes perfect sense for nurses to become involved politically. But more importantly, it is important for nurses to become engaged in policy development that can benefit and drive changes for communities as well as the profession.

APNs have the most to gain by developing political competence, because this skill can help to drive effective policy for scope of practice changes within the State, thereby impacting the ability of disparate populations to have increased access to care. The IOM (Institute of Medicine, 2010) has long called for nurses to be permitted to work fully to the scope of their education. Sadly, today's nurse practitioners have full practice authority in a little more than 20 states in the United States (American Association of Nurse Practitioners, n.d.). However, the list of states that allow full practice authority for nurse practitioners continues to grow because of the efforts of nurses who are politically aware and engaged with this important issue at the local, state, and national level. APNs engaged in political advance of scope of practice needs have found a passion to advance the profession and work day to day to make this happen. The development of a political competency plan helps to drive this passion and improve confidence.

Politically novice nurses may wonder how they develop a passion for an issue that is outside of their work environment. To answer this question, one needs only to look to the discipline of nursing relating to scope of practice issues, the community, or the population for urgent care needs that must be addressed to improve quality of life. Is the care within your community meeting the needs of the community? Does your community align with the goals established for Healthy People 2020 (U.S. Department of Health and Human Services, 2017)? Issues include, but are not limited to, school lunches, gender equality, diabetes, access to care for disparate populations, childhood immunizations, and health insurance coverage. APNs need to look to what they know and capitalize on this skill to seek out an issue that needs attention or needs to be changed to promote healthier living within the community. For some APNs, issues relating to access to care are very important and cause for passion. For others, it may be practice barriers that prevent full practice authority. Regardless of the issue, APNs are well prepared to address the issues head on as political advocates (Brokaw, 2016).

As you look to what you know as an APN, define what you are passionate about and what you think about healthcare policies that are impacting your work, family, and community. From this vantage point, you will find your issue and develop a passion for change.

*Case Vignette*

Sarah has been a registered nurse for the last 15 years and has returned to school to earn her master's degree as a family nurse practitioner. She understands the important role she will play in relationship to advancing healthcare policy priorities for her community. She is admittedly overwhelmed with the entire idea of becoming politically involved. Sarah's professor encourages her to develop a political competency plan.

*Reflect on your reading*: Political astuteness is developed by becoming aware of political issues within the community, developing relationships with policymakers, defining experiences that promote confidence in the advancement of a policy platform, and understanding how to develop policy recommendations that are based in evidence and can promote change. To help Sarah develop her political competency plan, what are the first two important leaning experiences that Sarah needs to include in her competency plan and why are these two experiences important? Describe why APNs are considered healthcare experts and why the APNs perspective will be a valued contribution to the policymaker. Define at least three reasons why establishing relationships with policymakers is an important part of the political competency plan. Finally, describe three rational approaches to effectively communicating with a policymaker in relationship to advancing a policy platform that is important to the community.

*Case Vignette*

Tim Sullivan has been an APN in the school setting for 10 years. He is focused on prevention and early intervention services, and he is pleased to have done so much with grants being secured in the past. He notes that many politicians at the national, state, and local levels are seeking cutbacks on prevention services.

Nurse Sullivan notices that students are getting little or no exercise on a regular basis. He has connected this dynamic to a plethora of health issues and has targeted the middle school population to begin a prevention and intervention program.

What are the first things that Nurse Sullivan needs to do in developing this intervention? What current grants and national supports for school nurses are available to support his concern for student health? What political avenues might Nurse Sullivan consider as a means to achieving his overall goal?

## Advocating for Healthcare Policy Changes

You have graduated from your nurse practitioner program and have a passion for full practice authority or perhaps you have found an issue that is important to you as a citizen and as a new APN. Now it is time to develop your platform for change. But first, there are a number of items that need to be accomplished before you are ready to change the world. Let us begin by first talking about the issue. What is your healthcare issue? Are you well versed in all aspects of the issue? Do you have knowledge about the origination of the policy? Is the policy current law and is it effective (meeting the intended purpose)? What about the policy needs to change?

Discovering an issue that needs attention is the first step in promoting change that can better meet the needs of the population served within the community. Maybe you have discovered an issue that is not currently addressed in law but needs to be. Moving forward with development of a new policy can be different than advocating for policy changes.

Advancing an agenda of change for an existing policy requires dedication to exploring alternatives and assembling empirical evidence that supports the policy recommendations. For example, if you want to change the school lunch menu for the children that attend the local elementary school, this policy change requires data to support the current nutritional value of the menu and evidence to support the proposed nutritional value of the new menu. As another example, maybe you are concerned with the lack of paid medical leave for female employees who take time off from work for maternity leave. Each of these issues requires an initial foundation and background understanding. Who is the population impacted by the policy? Who are the side stakeholders that would be impacted by the policy change? What is wrong with the current policy and why does it need to be changed? What changes would make the policy more effective? What does the empirical evidence on this issue and is the evidence driving this overall change?

The initial steps in policy formulation reflect the ability to know what must change about the existing policy and to work toward development of policy revisions that would increase the overall effectiveness of the policy. This process begins with assembling and reading the available empirical research on the issue to ascertain what the research recommends in terms of policy development. This initial step can be rather tedious and requires time involvement with locating empirical research, critiquing the research for relativity to the issue at hand, and determining if the research is reliable for the given purpose (Benton, 2012). After the discovery stage, the nurse can begin to formulate solutions to the healthcare policy issue by providing empirically based recommendations for policy improvement. This is the beginning stage in developing a policy platform that helps to inform others about the origins of the policy, the reasons behind why the policy is generally ineffective, what research says about the issue at hand, and finally, recommendations for policy improvement.

Policy formulation can be a challenging task but one that, when completed accurately, can provide a strong foundation for political advocacy. Upon completion of the revised policy, the nurse needs to seek out partnerships and coalitions that can help advance the political platform.

Kostas-Polston *et al.* (2015) say, "Building partnerships and working with strong coalitions are strategies that are useful when moving policy issues" (p. 18). Nurses are excellent collaborators because this is a skill that nurses use every day managing and coordinating care for their patients. The central idea of building partnerships and coalitions is to receive support for the policy proposal. The more groups engage in supporting the policy, the more likely the policy issue will be credible to the policymaker, and he or she will want to support the initiative.

If you are proposing a healthcare policy that is new and not a revision to an existing policy or law and you hope to see this policy become law, you will need to solicit the support of a legislator to develop a public house bill. A public house bill is a proposed change in the law to reflect the healthcare policy that is being proposed. An elected representative and member of Congress is the only individual who is permitted to introduce a house bill to Congress (Lucas, n.d.). If a nurse wants to introduce a new healthcare policy that will eventually become law, he or she needs to select a member of the legislature who can sponsor the bill and is willing to introduce the proposed house bill to the legislature. For this text, we will not go into detail about this except to say the process for formulation of a new house bill requires many of the steps one would use to revise an existing healthcare policy. The large difference, of course, is the requirement for sponsorship by a member of the legislature.

*Case Vignette*

You are interested in having a bill be put forth before Congress. You have gathered the information necessary, and you have determined that a bill is required at the National level to make an impact on this health concern. As you work to develop your policy platform, describe the important role a member of Congress would play in helping you introduce a public house bill.

**Meeting with a Policymaker**

Once revisions to the healthcare policy are completed, research that supports the policy platform is assembled, it is time to meet with the policymaker. Policymakers are very busy people, which make it difficult at times to schedule a face-to-face meeting. Your meeting may be delegated to a legislative aide, or they may schedule you for a phone interview rather than a face-to-face meeting. Do not be discouraged.

According to Kostas-Polston *et al.* (2015), the best way to ensure an appointment is to provide the scheduler with your contact information and confirm the appointment the day before. It is best to work with the scheduler and get to know this person well. When scheduling your meeting with the policymaker, be sure to be succinct with your topic so the legislator knows what you will be presenting. Secure the email address for the scheduler and the policymaker. This will enable you to send talking points to the office so the policymaker can be prepared for your meeting (Kostas-Polston *et al.*, 2015).

Remember that APNs are held in high esteem by many in the community. This same sentiment is true with an elected official. Although you may not be a policy guru, your honesty and genuine approach to your policy proposal will come across to the policymaker. However, to ensure your meeting goes without any trouble, it is important to consider a few important items, such as communication strategies, formalized etiquette when meeting with an elected official, time, and what your goals are for the meeting.

Let's start with communication as this is a central issue when presenting to a policymaker. Chances are your communication style is good as you were successful in establishing the meeting. Communicating in the meeting is equally as important and requires a plan. Kostas-Polston *et al.* (2015) suggest the nurse read about the legislator prior to the meeting. Get to know his or her platform, how long he or she have been in office, what he or she is most passionate about, his or her voting record, and the issues that have defined his or her office. These items will provide you with a well-rounded understanding of the elected official and may even make you feel more confident in your approach and communication style with the policymaker. Understand the required etiquette when meeting with an elected official. Address the legislator with the terms "Congressman/woman" or "Senator" depending on his or her formal title. Be mindful of your time. Practice your presentation with friends, family, or nurses who are involved with your policy platform. Practice in front of a video camera and record your presentation. This will allow you to critique your presentation and the time involved with presenting the important aspects of your platform. It will also allow you to trim information that might not be necessary in soliciting support. Dress professionally and evaluate how you look when you critique your presentation on video.

One of the most important aspects of preparing to meet with an elected official is defining what you want to gain because of the meeting, that is, define your meeting goals. Having a goal in mind when meeting with the policymaker helps you to remain focused on the message and describes the type of support you hope to gain from the policymaker. If you are proposing a change to an existing policy, your goal may be to gain support from the policymaker and direction in terms of defining the next steps to take. If you are proposing a house bill for a new legislative initiative, you want the policymaker to agree to sponsor a new house bill or at the very least describe to you the changes you need to make to your policy platform to receive his or her support. Preparations for this meeting can be exhausting, but the time taken on the front end will yield many positive benefits as the policy begins to move from inception/revision, to a viable piece of legislative policy.

As you begin to meet with the elected official, thank him or her for taking time from his or her schedule to meet with you on this very important issue. It is also a good idea to thank him or her for his or her service to your community, state, etc.; this breaks the ice and lets the policymaker know you are respectful and appreciative of the time he or she is taking with you. It is very important for you to share your background and experience as a registered nurse and/or APN as this lends additional credibility to your cause. Remember to share that you are a constituent in the voting district of your policymaker, because this will help him or her to understand you have a vested interest in the district and your opinion is valuable. When you begin your presentation, stay on task by referencing your talking points. There are times when the policymaker may go off track. Be polite, answer questions, and then stay focused on your mission and goal. Remember your critique with the video and be sure to be concise and accurate in your data reports and policy recommendations. Above all, remember to identify the support you have for your platform from special interest groups, your coalitions, and maybe even your professional organization. This not only lends credibility to your argument, but also lets the policymaker know this issue is important for a number of vested stakeholders.

As you come to the completion of your presentation and meeting, be sure to ask the policymaker for his or her support of your policy platform. Ask about the next steps he or she would recommend and ways in which the policy could be improved. Far too often, nurses will not ask for the support needed and assume this was inherent and implied within the presentation. Asking for support speaks to your commitment to the issue, support for the cause, and respect for the policymaker's office and what he or she can do to help advance your policy proposal.

As you complete your formal presentation, be sure to again thank the policymaker for taking the time from his or her schedule to meet with you. Leave your business card or contact information to make follow-up easier for both parties involved and the policymaker's staff (Kostas-Polston *et al.*, 2015). Remember to leave any handout material along with a summary of your assembled research so the policymaker can reflect and reference your material after you leave. This is an important step because the policymaker may resonate on your policy issue and want additional information. As a last point, offer your assistance to the policymaker as a point person for future healthcare policies in which he or she may need assistance interpreting healthcare policies. As healthcare experts, nurses are uniquely qualified to provide this form of assistance to policymakers (Webber, 2011). Your offer of assistance provides the policymaker with a new and well-qualified resource, and it serves to provide the nurse with repeated exposure to the political process, increasing knowledge, confidence, political competence, and increased accessibility to the policymaker.

Consider the vignette in the previous section. What did you learn in this segment that will assist you in refining your quest to get an item considered as a possible bill at a National level? What specifically will change in how you will broach this issue?

**Time for Reflection**

After the meeting with the policymaker has concluded, reflect on the entire process and determine what was effective with the presentation and what needs to be changed. Typically, the meeting with the policymaker is the first step in securing support for the advancement of your political platform. Rest assured, you will be giving this presentation again to gain support from interest groups, coalitions, and other parties that want to help you advance your policy platform. Reflection also provides one with the ability to process through the feelings associated with doing something new, different, and often exciting. The opportunity to embrace and enjoy the success of your first political encounter is cause for great celebration. It is an accomplishment for most nurses to arrive at a place in which they have faced the fear of becoming engaged in the political process and made a difference. This is a time to celebrate the effort, hard work, patience, and perseverance that comes from doing something that is outside of one's comfort zone and being successful.

## Summary

Over the course of this chapter, we have talked about the important role nurses can play in advancing healthcare policy. Nurses have a moral and ethical responsibility to become more engaged in political activism that will allow them to become involved in healthcare reform and the national conversation on healthcare reform. Sadly, most nurses are not well prepared to play a significant role in political advocacy and need additional education and training on the subject. Establishing competency that fosters the advancement of healthcare policy requires the nurse to reflect on the knowledge and experiences needed to be successful. Through this reflection, nurses can develop a strategic plan that provides for professional growth and development of skills needed to build confidence, understand the political geography within a community, and understand how to read and interpret healthcare policy, evaluate healthcare policy for effectiveness, and development of an overall awareness. Awareness of the political arena and the valuable contribution nurses can make to their communities is very important not only to the community they service, but to the profession of nursing as a discipline.

The steps to becoming more politically competent require hard work and dedication. Joining a professional organization and becoming part of the lobbying and legislative arm of this organization can help to expose the nurse to experiences that will build confidence. Equally as important is working with more politically experienced nurses as mentors and modeling this behavior. Today's healthcare system is complex and requires the involvement of nurses to bring real-life perspective to the policy development process. Nurses work on the front lines of healthcare within this country every day, understand the complexities of care, and can be part of the collaborative effort to improve healthcare locally, nationally, and globally (Webber, 2011).

## Tool Kit and Resources

*Important Websites and Links*

American Nurses Association—Policy & Advocacy: http://www.nursingworld.org/MainMenuCategories/Policy-Advocacy

AANP Legislation & Regulation: https://www.aanp.org/legislation-regulation

Congress—the 115th Congress: https://www.congress.gov/browse/115th-congress

The American Nurse: Lobbying Day: http://www.theamericannurse.org/2013/04/03/nurses-expertise-valued-and-needed-in-policy-development/

*Discussion Questions*

What makes an advance practice nurse (APN) a healthcare expert? For this discussion, provide at least three evidence-based characteristics that demonstrate the APN has the skills to be a healthcare expert.

1. Reflection—as you look to become more politically savvy, define your political competency plan to include at least three evidence-based learning experiences that would help you gain political confidence defining a healthcare policy issue, meeting with a policymaker, and gaining support for a healthcare policy change within your community.
2. Describe effective communication strategies that would be used when meeting with an elected official.
3. Taking an example from your practice as a registered nurse, describe an ineffective healthcare policy that has impacted your practice. Provide details on this policy and why you believe it to be ineffective. Provide at least three solutions that would make the policy more effective and support your assertion with empirical evidence.

**Case Study 1**

Renee is an advance practice registered nurse in family practice (family nurse practitioner [FNP]). She works for a large community-based hospital as a hospitalist and has been asked by a peer if she would be interested in participating with a grass roots committee to address the issue of childhood obesity (CO) in her community. It would be Renee's responsibility to identify causative factors for CO in the community and, with the school nutrition program, develop a policy platform that would help to inform members of the committee about the issue and ways in which healthcare policy might be developed to help educate parents, school board members, teachers, and principals. Renee has been told she will need to present her findings to the committee, as well as her policy recommendations and advocacy platform at the next scheduled school board meeting in 45 days.

• What is the first set of priorities for Renee as she works to develop her policy platform?
• Childhood obesity is a very broad topic. How should Renee narrow her focus?
• What type(s) of evidence should Renee collect?
• What is the process Renee should use to develop a policy platform?
• How will Renee want to frame her presentation to the school board members? ·
• What should Renee's goal be when presenting to the school board members?

**Case Study 2**

Meredith is a certified nurse midwife (CNM) and works with a small obstetrics practice in the community. She frequently serves as the CNM for nurses having babies that work for the local hospital where she practices. Over the years, Meredith has heard complaints from the nurses and other female employees of the hospital that the hospital does not have any place for new mothers breastfeeding to pump while they are on duty. Initially, the complaints about this problem were few and Meredith helped each new mother figure out an alternative solution.

Over the last few months, she has seen a dramatic increase in the number of new mothers raising the issue of returning to work while still breastfeeding and not having a private place in which to pump. Meredith decides she wants to explore this issue a little further and speaks with the nurse manager on the postpartum unit of the hospital. The nurse manager confirms that the hospital does not have a policy regarding new mothers coming back to work while breastfeeding and says her nurses find an empty room where they can pump in private. However, the nurse manager readily admits that when the unit is full, there is no private area for this activity to occur.

Meredith is growing concerned with this issue as she knows new mothers are often hesitant to continue breastfeeding after they return to work and this issue has the potential to dissuade new mothers from continuing to breastfeed. Meredith is passionate about mothers breast-feeding, and this passion is supported by the literature. She wants to influence change within the hospital to encourage hospital leadership to take this issue seriously and develop policy that provides female employees with the time and a private space to pump.

- Meredith understands the hospital does not have an existing policy that governs breastfeeding employees. What is Meredith's first priority when establishing a new healthcare policy?
- What type of support should Meredith seek out from like-minded groups?
- Describe the necessary elements to a newly formed healthcare policy. What would Meredith's policy include to make the policy credible?
- Organizational policy is generally governed by hospital leadership. If Meredith wanted to make her new breastfeeding policy a requirement for all hospitals in her district, how would she go about advocating for this change in her community?

**Case Study 3**

Tom is a certified registered nurse anesthetist (CRNA) and works with the ambulatory surgical center that is associated with the local community hospital. Tom has been a CRNA for several years and wants to explore becoming more politically savvy in order to help influence positive trends for CRNAs. In order to do this, Tom decided to join the board of a local company as a trustee. Tom figures he is well-educated, professional and has been a member of the community both personally and professionally for the last 10 years, and he believes he is a shoo-in for the opportunity. He thinks to himself, "Heck I am not getting paid; they should love to have someone like me on the board."

Tom reaches out to a friend of his about an opening on the board of trustees for a local bank. The bank recently had a member of the board retire, and there are a few other board members who will be ending their terms in the next year. Tom's friend explains to him that it is unlikely he will get a board appointment, because he has no general board experience. Tom encourages his friend to put in a good word for him as he begins to draft his letter of application to the Chairman.

That same afternoon, he receives a call from the Council of Aging. The executive director speaks with Tom about a board appointment opportunity for Meals-on-Wheels. The executive director is very excited to talk with Tom, because she heard through a friend that Tom might have an interest. Tom thanks the executive director for reaching out to him but declines the opportunity, citing he will be taking a board appointment with the local bank and will not have time to serve on two boards. Tom thinks to himself, "A Meals-on-Wheels board position is not exactly what I had planned. I am so glad I will be taking the appointment with the bank."

A few days later, the bank calls Tom and thanks him for his letter of application to become a board member. They regretfully inform Tom that, with his limited board experience, they went with an individual that brought more experience to the table. Tom is in shock.

- Where did Tom go wrong in his thinking and why?
- Compare and contrast the two different types of board appointments and determine why you think Tom preferred the bank appointment over the Meals-on-Wheels appointment.
- Describe why starting out with a smaller board might be beneficial to a nurse seeking a board appointment.
- What should Tom do as a result of his rejection with the bank?

**Case Study 4**

Nancy has been a registered nurse for the last 12 years. She returned to school to earn her degree in nursing education. It is her goal to teach nursing to undergraduate students in a prelicensure program. Until she graduates, she is still working for a busy intensive care unit (ICU). Her nurse manager asked her to chair the practice council for the hospital. The hospital is planning for Magnet status in the next three years and established a practice council last year as a means to integrate empirical evidence from research into the practice standards and clinical policies in the hospital.

Nancy is very excited about leading the practice council but wishes she had participated in some of the meetings before assuming such a senior leadership role. She wonders if she has the skills, experience, and education to be directing such a high-level council with her hospital.

Nancy hosted her first meeting with the council and was simply not prepared for the meeting. She did not provide an agenda, was unaware of what the council had been discussing at previous meetings, and was not informed of the priorities the council had set from the previous year. This was the first meeting of the council for this practice year.

Nancy apologized to the council members and rescheduled the meeting for later in the month in an effort to ensure the council had an initial meeting that was productive and addressed the defined priorities from the previous year.

- Nancy did not have the confidence necessary to lead a group of nurses on this practice council. As a part of developing political competency, what steps should Nancy take (prior to the next meeting later in the month) to ensure she has the confidence and ability to lead these nurses and make meaningful change?
- Reflecting on the steps addressed above, define specific learning experiences that will help Nancy be more successful in the next meeting.
- What role did the nurse manager play in the failure of Nancy with the practice council?
- What steps can Nancy take to gain respect from members of the practice council so she can be successful in getting things done?

## References

American Association of Colleges of Nursing. (2006a). *The essentials of doctoral education for advance practice nursing.* Retrieved from http://www.aacn.nche.edu/dnp/Essentials.pdf

American Association of Colleges of Nursing. (2006b). *The essentials of master's education for advanced practice nursing.* Retrieved from www.aacn.nche.edu/education-resources/MasEssentials96.pdf

American Association of Colleges of Nursing. (2008). The consensus model for APRN regulation: Licensure, accreditation, certification & education (2008). Retrieved from http://www.aacn.nche.edu/education-resources/APRNReport.pdf

American Association of Nurse Practitioners. (n.d.). State practice environment. Retrieved from https://www.aanp.org/legislation-regulation/state-legislation/state-practice-environment

American Public Health Association. (2017). What is public health? Retrieved from https://www.apha.org/what-is-public-health

Benton, D., (2012). Advocating globally to shape policy and strengthen nursing's influence. *OJIN: The Online Journal of Issues in Nursing, 17*, 1, Manuscript 5. doi: 10.3912/OJIN.Vol17No01Man05

Brokaw, J. J. (2016). The nursing profession's potential impact on policy and politics. *American Nurse Today.* Retrieved from https://www.americannursetoday.com/blog/nursing-professions-potential-impact-policy-politics/

Byrd, M. E., Costello, J., Gremel, K., Schwager, J., Blanchette, L., & Malloy, T. E. (2012). Political astuteness of baccalaureate nursing students following an active learning experience in health policy. *Public Health Nursing, 29*(5), 433–443. doi:10.1111/j.1525-1446.2012.01032.x

Des Jardin, K. (2001). Political involvement in nursing—politics, ethics, and strategic action...second article in a two-part series. *AORN Journal, 74*(5), 613–626. doi:10.1016/S0001-2092(06)61760-2

Evans, K. A. (2013). Health policy: What's your role? *Advance Health Care Network.* Retrieved from http://nurse-practitioners-and-physician-assistants.advanceweb. com/Columns/Role-Growth/Health-Policy-Whats-Your-Role.aspx

Fackler, C. A., Chambers, A. N., & Bourbonniere, M. (2015). Hospital nurses' lived experience of power. *Journal of Nursing Scholarship, 47*(3), 267–274. doi:10.1111/ jnu.12127

Gallup. (2016). American rates healthcare providers high on honesty, ethics. Retrieved from http://www.gallup.com/poll/200057/americans-rate-healthcare-providers-high-honesty-ethics.aspx?g_source=Social%20Issues&g_medium=newsfeed&g_campaign=tiles

Gleeson, J., Hemingway, A., & Rosser, E. (2015). To what extent do health visitors and school nurses have a voice in the policy process? *Community Practitioner, 88*(6), 38–41.

Institute of Medicine (2010). The future of nursing: Leading change, advancing health. Retrieved from http://books.nap.edu/openbook.php?record_id=12956&page=R1#

Kindig, D ., & Stoddart, G. (2003). What is population health? *The American Journal of Public Health, 93*(3), 380–383.

Kostas-Polston, E. A., Thanavaro, J., Arvidson, C., & Taub, L. M. (2015). Advanced practice nursing: Shaping health through policy. *Journal of the American Association of Nurse Practitioners, 27*(1), 11–20. doi:10.1002/2327-6924.12192

Kung, Y. M., & Lugo, N. R. (2015). Political advocacy and practice barriers: A survey of Florida APRNs. *Journal of The American Association of Nurse Practitioners, 27*(3), 145–151. doi:10.1002/2327-6924.12142.

Lucas, F. (n.d.). How a bill becomes law. Retrieved from https://lucas.house.gov/legislative-work/how-bill-becomes-law

Manning, J. E. (2017). Membership of the 115th Congress: A profile. *Congressional Research Service.* Retrieved from https://fas.org/sgp/crs/misc/R44762.pdf

Mason, D. J., Gardner, D. B., Outlaw, F. H., & O'Grady, E. T. (Eds.). (2016). *Policy & politics in nursing and healthcare* (7th ed.). Saint Louis, Missouri: Saunders Elsevier.

Molina-Mula, J., & De Pedro-Gómez, J. E. (2013). Impact of the politics of austerity in the quality of healthcare: ethical advice. *Nursing Philosophy, 14*(1), 53–60. doi:10.1111/nup.12000

Morales, K. (2017). Politics and nursing: get involved! *Georgia Nursing, 77*(1), 4.

National Nurse Act. (2017). Retrieved from http://nationalnurse.org/faq.pdf

Nurses on Boards Coalition. (2017). Retrieved from http://nursesonboardscoalition.org/

Webber, J. (2011). Nurses must influence governments and policy. *International Nursing Review, 58*(2), 145-146. doi:10.1111/j.1466-7657.2011.00908.x

Weston, M. J. (2010). Strategies for enhancing autonomy and control over nursing practice. *OJIN: The Online Journal of Issues in Nursing* (15), 1, Manuscript 2. doi: 10.3912/OJIN.Vol15No01Man02

U.S. Department of Health and Human Services, Office of Disease Prevention and Health Promotion. (2017). Healthy people 2020. Retrieved from http://www.healthypeople.gov/2020/about/default.aspx

## CHAPTER 5

# The Nurse Executive Role in Population Health

GRACE SOTOMAYOR, DNP, MSN, MBA, FACHE, NEA-BC

## Nurse Executive Role in Population Health Overview

**E**FFORTS to define what exactly is meant by the term "Population Health" continue as scholars and researchers in healthcare attempt to parse its various components. Two of the most articulate and quoted writers on this topic, Kindig and Stoddart, stated initially in the American Journal of Public Health that population health consisted of 3 components, "health outcomes and distribution in a population (dependent variables), patterns of health determinants over the life of the course (independent variables), and policies and interventions at the individual and social level" (Kindig & Stoddart, 2003, pp 380–383).

In 2015, Kindig further refined this thinking and described population health as having two definitions, "*Population health management or population medicine* when referring to patient populations, and *Population health or preferably total population health* when referring to the health for geographic populations, which are the concern of public health officials, community organizations, and business leaders".

Although it is important for clarity of understanding that dialogue continue to better define what population health means, recognition of the foundational work that nurse leaders have done and are continuing to do in this space is long overdue.

Historically, there have been visionary and effective nurses leading the improvement of health in patient populations. They have also impacted quality of care of patients within specific geographic regions,

103

and their contributions have withstood the test of time. Florence Nightingale's contribution to the health of the military patient population and infection prevention, for example, is well known and her method of demonstrating relationships between data and care improvements by conducting statistical analyses and depicting results graphically is still used worldwide (Lewenson, McAllister & Smith, 2017).

In 1893, using Nightingale's principles as a model for her work, Lillian Wald established the Henry Street Settlement in the Lower East Side in New York to help the poor and sick inhabitants of that geographic area. Building coalitions wherever she could and advocating for the needs of the community, Wald achieved changes in health, industry, education, recreation, and housing. The settlement later evolved into the Visiting Nurse Service of New York, laying the foundation for modern day Public Health Nursing (Curley & Vitale, 2016).

Year after year, the United States (U.S.) has made enormous strides in illness care. However, there has not been a disciplined focus on prevention and on building seamless cross-continuum systems of care nation-wide from acute inpatient to outpatient and community. This has resulted in an unsustainable trajectory of growth in healthcare costs fueled by expensive hospital care, medications, and procedures (Stanhope & Lancaster, 2016). Currently, the Centers for Medicare and Medicaid Services (CMS), reports that national health expenditures are consuming greater than 17% of U.S. Gross Domestic Product (GDP) and will rise to 19.9% by 2025 (CMS, 2017). At the same time, population health benefits seen in other developed countries with lower healthcare costs remain elusive. As reported by the Commonwealth Fund the U.S. continues to be challenged with lower life expectancy and worse health outcomes (Commonwealth Fund, 2015).

It has been well-recognized that because of nursing's holistic focus and large numbers, clinical improvements in the health of the population cannot be achieved without the contributions of nurses (Institute of Medicine, 2010). Population health, however, is concerned not only with public health (i.e., what we can do to keep people healthy (Institute of Medicine, 1988), but also with a broader construct that includes evaluation of the determinants that affect health, such as medical care, public health interventions, genetics, and individual behavior, along with components of the social (e.g., income, education, employment, culture) and physical (e.g., urban design, clean air, water) environments, (Kindig & Stoddart, 2003). Nursing leadership in population health, therefore, demands skilled executives who can lead clinical nurses, and build effective cross continuum care models and inter professional teams. These executives also need to be courageous and comfortable using business tools to quantify and drive change. Because nurses themselves constitute a population with unique educational, psychosocial, and developmental needs, attention to the growth of the nursing profession and the environment within which nursing is practiced is likewise essential.

Leaders exist at every level of nursing in practice, education and administration. However, this chapter is devoted to the nurse leader who serves at the executive level in health systems or hospitals. This role has evolved from a focus on inpatient care to extensive accountability for patient care across all venues. The increase in role responsibilities has shifted the concept of the nurse executive as *administrator* (a leader managing functions and processes) to *executive* (someone with accountability for such broader activities as strategic planning).

Mosby's Medical Dictionary describes a certified *nurse administrator* as "a nurse who supervises nursing staff, establishes work schedules and budgets, maintains medical supply inventories, and manages resources to ensure high-quality patient care" (Mosby, 2009). A *nurse executive*, however, is described as playing a "central role in providing strategic, expert, evidence-based advice to boards and ensures that policy, macro decision-making, purchasing, reporting and monitoring are contextualized within the realities of individual patient care and population health settings" (Lúanaigh & Hughes, 2016, p. 133). Expansion of the nurse executive's responsibilities from administration to strategy and from being primarily hospital based to leadership across the continuum of care, has paralleled widespread appreciation of the value that nurses who are prepared at the executive level bring to population health. This has become intensified because of ongoing research showing that that the environment within which clinical nurses practice contributes significantly to the quality of healthcare and that executive nursing leadership is essential to the health of this environment, (Aiken *et al.*, 2011).

In 2007, the term *Triple Aim* was coined by Dr. Donald Berwick and other leaders at the Institute for Healthcare Improvement (IHI) in response to the rising cost of healthcare in the United States. It describes the necessity of building health programs that simultaneously pursue improvements in patient experience of healthcare, the health of populations, and reductions in per capita cost (IHI, 2007). Specific health outcomes and behavioral and physiological metrics subsequently recommended by the IHI in 2012 to measure success with Triple Aim efforts have historically been the focus of nurses. These include disease prevention through patient education, motivation, and behavior modification (IHI, 2012).

Meanwhile, in the Institute of Medicine (IOM) publication *"The Future of Nursing: Leading Change, Advancing Health,"* the authors stress that the need to support the development of nurses is integral to improving quality and transforming healthcare in the U.S. The report clearly indicated that:

Nurses should practice to the full extent of their education and training, that they should achieve higher levels of education and training through an improved education system that promotes seamless academic progression, they should be full partners, with physicians and other healthcare professionals, in redesigning healthcare in the United States and that data collection and information systems infrastructure should be redesigned to support policy and workforce planning. (IOM, 2010)

Private sector investments in nursing, such as the Robert Wood Johnson Foundation (RWJF) Executive Nurse Fellows Program, have further signaled that support for nursing, and the preparation of emerging nurse leaders, are necessary initiatives to improve population health. The Fellows program is transitioning in 2017 to include healthcare leaders from all professions; however, the recognition of the role that nurses play as part of a multi professional leadership team has been well established (RWJF, 2014).

### Nurse Executives

Nurse Executives operate at health system and hospital levels. Many of them serve as chief nursing officers at the assistant vice president (AVP) or director level or may function as chief nursing informatics officers (CNIO)s or chief quality officers.

Recognizing the need for these leaders to be competent to lead population health efforts, graduate level preparation programs and leadership organizations are spending significant effort defining the requisite education and competencies. For example, the American Organization of Nurse Executives (AONE) was created in 1967 as a professional organization for nurse leaders. It has aligned itself with the American College of Healthcare Executives (ACHE) and has seen its membership increase to 9,000 in 2016, as nurse executives saw benefit in networking and group learning. AONE's work has included periodic analysis of nurse leader jobs and the creation of general and specific competencies for the nurse executive. Noting the growing trend toward health systems integration and the focus on improving health for populations and individuals, the AONE published its Nurse Executive Competencies for Population Health. The following elements were added to the general competencies and were cited, along with graduate level educational preparation), as essential for nurse executive success: "Communication and relationship building, knowledge of the Healthcare environment, leadership, professionalism and business skills" (AONE, 2015).

AONE has organized a partnership with the Healthcare Financial Management Association (HFMA) to assist nurse executives with better understanding of value based purchasing and methods to quantify the dollar value of clinical outcomes. Furthermore, recognizing that population health demands teamwork in developing and executing necessary changes, the AONE and HFMA have joined with ACHE, the American Association for Physician Leadership, the Healthcare Information and Management Systems Society, and the Medical Group Management Association to form the Healthcare Leadership Alliance. The goal of this alliance is to advance the healthcare management profession by sharing inter professional best practices (AONE, 2017).

Nurse leaders who are clinically focused contribute to population health through their management of health outcomes for individuals and groups. Nurse leaders who are educators work to ensure that nursing curricula are flexible enough to adapt to the needs of population health practice settings. The contributions of nurse executives to population health, however, result in changes to both education and practice, because they may involve policy or care model redesign. Success depends heavily on nurse executives' ability to advocate for and lead efforts to do the following:

1. Support a population health focus by collaborating with other stakeholders
2. Optimize informatics across the healthcare continuum
3. Position nursing to contribute and lead population health initiatives
4. Strengthen the health of the nursing population itself

Present-day examples from high-profile systems such as the Veterans Affairs and Geisinger Health Systems describe the successes that nurse executives are achieving in population health by paying attention to these elements.

## Department of Veterans' Affairs

In the 1990s, in response to the increased demand for care of aging World War II veterans and large numbers of wounded soldiers from Afghanistan and Iraq, Cathy Rick, RN, PhD(h), Chief Nurse Executive of the Veterans Administration (VA), with other colleagues at the VA, began to position the nursing service away from a hospital-based focus to a healthcare system providing care closer to where veterans lived. This was achieved by assigning experienced VA RNs to coordinate care and provide chronic disease management and by investing heavily in the recruitment of nurse practitioners as primary care providers across all settings. Ms. Rick built collaborative partnerships with physicians and governmental administrators to enable nurse practitioners to educate, conduct research, and apply their findings in their clinical settings. At the same time, she encouraged a professional, mutually appreciative culture with physicians and other disciplines and advocated for active nursing involvement in the development of an information technology system to link all the VA's services. Results of these efforts are impressive, with outcome data showing that VA patients in general receive better healthcare than patients enrolled in the Medicare fee-for-service program (Ibrahim, 2007; VA, 2010).

Over the last 10 years, Ms. Rick has also implemented the use of the Clinical Nurse Leader (CNL), a masters prepared nurse generalist, to bring evidence based practice to population health (VA, 2013). She has been vocal in her support for nurses' career development and expanded practice for the close to 6000 advanced practice registered nurses (APRNs) employed by the VA. Working with physicians and administrators, she has built the coalitions and laid the groundwork for sweeping change that will most likely impact other healthcare systems. In December 2016, the VA declared that regardless of state barriers, VA APRNs who are clinical nurse specialists, nurse practitioners, and nurse midwives would be granted full practice authority and that the scope of certified registered nurse anesthetists (CRNA's) was being similarly reviewed. Making the announcement about this evolution, Dr. David J. Shulkin, VA Under Secretary for Health, stated the following:

Amending this regulation increases our capacity to provide timely, efficient, effective and safe primary care, aids VA in making the most efficient use of APRN staff capabilities, and provides a degree of much needed experience to alleviate the current access challenges that are affecting VA. (VA, 2016)

## Case Vignette

The chief nurse executive in a Level 1 trauma academic center in the south is aware that employed CRNAs in the organization are not being allowed to practice to the top of their license as permitted by state law. This has resulted in CRNA dissatisfaction, student CRNAs having to complete clinical rotations at other facilities, and delays in completing radiology and other procedures because of waiting for an anesthesiologist to respond. The barrier is the independent anesthesiology group who supervises the CRNAs and bills patients for services provided. The leader of the group has cited evidence showing that anesthesiologists have more years of training than CRNAs but can point to no safety concerns. The academic center has a contract with the group, and the contract is now up for renewal. The nurse executive has been asked by the hospital president for input into terms of a new contract.

*Question*: From your previous reading, how would you recommend the nurse executive respond? What rationale could be cited to support appropriate CRNA practice?

## Geisinger Health System

Geisinger Health System's chronic care management system is often described as an example of a successful population health model (Nash, Reifsnyder, Fabius & Pracilio, 2011). Janet Tomcavage RN, MSN, is the Chief Population Health Officer for Geisinger Health System. Over the past 18 years, Ms. Tomcavage and her colleagues have been experimenting with ways to reduce cost of care while improving quality for patient populations. Initially focusing on patients with multiple conditions such as diabetes, congestive heart failure, and chronic obstructive pulmonary disease, Geisinger has achieved remarkable decreases in hospital admissions and readmissions by embedding nurse case managers in primary care practices (Steele *et al.*, 2010). Its ProvenCare® system of standardizing acute care for patients with chronic disease has been widely recognized as successful (Goudreau & Smolenski, 2014). Ms. Tomcavage leads strategy development and oversight for Geisinger's systemwide value based reengineering work, including ProvenHealth Navigator, which is Geisinger's advanced medical home. She has evolved the nurse case manager role from having primarily a utilization review acute care focus to one with responsibility for patients' health across the care continuum. Ms. Tomcavage is also responsible for other important population health functions, including clinical informatics and population health systems development.

In April 2015, Ms. Tomcavage and her colleagues at Geisinger reported an approximately 8% decline in total costs of care for the Medicare population enrolled in their patient centered medical home, (Maeng et al, 2015). The largest source of the decrease was noted to be in the cost of inpatient care due to a drop-in hospital admissions for this patient group. It clearly indicated that the strategy of using nurse practitioners and case managers to manage patient care in Geisinger's clinics is leading to sustainable care improvements and lower cost.

*Case Vignette*

The Assistant Vice President (AVP) of Women's Services in the flagship hospital of a fully integrated healthcare system is frustrated with the lack of integration between the corporate home health division and obstetric care for high-risk pregnant women. These women are admitted to the maternity unit and can stay upwards of 3 to 4 weeks to get their diabetes, hypertension, or other comorbid conditions under control. It is disruptive to families, costly, and reduces capacity for postpartum patients in this busy service, which delivers more than 6500 babies annually. The AVP is aware of studies done elsewhere showing that home visits from maternity nurses can reduce hospitalizations in high-risk antepartum women; however, Women's Services is not a strategic priority for the system and the home care division will not invest in an antepartum service.

*Question*: From your prior reading, what steps can the AVP take to solve this problem?

**Informatics and Technology**

The growth of the internet and the proliferation of mobile technology offer exciting opportunities as tools for improving population health. Besides the need for nurse executives to maintain competency in office technology to communicate with nurses of all ages and disciplines, it is imperative that they stay abreast of optimization opportunities for electronic medical records (EMRs), applications that can promote population health, and virtual systems that negate the need for nurses or patients to travel to care locations. Serving as the advocate for clinical nursing involvement in evaluations of information systems, revision of patient care processes and planning, design, choice, and implementation of information systems in the practice setting is an essential role for the nurse executive who leads population health efforts.

In addition, data integrity and security are areas that have gained popular attention because of well-publicized data breaches that have startled the healthcare industry over the last 5 years. Ability to demonstrate proficient awareness of legal and ethical issues related to client and employee data are necessary competencies for the nurse executive and further evidence of nursing leadership in a culture of safety. Perhaps the most challenging aspect of informatics is making sense of the enormous amount of data that are now available to healthcare leaders. If integrated across care settings, data from the EMR, although not perfect, can be used to track, trend and determine factors that are impacting the health of populations. However, because much of this capability is still in development, knowing what questions to ask and establishing meaningful relationships between pieces of data to make good decisions is a nurse executive competency that will need ongoing work.

Vendors of technology appreciate the perspective that nurse executives have on population health and practically all major EMR and healthcare software vendors, such as Epic, Cerner, or Press Ganey, employ a nurse executive. These individuals serve as part of the company's leadership team, providing input and functioning as iterative boundary spanners between technology products and the patient care arena.

In their 2016 article, *The Role of the Chief Nurse Executive in the Big Data Revolution*, Englebright and Caspers describe the American Nurses Association's Social Policy Statement as the "framework for the leadership role that the Chief Nurse Executive can provide in big data analysis" (p. 282). They also emphasize that in two specific areas, ensuring the presence of nurse sensitive data and research across the healthcare enterprise, and advocating for a robust, interoperable data infrastructure supportive of the patient, community and inter professional team, the nurse executive must take the lead.

### Case Vignette

While attending a leadership development seminar with physicians and other administrative colleagues, the chief nurse executive of a hospital learns about a program that can be used to educate hospitalized patients on diet, medications, and treatments using prompts on their televisions. It can also be used to alert and prepare them for discharge, and when they leave the hospital, they can continue to have access to its content. Nurses can document in the program and documentation flows to the patient's medical record. The program interfaces with all the hospital's disparate documentation systems and can pull all patient information to one location.

Some physicians present at the seminar are concerned that they will not be able to approve information shared with their patients. The chief financial officer is concerned about the cost of the system but is acutely aware of the importance of reducing length of stay and preventing readmissions.

*Question*: How would you advise the nurse executive to prepare a case for purchasing or at least obtaining support for a trial of the system?

### Nursing Education

Similar to physician practice, nursing practice has evolved into specialties that are primarily hospital based. Direct care nursing in the community setting, while a specialty unto itself, has not yet fully risen into its own as a major contributor to population health apart from gains demonstrated by APRNs. Strong linkages between inpatient and outpatient nursing, with the exception of some case management models, have not widely evolved to benefit the health of patient populations. The nurse executive plays a significant role in evaluating what direct care nurses in all settings need to understand about population health. This makes working with academic partners to ensure that nursing curricula and clinical rotations reflect this knowledge essential, since nurses' competency now needs to include ability to work in inter professional teams with patients and families to set and meet goals of care across the continuum.

One of the most promising largescale partnerships between nurse executives and nurse leaders in education has been the collaboration to develop the role of the clinical nurse leader (CNL) (Stanley, Hoiting, Burton, Harris, & Norman, 2007). Recognizing that, for population health efforts in nursing to succeed, gaps in care needed to be closed, the American Association of Colleges of Nursing (AACN) convened a task force consisting of stakeholders from both education and practice. Out of this collaboration has come a masters prepared nurse generalist, educated in the recognition and resolution of system issues that interfere with health outcome achievement. CNLs are taught to apply systems theories and to use assessment, planning, and implementation tools that are adaptable to microsystems, mesosystems, or macrosystems in healthcare, (Nelson, Batalden, & Godfrey, 2007; Nelson, Batalden, Godfrey, & Lazar, 2011).

One of these tools is the 5P assessment developed by clinicians at Dartmouth Hitchcock in 2010 to evaluate the functioning of clinical microsystems. They described the clinical microsystem as the place where "patients, families and the care team meet" (Dartmouth Institute for Health Policy & Clinical Practice, 2010). Extrapolating this concept to population health, a clinical microsystem may be a clinic, a doctor's office, the patient's home, an emergency department, a hospital, a community center, or a church. This makes their tool adaptable to any care venue and completion of its five dimensions of evaluation: **Purpose** (i.e., goal of the specific environment), **Patients** (i.e., characteristics of the people with healthcare needs [describing the population]), **Processes** (i.e., steps used in the process of providing care), **Professionals** (i.e., healthcare members providing care), and **Patterns** (i.e., trends of performance), provide a comprehensive framework for assessment. This results in a profile from which the CNL can identify and prioritize issues for resolution to improve the health of populations of patients or individuals inhabiting specific geopolitical areas.

After the completed 5P Assessment, the CNL and other members of the healthcare team evaluate opportunities for improvements then develop a global aim statement. The statement is expected to be clear and concise so that required actions can be precisely identified. Changes are implemented continually using a structure called an improvement ramp. The goal is to achieve consistent incremental improvements. Measuring outcomes is a key part of the process, and answering the question, "How do you know that what you changed added value (e.g., lowered cost and improved quality)?" is expected with every change. This disciplined approach is similar to the Plan, Do, Study/Check, Act (PDSA/PDCA) cycle used in performance improvement in many healthcare settings.

Nurse executives should assess whether the addition of the CNL role can strengthen existing care delivery models across the care continuum. For systems with CNLs already in place, the nurse executive may require completion of the 5P assessment to assist in the development of new programs or periodic evaluation of existing programs to determine areas for improvement. The tool can also be used to determine the extent of individual clinical microsystem contribution to overall population health goals for groups of patients.

Figure 5.1 shows a picture of the 5P assessment tool and Figure 5.2, the Dartmouth Microsystem Improvement Ramp.

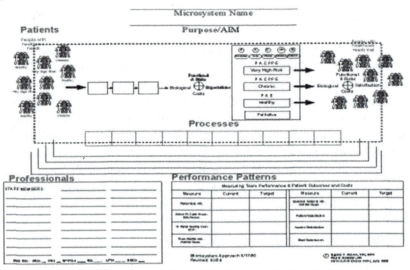

**FIGURE 5.1.** *Dartmouth Institute 5P Assessment Tool Used by CNLs.*

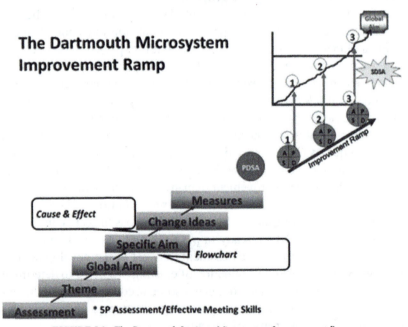

**FIGURE 5.2.** *The Dartmouth Institute Microsystem Improvement Ramp.*

## Process Improvement and Lean Management Systems

Originally pioneered by W. Edwards Deming, tools for process improvement such as lean management systems, 6 Sigma, and the Plan Do Check Act (PDCA) cycle have been evolving over the last 70 years. Their concepts are based on three fundamental elements: waste removal, continuous improvement, and recognition that the people closest to the work are the best able to identify processes that can be done better. Used extensively in manufacturing, these systems have found their way into healthcare, most significantly championed by organizations such as Theda Care and Virginia Mason (Mannon, 2014; Kenney, 2011) and by cross-service healthcare functions such as the pharmacy and laboratory (Clark, Silvester, & Knowles, 2013). The nurse executive plays a vital role in the identification of opportunities for improvement across the continuum of care and in the standardization of best practices once identified. Consistent communication about the need for change and engaging staff who work with patients to be actively involved in performance improvement is essential. The eight wastes of healthcare—waiting, overproduction, defects, nonutilized talent, motion, over/excess productions, transportation, and inventory—are present in all locations at which care is provided. It is important for the nurse executive to Gemba (go to where the work is done), observe and understand processes, and seek input for improvements.

## Change Management

The nurse executive leads and drives necessary change to advance care delivery, enhance patient experience, improve quality, support teammate engagement, and achieve multiple other organizational operational goals. A variety of change theories and change management tools exist in the healthcare business literature. Population health efforts demand supporting the nursing workforce through transition from an episodic focus to a care continuum and from siloed practice to whole system care, which requires a significant culture shift. The ability of nurse executives to communicate a compelling reason for these changes and to translate what is often an ambiguous message is extremely important. Sinek's work on the necessity of continuously explaining the reason for changes (Sinek, 2011), is a valuable resource as is Patrick Lencioni's model on strengthening teams (Lencioni, 2002). The focus in Lencioni's leadership development model is perfecting the skill to work with teams to develop trust, engage in healthy conflict, commit to agree upon goals, accept accountability for outcomes, and produce results. Developing the skill to paint a compelling picture of changes that need to be accomplished to achieve population health goals is one of the most important tasks for the nurse executive.

## Challenges Faced by Nurse Executives in Population Health

### Registered Nurse Supply and Demand

Nurse executives continue to face challenges in leading population health efforts. An important one is having enough qualified staff to meet healthcare needs. The United States is in the throes of a national shortage of experienced nurses, a situation that Buerhaus (2016) described as a "knowledge shortage." This has been primarily created by older nurses retiring, increased care demands of an aging U.S. population and the plethora of nonclinical choices available to nurses (Juraschek, Zhang, Ranganathan, & Lin, 2012. Studies also indicate, however, that nursing performance and retention are related to leadership behaviors (Germain & Cummings, 2010); therefore, the culture within which nurses work and the support and leadership that they receive are critical to their ability to effectively contribute to population health.

Nurse executives are vital to ensure that adequate resources and support are available to enable nurses to practice at their optimal skill level. Using business tools such as return on investment (ROI) analyses to demonstrate, for example, why appropriate registered nurse (RN) staffing is cost effective will continue to need refinement for the long term. Labor is the largest expense for healthcare organizations and nursing generally constitutes the largest labor component. Attempts to reduce labor costs without redesigning work are a constant challenge as reimbursements for healthcare continue to be reduced.

### Nurse Retention

On the nursing retention front, programs such as new graduate residency and transition to practice have been well studied in the literature for their contributions to nurse retention and satisfaction (National Council of State Boards of Nursing, 2017). At the same time, how errors are managed and the culture that is fostered around quality and safety contribute to nurses' perception of their work environment as either supportive or punitive. Several specific interventions can be put in place by the nurse executive to improve the nursing work environment.

*Accountability*

Work done on understanding how errors occur, such as familiarity with Reason's model of accident causation (Reason, 1990) and methods of evaluating errors in a fair and consistent manner are important to establish and maintain a "Just Culture" (Khatri, Brown, & Hicks, 2009). The principle behind a "Just Culture" is that discipline needs to be tied to the behavioral choices of individuals and the potential risks these choices present rather than be dependent upon the actual outcome of actions. Several boards of nursing provide guidance on this topic. For example, a "Just Culture," as summarized by the North Carolina Board of Nursing, contains these 7 specific elements:

1. Places focus on evaluating the behavior and choices made by an individual, not on the outcome of the event
2. Requires leadership commitment and modeling
3. Distinguishes among normal human error, unintentional risk-taking behavior, intentional risk-taking behaviors, and reckless behaviors
4. Fosters a learning environment that encourages reporting (including selfreports) of all near misses, mistakes, errors, adverse events, and system weaknesses
5. Lends itself to continuous improvement of work processes and systems to ensure the highest level of client and staff safety
6. Encourages the use of non-disciplinary actions whenever appropriate (including coaching, counseling, training, and education)
7. Holds individuals accountable for their own performance in accordance with their job responsibilities but does not expect individuals to assume accountability for system flaws over which they had no control (NCBON, 2011).

Using the elements, the NCBON has developed an algorithm that can be a helpful tool for nurse executives when dealing with practice issues, because it clearly demonstrates support for the nurse yet does not disregard professional accountability for practice.

Another strategy for improving the work environment for nurses is for the nurse executive to advocate for investments in building team health. Some organizations have robust organizational development departments that can conduct assessments and deliver programs to strengthen the ability of the healthcare team to manage conflict. If this is not the case, competent management consulting firms are available to assist, such as the Table Group, led by well-known executive consultant Patrick Lencioni. Mr. Lencioni offers tools for building healthy organizations that the executive team can use (Lencioni, 2012), as well as tools for identifying, hiring, and developing team members who will optimize teamwork (Lencioni, 2016).

### Succession Planning and Talent Management

Succession planning and talent management are other important strategic activities that the nurse executive must undertake to ensure a pipeline of leaders prepared at all levels to deliver population health. Although most of the literature on succession planning focus on the role of the chief executive officer (CEO), it is important for sustainability of leadership direction and organizational culture that plans for development and advancement of nursing leaders at all levels be developed and executed. Yet healthcare lags behind other industries in succession planning (Blouin, McDonagh, Neistadt, & Helfand, 2006; Collins & Collins, 2007).

In 2009, Carriere, Muise, Cummings, and Newburn Cook conducted a review of articles addressing succession planning in healthcare to determine whether strategies utilized were like those used by the business community and whether any best practices for implementation were noted. The authors found similar frameworks as in business and no identified best practices. However, a common thread was found linking strategic planning to succession planning to ensure that the type of talent being developed would meet organizational goals.

In terms of population health, as organizations forecast needs for physicians and other providers based on new programs and program growth, it is incumbent on the nurse executive to assess the implications of these forecasts for nursing and use the information to structure succession plans. The American Hospital Association (AHA), has published a white paper in 2013 on workforce planning. This can be a helpful model for the nurse executive to use in forecasting nursing resources required for future population health needs.

Finally, as nurse executives seek to assess whether an appropriate cultural environment exists in their organizations to enable nursing to contribute to population health, the Practice Environment Scale of the Nursing Work Index (PES-NWI), developed by Lake in 2002, can be used as an objective measure. Lake's tool has been endorsed as an evaluation of nursing practice environments by influential organizations such as the National Quality Forum (NQF, 2008) and the American Nurses Credentialing Center (ANCC). The ANCC administers the Magnet

Recognition Program, which uses several elements of performance including indicators of transformational leadership to identify healthcare facilities that provide healthy work environments for nurses. Currently, about 6% of hospitals in the United States have earned this designation (ANCC, 2017). Most organizations already have access to PES-NWI items as part of their employee satisfaction survey tool, because one of the largest staff satisfaction survey vendors in the country, Press Ganey, has incorporated the PES-NWI into its RN survey.

*Nursing Education and Practice*

Although there have been multiple national and international nursing research studies that show strong relationships between a baccalaureate prepared nursing workforce and better patient outcomes (Robert Wood Johnson Foundation, 2014), support for changing the RN entry into practice to a bachelor of science in nursing (BSN) has not been widespread. IN 2010, the IOM added weight to this issue by recommending that, by 2020, 80% of practicing RNs should be at the BSN level (IOM,2010). In response, nurse executives in several states have developed regionally increasing baccalaureate nursing (RIBN) programs by building coalitions between community colleges and universities (Robert Wood Johnson Foundation, 2014). Some nurse executives were able to garner support in their organizations for only hiring BSN graduates and for instituting policies to move incumbent non-BSN nurses along the BSN path (AACN, 2015). In 2015, the IOM issued a progress report on its 2010 recommendations indicating that, while barriers still existed, many states and organizations were well on their way to achieving the 80% goal (IOM,2015). Nurse executives are encouraged to continue partnerships with academia to strengthen the entry level BSN as well as the BSN completion programs.

The absence of a well-educated nursing workforce to align public health efforts with population health is a particularly serious dilemma. In its 12th annual report to the U.S. Congress in 2014, the National Advisory Council on Nursing Education and Practice (NACNEP) highlighted this dilemma in the following statement:

> Shortages in nurses with advanced training as mid and executive-level public health nurses compromise a high functioning national public health workforce. For example, only a small proportion of nurses working in state (6 percent) and local health departments (10 percent) have graduate or doctoral degrees in nursing (RWJF, 2013). This is also reflected in academic institutions where shortages in faculty with advanced public health training may result in unqualified or

under qualified faculty teaching public health nursing courses. Greater emphasis is needed for advanced practice registered nurse (APRN) roles in public health nursing. The care of populations hinges on collaboration and partnering and no one discipline or entity can be solely responsible for population health outcomes. While nursing should can take the leadership role, this collaborative emphasis mitigates the notion of role overburden and opens new opportunities for APRN roles including dual degrees such as the Doctor of Nursing Practice and Master of Public Health (DNP/MPH) and Doctor of Philosophy in Nursing with an emphasis on public health. These advanced practice roles are especially needed to lead inter professional public health teams and efforts that address population health (NACNEP, 2014).

## Additional Barriers

Other barriers faced by nurse executives as they work to prepare and support the nursing workforce to serve in population health are state and institutional policies that inhibit full scope of nursing practice. These policies demand focused efforts from nurse executives to galvanize advanced practice nurses, professional organizations, educators, policy makers, and payers to effect change (Hain & Fleck, 2014).

### Case Vignette

A large integrated healthcare system in the South has owned and operated a school of nursing that has prepared graduates at the associate degree level for the last 20 years. The school's program was wisely supported by the system CEO, who saw the new graduates as an annual source of RN recruits and a hedge against future nursing shortages. The new nurse executive of the system's flagship hospital sits on the school's executive board and has begun to advocate for the program to be transitioned to a baccalaureate program, because she sees the need for more highly educated nurses to assist with population healthcare continuum demands. Her hospital's percentage of BSN prepared nurses is at 53%, and it is not likely to achieve the 80% goal by 2020, since it hires 85% of its RNs from the associate degree program. The president of the school is eager to move in the baccalaureate direction and views it as something that would increase the school's status in the community. However, the CEO is concerned that this action could impact the annual supply of nurses because of the comparative length of the BSN program.

*Question*: From your previous reading, what steps can the nurse executive take to successfully increase the percentage of BSN prepared RNs in her facility?

## Substance Abuse and Drug Dependency in the Nursing Population

Nurses as a population group have been noted to suffer from a variety of disorders, including stress from exposure to downsizing and restructuring (Bourbonnais, Brisson, Malenfant, & Vézina, 2005), obesity (Miller, Alpert, & Cross, 2008), and addiction to nicotine (Bialous, Sarna, Wewers, Froelicher & Danao, 2004) among other substances. One of the most serious and perhaps underestimated issues impacting the health of the nursing population is the incidence of substance abuse. Nurses are reluctant to self-report due to fear of job loss and stigmatization and may feel as though they are failing the profession (Copp, 2009). It has been thought that about 10% (Dunn, 2005) and as high as 20% (Monroe, Pearson, & Kenaga, 2008) of nurses are addicted to controlled substances. Predisposing factors may include the presence of alcoholic parents and certain risk behaviors (West, 2002) or working as part of a specific provider group, such as anesthesia (Luck & Hedrick, 2004). Although most employers screen nurses on hire for substance abuse and conduct periodic random screenings, the nurse executive cannot simply rely on these basic tactics to manage this health issue in the nursing population. Other tools such as pharmacy information management systems, which contain software that can spotlight unusual trends in individual nurses' medication administration patterns, can be used. The nurse executive can also partner with pharmacy and information systems staff to link data from medication dispensing systems to medication administration documentation to determine whether drug diversion is occurring (Brenn, Kim, & Hilmas, 2015). This can enable earlier detection and assistance for the impaired nurse.

On a broader scale, nurse executives can facilitate coalitions of such stakeholders as state health departments, hospital associations, providers, law enforcement, and boards of nursing to address this important issue. One example of such an effort is the work done by nurse executives in the Minnesota Department of Health and the Minnesota Hospital Association. Working together to prevent and respond to drug diversions, they have developed a roadmap and tool kit that other leaders can use (Minnesota Hospital Association, 2017).

## Summary

Nurse executives play an integral part in improving the health of patient populations as well as total population health. They do so by supporting and guiding nurses toward a population health focus and include the optimization of information systems across the care continuum. Nurse executives also position nurses to lead population health initiatives by developing key inter professional partnerships, planning succession, and strengthening the nursing practice environment. Finally, they improve the health of the nursing population itself by being sensitive to risk factors for disease and disability in nurses and taking appropriate steps to mitigate and manage them. Incorporating concepts of strategic planning, quality improvement, and change management across the continuum of healthcare holds significant promise for nurse executives to lead the improvement of population health, as is evidenced by the nurse executives who have been successful. The caution is that, although there are many tools available to the nurse executive, they will only be successful if they are a part of a holistic management system and leadership culture committed to investment in ongoing improvement (Kaplan, Patterson, & Blackmore, 2014).

## Tool Kit and Resources

*Advanced Practice Program Development Resources*
http://www.carolinashealthcare.org/center-for-advanced-practice

*Clinical Nurse Leader Quality Improvement tools*
5P assessment and Dartmouth microsystem improvement ramp: http://clinicalmicrosystem.org/worksheet

*Drug Diversion Prevention Resources*
Roadmap and toolkit—www.mnhospitals.org

*Nursing Practice Environment evaluation*
Engaging nurses to achieve safe high quality care—nursing survey incorporating the PESNWI tool- www.press ganey.com

*Population Health Improvement Tools*
Tools for reducing Medicaid readmissions—www.ahrq.gov
Project BOOST implementation toolkit—www.hospitalmedicine.org
LACE readmission tool—https://www.ncbi.nlm.nih.gov

*Return on Investment (ROI)*
ROI estimator tool—www.ahrq.gov
The ROI of real time intelligence—www.hp.com

*Discussion Questions*

1. How can a nurse executive best prepare acute care nurses to contribute to population health outcomes?

2. What role should a nurse executive play in policy making with state boards of nursing to ensure that advanced practice nurses are working at top of their license?

3. What type of partnerships would be helpful for nurse executives to engage in to manage substance abuse in the nursing population?

4. Why should nurse executives position nursing to have an ongoing leadership role in informatics?

*Assignments*

1. Identify a challenge that a nurse executive may encounter in developing a return on investment for a proposed program to allow inpatient maternity nurses to make home visits to high-risk mothers after discharge. Investigate a tool that can be used to support the proposal. Explain why you would use it.

2. A nurse executive has recently moved to a new state for a position leading population health management efforts for elderly patients in a poor community. Identify key partners with whom you would advise the executive to promptly build alliances. Explain your rationale.

3. Nurses in a community clinic of an integrated healthcare system report to the nurse executive that Hispanic patients discharged from system hospitals are unprepared to manage their care needs at home. Determine what actions the nurse executive should take to evaluate and if necessary address this issue.

## Case Study 1

*Management of Patients with Sickle Cell Disease*

Sickle cell disease (SCD) is a low volume high risk condition affecting about 70,000 to 100,000 individuals in the United States (National Institutes of Health, 2014). It causes significant disruption within healthcare primarily because of lack of knowledge about the disease and biases toward the population the disease affects, mainly African American people. Pain management is an important competency for healthcare providers to demonstrate, as well as knowledge of community resources, because patients with SCD often have significant pain management and psychosocial needs.

In a comprehensive healthcare system in the south, its population of patients with SCD was primarily concentrated in urban areas. Eight percent of these patients received care in the emergency department (ED) at the system's Level 1 Academic Center. However, a proportion of these patients were lower acuity and could be managed in the Academic Center's community hospital. Barriers were nursing and provider discomfort at the community hospital with managing these patients. As the facility paid more attention to value based purchasing and examined its data on average length of stay (ALOS) and readmissions, patients with SCD were noted to be major contributors to readmission rates and ALOS outside of that expected in the Medical Service Line. Hematologists within the hospital's oncology department had tried for years to effectively manage these patients with little success. There was widespread frustration in the ED and medical and oncology units and among the patients themselves. Lack of consistency from provider to provider, absence of a process for patient engagement, and a need for aggressive psychosocial care coordination characterized the situation. In 2015, as capacity constraints intensified at the Academic Center, the nurse executive partnered with a new hematologist who was hired by oncology leadership to focus on SCD. She saw the opportunity to use the skills of the clinical nurse leader (CNL) role, a generalist master's prepared nurse that the CNE had added to the medical surgical care delivery model in 2010. Initially assigned to each medical surgical inpatient unit as its microsystem, the nurse executive had encouraged and enabled expansion of the CNL's role to include pre- and post-hospital venues for care. The focus of the CNL was to identify evidence based practices for the care of patients, coordinate clinical care, and develop and implement systems to close gaps that were contributing to poor patient experience, low quality, and increased cost.

A CNL from the Academic Center's general oncology inpatient unit worked with the hematologist to develop standard care plans and order sets for the ED and hospitalist providers. The CNL and the hematologist conducted education sessions for nurses and physicians over a one year period in 2016 in the community hospital. Patients were included in their plans of care, and complex patients were referred to the hematologists at the Academic Center. Specific inpatient hospital care units were identified for when patients needed to be admitted, and the nursing, case management and pharmacy team received focused education. The

TABLE 5.1. Sample Items Measured to
Evaluate SCD Population Health Improvement.

| Item | Pre-Nursing Intervention | Post Nursing Intervention |
|---|---|---|
| % SCD standard care plans and order sets in place | | |
| Average length of stay of SCD patients | | |
| Readmission rates of SCD patients | | |
| % SCD patients admitted to community hospital | | |
| % SCD patients admitted to Academic Center | | |
| % SCD patients returned from community hospital to academic center | | |
| % SCD patients reporting ability to consistently go to work and/or school | | |

CNL served as expert resource for all members of the team and used information such as that in the sample, Table 5.1, to assess program effectiveness.

*Question*: A new chief financial officer (CFO) in the organization is concerned that clinical nurse leaders may be driving up the cost of patient care since they are not providing care at the bedside but are counted in nursing costs. As a nurse executive, what population health rationale would you use to address the CFO's concern?

## Case Study 2

*APRN Supply and Demand*

The chairman of the department of urology in a Level 1 Trauma academic center has contacted the nurse executive because he is unable to recruit advanced care practitioners to join his growing service. When the recruitment department does occasionally find a nurse practitioner or physician's assistant, the candidate is either a brand-new graduate or an experienced provider but always unfamiliar with the specialty of urologic practice and the demands of a complex inpatient practice Operating Room (OR), and outpatient practice. This has resulted in long patient waits for outpatient appointments and delays in OR procedures. Physicians in the urology department are frustrated and would preferably to train their own teams of advanced care practitioners.

The nurse executive coordinates several planning sessions with the urologists, a respected APRN from the trauma service, and administrative leaders from the local university. An assessment of needs is done for other clinical departments in the Academic Center, and similar needs are confirmed for several specialties. The planning team develops a proposal whereby the university agrees to expand its nurse practitioner program and the Academic Center agrees to provide paid hands on postgraduate fellowship in urology.

*Question*: How would you assess the effectiveness of this proposal? How would you decide whether to expand it to other specialties?

## Case Study 3

*Substance Abuse in the Nursing Population*

The nurse executive at a community hospital that is part of a large integrated healthcare delivery system is contacted by the local police chief after a post anesthesia care nurse, who worked at her facility, was found dead at home. The nurse's colleagues became concerned when she did not report for work and called her son, who called the police. On arrival at her apartment, officers were alarmed because several empty labeled vials of controlled substances bearing the hospital's name, as well as patient identifiers, were found in her apartment.

The nurse executive is active in her state's practitioner remediation program and has referred several nurses for assistance over the years. She is familiar with recognition and treatment of drug diversion but has never dealt with an employee dying from an overdose before.

*Question*: What steps do you recommend the nurse executive take? How can she use this tragic event to impact the health of the nursing population in her hospital, system, and community?

## References

Aiken, L.H., Cimiotti, J.P., Sloane, D.M., Smith, H.L., Flynn, L., & Neff, D.F. (2011). The effects of nurse staffing and nurse education on patient deaths in hospitals with different work environments. *Medical Care, 49* (12), 1047–1053 doi:10.1097/MLR.0b013e3182330b6e

American Association of Colleges of Nursing. (2015). *Employment of new nurse graduates and employer preferences for baccalaureate prepared nurses*. Retrieved from http://www.aacn.nche.edu/leading_initiatives_news/news/2015/employment15

American Association of Nurse Executives. (2015). *AONE nurse executive competencies: Population Health*. Retrieved from http://www.aone.org/resources/population-health-competencies.pdf

American Association of Nurse Executives. (2017). *About the Healthcare Leadership Alliance*. Retrieved from http://www.aone.org/resources/hla-directory.shtml

American Hospital Association. (2013). *Developing an effective healthcare workforce planning model*. Retrieved from http://www.aha.org/content/13/13wpmwhitepaperfinal.pdf.

American Nurses Credentialing Center. (2017). *Magnet Recognition Program overview*. Retrieved from http://www.nursecredentialing.org/

Bialous, S.A., Sarna, L., Wewers, M.E., Froelicher, E.S., & Danao, L. Nurses perspectives of smoking initiation, addiction and cessation. *Nursing Research, 53*:387–395. PMI 015586135

Blouin, A.S., McDonagh, K.J., Neistadt, A.M., Helfand, B. (2006). Leading tomorrow's health care organizations: strategies and tactics for effective succession planning. *Journal of Nursing Administration*, Jun: 36(6), 325–330.

Bourbonnais, R., Brisson, C., Malenfant, R., Vézina, M. (2005). Health care restructuring, work environment, and health of nurses. *American Journal of Industrial Medicine, 47*: 54–64. doi:10.1002/ajim.20104

Brenn, B.R., Kim, M.A., Hilmas, E. (2015). Development of a computerized monitoring program to identify narcotic diversion in a pediatric anesthesia practice. *American Journal of Health -System Pharmacy, 72*:1365-1372

Buerhaus, P. (2016). The 4 forces that will reshape nursing. *Hospitals and Health Networks*. Retrieved from http://www.hhnmag.com/articles/7522-the-4-forces-that-will-reshape-nursing

Carriere, B. K., Muise, M., Cummings, G., Newburn-Cook, C. (2009) Healthcare succession planning: an integrative review. *Journal of Nursing Administration*, Dec; 39(12):548–55. doi: 10.1097/NNA.0b013e3181c18010

Centers for Medicare and Medicaid Services (CMS) ,2017. *National Health Expenditures*. Retrieved from https://www.cms.gov/research-statistics-data-and-systems/statistics-trends and reports/nationalhealthexpenddata/Downloads/proj2016.pdf

Clark, D. M; Silvester, K.; Knowles. S. (2013) S. Lean Management System: Creating a Culture of Continuous Quality Improvement. *Journal of Clinical Pathology, 66*:638–643.

Collins, S. K., Collins, K. S. (2007). Changing workforce demographics necessitates succession planning in healthcare. *Health Care Management 26*(4). 318-325 Doi10.1097/01.HCM.0000299249.61065.cf

Commonwealth Fund (2015). *International profiles of health care systems 2015*. Retrieved from http://www.commonwealthfund.org/publications/fund-reports/2016/jan/international-profiles-2015

Copp, M.A.B. (2009) *Drug addiction among nurses: confronting a quiet epidemic*. Retrieved from http://www.modernmedicine.com/modernmedicine/news/modernmedicine/modern-medicine-feature-articles/drug-addiction-among-nurses-con?page=full

Curley, A.L., Vitale, P.A. (Eds.). (2016). *Population Based Nursing*. (2nd ed.) New York. N.Y: Springer Publishing.

Dartmouth Institute for Health Policy &Clinical Practice. (2010). In M. Godfrey (Ed.), *Microsystems at a glance*. Retrieved from www.clinicalmicrosystem.org

Dunn, D. (2005). Substance abuse among nurses- defining the issue. *AORN Journal,* *82*(4),572–596 http://doi.org/10.1016/S0001-2092(06)60028-8

Englebright, J., & Caspers, B. (2016). The role of the Chief Nurse Executive in the Big Data Revolution. *Nurse Leader, 14*(4), 280–284

Germain, P. B., &Cummings, G. G. (2010). The influence of nursing leadership on nurse performance: A systematic literature review. *Journal of Nursing Management* *18*(4), 425–439. doi: 10.1111/j.1365-2834.2010.01100.x

Goudreau, K.A., & Smolenski, M.C. (Eds.) (2014). Health policy and advanced practice nursing. New York. NY: Springer Publishing

Hain, D., & Fleck, L., (2014). Barriers to Nurse Practitioner Practice that Impact Healthcare Redesign. *OJIN: The Online Journal of Issues in Nursing, 19*(2) doi: 10.3912/OJIN.Vol19No02Man02. Retrieved from http://www.nursingworld.org/MainMenu-Categories/ANAMarketplace/ANAPeriodicals/OJN/TableofContents/Vol-19-2014/No2-May-2014/Barriers-to-NP-Practice.html

Ibrahim, S.A. (2007). *The Veterans Health Administration. A domestic model for a national health care system?* Retrieved from https://www.va.gov/opa/pressrel/pressrelease.cfm?id=2847

Institute for Healthcare Improvement. (2007). *The Triple Aim: Optimizing health, care and cost.* Retrieved from http://www.ihi.org/engage/initiatives/TripleAim/Documents/BeasleyTripleAim_ACHEJan09.pdf

Institute for Healthcare Improvement. (2012). *A guide to measuring the Triple Aim.* Retrieved from http://www.ihi.org/resources/Pages/IHIWhitePapers/AGuidetoMeasuringTripleAim.aspx

Institute of Medicine. (1988). *The future of Public Health.* Retrieved from http://www.nationalacademies.org/hmd/Reports/1988/The-Future-of-Public-Health.aspx

Institute of Medicine. (2010) *The Future of nursing: Leading Change, Advancing Health.* Retrieved from https://www.nationalacademies.org/hmd/~/media/Files/Report%20Files/2010/The-Future-of-Nursing/Future%20of%20Nursing%202010%20Recommendations.pdf

Institute of Medicine. (2015) *Assessing progress on the IOM report the future of nursing.* Retrieved from http://www.nationalacademies.org/hmd/Reports/2015/Assessing-Progress-on-the-IOM-Report-The-Future-of-Nursing.aspx

Juraschek, S. P; Zhang, X.; Ranganathan, & V.; Lin, V. W. (2012). United States Registered Nurse Workforce Report Card and Shortage Forecast *American Journal of Medical Quality* May/June 27: 241–249.

Kaplan, G; Patterson, S; & Blackmore, C. (2014). Why Lean doesn't work for Everyone. *British Medical Journal of Quality and Safety,* doi: 10:1136/BMJQS 2014 –003248

Kenney, C. (2011). *Transforming Health Care Virginia Mason Medical Center: Pursuit of the perfect patient experience.* Boca Raton, Fla: CRC Press.

Khatri, N., Brown, G.D., Hicks, L.L. (2009). From a blame culture to a just culture in health care. *Health Care Management Review: 34*(4) 312-322 doi: 10.1097/HMR.0b013e3181a3b709

Kindig, D., & Stoddart, G. (2003). What is population health? *American Journal of Public Health 93*(3),380–383.

Kindig, D. (2015). What are we talking about when we talk about population health? *Health Affairs Blog*. Retrieved from http://healthaffairs.org/blog/2015/04/06/what-are-we-talking-about-when-we-talk-about-population-health/

Lake, E.T. (2002). Development of the practice environment scale of Index. *Research in Nursing Health*, Jun 25(3), 176–188.

Lencioni, P. (2002). *The Five Dysfunctions of a Team*. San Francisco, CA. Jossey Bass.

Lencioni, P (2012). *The Advantage*. San Francisco, CA, Jossey Bass.

Lencioni, P. (2016). *The Ideal Team Player*. Hoboken, NJ. Jossey Bass.

Lewenson, S.B., McAllister, A.M., & Smith, K.M. Eds.). (2017). *Nursing history for contemporary role development*. New York, NY: Springer Publishing.

Lúanaigh P. & Hughes F. (2016). The nurse executive role in quality and high performing health services. *Journal of Nursing Management, 24*, 132–136.

Luck, S., Hedrick, J. (2004). The alarming trend of substance abuse in anesthesia providers. *Journal of Perianesthesia nursing, 19*(5), 308-311. http://doi.org/10.1016/j.jopan.2004.06.002

Maeng, D.D., Khan, M., Tomcavage, T., Graf, T.R., Davis, D.E., & Steele, G.D. (2015). Reduced acute inpatient care was largest savings component of Geisinger Health System's Patient Centered Medical Home. *Health Affairs, 34*(4),636–644. doi 10.1377hlthaff.2014.085

Mannon, M. Lean Healthcare and Quality Management. The experience of ThedaCare. *The Quality Management Journal*, 2014; 21.1: 7-10

Miller, S.K., Alpert, P.T., & Cross, C.L. (2008). Overweight and obesity in nurses, advanced practice nurses and educators. American Academy of Nurse Practitioners. doi 10.1111/j.1745-7599.2008.00319. Retrieved from ttp://onlinelibrary.wiley.com/doi/10.1111/j.1745-7599.2008.00319.x/full

Minnesota Hospital Association (2017). Quality and Patient Safety. Retrieved from www.mnhospitals.org/quality-patient-safety/collaboratives/drug-diversion-resources

Monroe, T., Pearson, F., Kenaga, H. (2008). Procedures for handling cases of substance abuse among nurses: A comparison of disciplinary and alternative programs. *Journal of Addictions Nursing, 19*(3), 156–161.

*Mosby's Medical Dictionary* (9th ed.). (2009), St Louis, Mo: Elsevier Publishing

National Advisory Council on Nursing Education and Practice (2014) 12th Annual Report to the US Congress. Retrieved from https://www.hrsa.gov/advisorycommittees/bhpradvisory/nacnep/

Nash, D. B., Reifsnyder, J., Fabius, R. J., & Pracilio, V. (2011). Population Health- Creating a culture of wellness. Sudbury, MA. Jones & Bartlett Learning. Retrieved from http://samples.jbpub.com/9780763780432/80432_FMxx_FINAL.pdf

National Council on State Boards of Nursing. (2017). Transition to Practice. Retrieved from https://www.ncsbn.org/transition-to-practice.htm

National Institutes of Health (2014) Evidence Based Management of Sickle Cell Disease. Retrieved from https://www.nhlbi.nih.gov/health-pro/guidelines/sickle-cell disease-guidelines

National Quality Forum (2008). National Voluntary Consensus Standards for Nursing

Sensitive Care. Retrieved from http://www.qualityforum.org/Publications/2010/10/National_Voluntary_Consensus_Standards_for_Home_Health_Care_—_Additional_Performance_Measures_2008.aspx

Nelson, E.C., Batalden, P.B., & Godfrey, M.M. (2007). *Quality by Design—A clinical microsystems approach.* San Francisco, CA. Jossey-Bass.

Nelson, E.C., Batalden, P.B., Godfrey, M.M., & Lazar, J.S.(Eds.) (2011). *Value by Design—Developing clinical microsystems to achieve organizational excellence.* San Francisco, CA: Jossey-Bass.

North Carolina Board of Nursing. (2011). Just Culture algorithm. Complaint evaluation tool. Retrieved from http://www.ncbon.com/dcp/i/discipline-compliance-employer-complaints-just-culture-resources

Reason, J. (1990). Human error: models and management. Retrieved from https://www.ncbi.nlm.nih.gov/pmc/articles/PMC1117770/

Robert Wood Johnson Foundation. (2013). Overcoming obstacles to health in 2013and beyond. Retrieved from http://www.rwjf.org/en/library/research/2013/06/overcoming-obstacles-to-health-in-2013-and-beyond.html

Robert Wood Johnson Foundation (2014). Building the case for more highly educated nurses. Retrieved from http://www.rwjf.org/en/library/articles-and-news/2014/04/building-the-case-for-more-highly-educated-nurses.html

Sinek, S (2011). Start with Why. London, U.K: Penguin Books.

Stanhope, M; Lancaster, J. (Eds.) (2016). *Public Health Nursing* 9th Ed. St Louis, Mo: Elsevier

Stanley, J. M., Hoiting, T., Burton, D., Harris, J., & Norman, L. (2007). Implementing innovation through education- practice partnerships. *Nursing Outlook, 55*(2) 67–73 Retrieved from http://doi.org/10.1016/j.outlook.2007.01.009

Steele, G. D., Haynes, J. A., Davis, D. E., Tomcavage, J., Stewart, W. F., …Shikles, J. (2010). How Geisinger's advanced medical home model argues the case for rapid cycle innovation. *Health Affairs, 29*(11). 2047–2053. doi: 10.1377/hltaff.2010.084.

Veterans Administration (2010). *Comparison of Quality of Care in VA and non VA settings- a systematic review.* Retrieved from https://www.hsrd.research.va.gov/publications/esp/quality.pdf

Veterans Administration (2013). *Clinical Nurse Leaders making a difference at VA.*

Retrieved from https://www.va.gov/health/newsfeatures/2013/october/clinical-nurse-leaders-making-a-difference-at-va.asp

Veterans Administration (2016). *VA grants full practice authority to advanced practice nurses.* Retrieved from https://www.va.gov/opa/pressrel/pressrelease.cfm?id=2847

West, M.M. (2002). Early risk indicators for substance abuse among nurses. *Journal of Nursing Scholarship, 34*(2), 187–193.

## CHAPTER 6

# Nursing Education for Population Health

PATRICK S. LaROSE, DNP, MSN, RN

## Nursing Education for Population Health

TODAY'S healthcare system remains in constant flux to reflect changing patient complexities, chronic illness, an aging population, emerging technologies, and changes to the drivers of high performance within healthcare. Changing population demographic reflects increases in diversity and cultural shifts within communities that require advance practice nurses (APNs) to adapt to a new normal within clinical practice. This rapid expansion, along with shifting healthcare priorities, continues to be driven by an aging population that requires more care than in any time in history. As healthcare improves through the use of cutting edge technology, populations are living longer and requiring more healthcare services. This new demand is predicated on overall improvements in lifesaving technology that has increased the need for expanded healthcare services and new need for chronic illness care. Today, more people are living with chronic illness that in any time in known history. The increasing complexity of care can be directly related to the growth in those aged 65 years and older within the population. According to Heller, Oros, and Durney-Crowley (2000), those ages 65 and older will represent at least 20% of the total population in the United States (U.S.) by 2020. The U.S. Department of Health and Human Services, Administration on Aging (2016), projects growth of those ages 65 and older will increase by 21.7% by the year 2040.

As the population ages, medical care must keep pace through improved technology to meet the everchanging landscape of those in need of this type of care. Technology advances over the last century, along with the focus on wellness care and illness prevention, have helped to improve life expectancy of the population. According to the Centers for Disease Control and Prevention (CDC; National Center for Health Statistics, 2015), average life expectancy in the United States is now projected at 78.7 years. To further add to this changing demographic, the baby boomer generation, long identified as the largest population explosion in the last century, has approached or will approach retirement age within the next 10 years. The baby boomer generation is best known for redefining the aging process, with the expectation of living a long and productive life. Born between the years 1945 and 1964 (Colby & Ortman, 2014), this generation is focused on health and well-being and is often recognized for healthseeking behaviors that are congruent with wellness and living an enriched life, with activities that promote the idea of fun.

The baby boomers (generation) continue to influence the healthcare dynamic within the country through increases in population need, the way in which healthcare is perceived by this population, and the mere numbers of people seeking care within the healthcare system. The baby boomers demand a more engaged and informed level of care. This population of patients is more educated, with 88% of the population holding at least a high school diploma and 28% holding at least a bachelor's degree (Colby & Ortman, 2014). The baby boomers continue to drive healthcare changes through their insistence on patient-centered care, development of relationships with healthcare providers, and the need to be informed and involved in care decisions beyond those of past generations.

As aging baby-boomers converge with an inflexible healthcare system, there is a shifting focus from hospital care of the past to a more modern view of healthcare where patients are provided care that is community-based. Acute stays in the hospital environment are now reserved for the very sick or those with chronic illnesses and complex care issues. As access to care becomes more of a visible issue in healthcare, hospitals and other healthcare organizations are looking at ways in which to meet the pressing needs within the community to improve access and drive quality care. This change in focus has the potential to provide a significant opportunity for nurse practitioners to develop nurse-led clinics for the management of chronic illness and care that is no longer focused within the hospital setting. The passage of the Patient Protection and Affordable Care Act (also referred to as the Affordable Care Act, or ACA) in 2010 provided opportunities for grants that helped to open nurse-led clinics as a means of providing community-based care (Van Vleet, & Paradise, 2015). With the support of hospital administrators and other stakeholders and with grants awarded by the U.S. Department of Health and Human Services, outpatient clinics are developing across the country. Many of these outpatient care organizations are increasingly being led by nurse practitioners (NPs). NPs can see patients on a nonacute basis to reduce readmission to the hospital and help improve the quality of care patients receive after discharge from an acute illness. These clinics also provide teaching and learning opportunities for students seeking to advance their nursing careers to become NPs (Van Vleet, & Paradise, 2015). Patient-centered care as well as improving access to care, reducing costs, and providing quality outcomes drives this major change in focus. NPs now provide primary care services in a number of settings that were once reserved for physicians, because NPs are a more affordable alternative and provide quality of care to their patients. According to Kaiser Family Foundation, the number of NPs is slated to increase by 30% by 2020 as a means to help meet the pressing shortage of primary care physicians (Van Vleet, & Paradise, 2015).

The education and preparation to become an NP is more expedient, and nurses who complete their education as NPs often have a number of years of clinical practice experience prior to finishing their NP education. Although NPs may be the answer to the primary care provider shortage, many NPs still face practice barriers that do not allow them to work to the fullest extent of their education and experience. In 2010, the Institute of Medicine (IOM) published a position paper on the future of nursing, which provided a strong recommendation that NPs should be allowed to practice to the fullest extent of their knowledge and education (Institute of Medicine, 2010). This same publication also called for third-party reimbursement groups to recognize NPs and afford reimbursement that was commensurate with the services rendered by these providers of care. Sadly, today, NPs continue the struggle with scope of practice issues, full practice authority issues and in one state, NPs still do not have full prescriptive authority (Van Vleet, & Paradise, 2015).

As the field of advanced practice nursing continues to grow, more work needs to be done to shape and balance issues such as reimbursement, scope of practice, and prescriptive authority. Nursing education plays a significant role in helping APNs work collaboratively to address these pressing issues, along with providing teaching and learning experiences that focus on community- and population-based care within a changing healthcare system.

## The APN as Nurse Educator in Population Health

Population health is impacted by a changing demographic of people who are growing older, by shifting national priorities from illness management to wellness and illness prevention, and by a need to increase access to care for populations that traditionally have had limited options for care within the community. Couple shifting priorities with national initiatives to combat the growing prevalence of diabetes, obesity, heart disease, and other health conditions, and population health education needs to be at the forefront of any nursing education program (including programs that lead to registered nurse [RN] licensure, degree completion programs, and APN programs). Population health is simply too important of a subject today and requires more attention in the nursing curriculum than in any other time in nursing history.

The importance of including a chapter on nursing education in a population health textbook speaks to the central idea, which confirms the important role APNs can play in the education of nursing students on population health. However, before we can translate the important role of the APN as a nurse educator for population health, we need to better understand the overall evolution of advance practice, educational standards for this level of practice in nursing, and ways in which the APN can leverage his or her clinical and educational knowledge as a means of bringing value and rich learning experiences for students engaged in population health education.

### Case Vignette

Consider you are a nurse educator with most of your students from the Millennial generation (those the age of 18–34 by 2015). What criteria would you include in your courses to assist these nurses in providing care to those from the Baby Boomer generation? What specific dynamics related to finances, policy, and understanding this generation would prove useful? How would you impart this information?

## History of the APN Evolution

The origins of the APN can be traced to the 1960s, when Loretta Ford and Henry Silver addressed prevalent healthcare concerns for disadvantaged communities with limited access to care (Hain & Fleck, 2014). Dr. Ford and Dr. Silver developed an educational program which focused on health promotion, disease prevention, and wellness for children and families (Hain & Fleck, 2014). Since then, the role of the APN has continued to evolve and grow to meet the pressing healthcare needs of communities across the nation. Today, APNs are recognized by all 50 states in the country, with full practice authority provided by at least 20 states (American Association of Nurse Practitioners, 2013). APNs function collaboratively as a significant member of the healthcare delivery system in many different roles that include nurse practitioners in family, pediatric, mental health and public health (NPs); nurse midwives (CNMs); certified registered nurse anesthetists (CRNAs); and clinical nurse specialists (CNSs) (Fitzgerald, Kantrowitz-Gordon, Katz, & Hirsch, 2012). The educational and curriculum standards for each practice area are different, but the philosophy of nursing remains at the core of this education.

APNs provide care to patients across the country and function in many different healthcare situations. Much of this success is attributable to the design and educational pedagogy of advance practice programs, in which NPs learn the art and science of advance practice. In addition to educational standards, national certification provides the foundation for the legitimacy of this class of APNs and provides assurances to the public of the APNs' competency.

## Standards for APN Education

Advanced practice nursing, as a profession, is rapidly expanding across the country, in part, due to the need for increased access to care and a shortage of primary care providers in rural areas. APNs have consistently stepped to the plate to meet the needs of the population to provide high quality, patient-centered care. Focused on maintaining this rich history, in 2004, nursing organizations and stakeholders came together with a vested interest in defining models of education and standards that would continue to promote advance practice and develop national standards to address education, accreditation, certification, licensure, and practice (National Council for State Boards of Nursing, 2014). In 2011, the APRN Consensus Model was adopted, receiving wide support from nursing organizations, to establish national standards to promote APNs in this country. The consensus model defines the practice of APNs, minimum educational requirements with a master's degree being the acceptable entry point, accreditation standards for programs educating advanced practice registered nurses (APRNs), requirements for board certification, and licensure standards that are consistent from state to state. The consensus model provides the framework from which advance practice nursing programs can build curricula to support the educational requirements for safe and competent practice (National Council for State Boards of Nursing, 2014).

Within the constructs of these standards, APNs receive education that is focused on the healthcare system, care of populations, advance health assessment, advanced pathophysiology, and advanced pharmacology (American Association of Colleges of Nursing, 2006b). Consistent with the consensus model, advanced practice nursing students have learning experiences that couple theory and evidence-based practice as a means to learn advance practice concepts. Through clinical experiences, students can demonstrate application of what is being learned, to establish competency with an APN mentor. APN mentors play a pivotal role in helping APN students learn critical skills that define practice. Preceptors or mentors for APN students can include NPs as well as physicians. Although it is desirable to have an APN preceptor or mentor, the use of physician-preceptor/mentor can also provide students with excellent learning opportunities. According to Donley *et al.* (2014), physician mentors need to be instructed on the importance of role modeling behaviors for practice and may need additional instruction on mentoring or precepting an APN student to bring meaning to the learning experience for the student. This notion speaks to the importance of having clear definition and scope for the preceptor that provides understanding of the expected learning experiences within each clinical course. Preceptors who understand the clinical objectives of the learning experience will have the opportunity to direct learning experiences that can help the student apply concepts that are learned in the class environment. Application allows the student to engage in clinical experiences that foster the development of critical thinking skills, enhances the client relationship, and allows the preceptor and faculty member to evaluate learning outcomes. Morin and Bellack (2015) assert that evaluation of learning outcomes is an ongoing process in which the student and faculty member are in agreement with the outcome expectations. Although the preceptor may be involved in the evaluation process and can report findings to the faculty member, the faculty member holds ultimate accountability for the final evaluation of performance and competency by the student. In addition, the faculty member holds accountability for the progression of the student in the program, which ultimately leads to graduation.

## Board Certification/National Recognition

Nursing education for the APN prepares graduates for entrance into clinical practice at the highest level for the profession of nursing. Graduates of these programs often assume significant roles on the healthcare team and, in some states, are recognized as the primary care provider within the community. As such, these nurses need to have legitimate credentials outside of the introductory education, to confirm knowledge and competency.

Board certification for the specialty area of practice for the APN is a requirement for both state licensure as an APN and the ability to practice within a state (National Council for State Boards of Nursing, 2014). According to the National Organization of Nurse Practitioner Faculties (NONPF, 2013), there are a total of five recognized bodies that provide certification for APNs, including NPs (with each specialization), nurse midwives, and clinical nurse specialists. National certification is an important element to the completion of an education program for the APN, because board certification validates the graduate has achieved the core knowledge requirements to enter safe practice as an APN, and this validation allows for licensing by the state of practice. According to the APRN Consensus Model (National Council for State Boards of Nursing, 2014, p.7), certification is defined as "the formal recognition of the knowledge, skills, and experience demonstrated by the achievement of standards identified by the profession."

The last step to entering practice is receiving a license to practice as an APN. According to the National Council for State Boards of Nursing (2014), licensure for APNs are standardized across the nation and require that those with the title designation of APRN be licensed in the state, with a population focus. This licensure will be based on successful completion of an accredited program and board certification as an APN with a specific population focus. The title APRN is protected and reserved for those who have the qualifications to hold such a title (NCSBN, 2014).

## From Practice to Academia

APNs are well situated to teach in an academic program at the graduate level, because the experience most APNs have translates exceptionally well. However, few APN programs offer pedagogy that is focused on teaching and learning and, in fact, few graduate nursing programs offer this focus unless the graduate student is enrolled in a degree program that specializes in nursing education. Postgraduate certification programs provide APNs with additional education on teaching and learning concepts that can help grow academic practice. Courses may include assessment and evaluation, curriculum development, teaching diverse populations, the role of the nurse educator, and other similar type courses designed to provide the APN with additional knowledge and education on the art of teaching.

Transitioning from a clinical position to an academic position will take time, but this time involves learning new and exciting skills that can help add to the portfolio of experiences by the APN. As with anything new, developing a plan for competence is an important part of this transition. Identifying specific goals to achieve additional education and learning that is needed, and exploring certifications that may be required as a part of the academic journey, will add to a continuing education plan. In many cases, APNs transitioning from a clinical role to that of nursing academic will be afforded a nurse educator mentor. This experienced nursing faculty member will provide the APN faculty member with oversight in teaching and learning and will help design a competency plan to promote the growth and learning of the new faculty member. The faculty mentor has an important responsibility to help transition and socialize the new APN faculty member as a member of the core teaching team within the faculty. Further, the faculty mentor will help the new APN faculty negotiate the culture of academia as he or she learns new responsibilities and becomes more aware of university policies. The APN faculty member, in cooperation with the mentor, will recognize that, within most schools of nursing, teaching, service, practice, and scholarship are central to the practice of an academic nurse.

Teaching refers to the development of pedagogy in which the nurse educator explores new and innovative ways to help students engage in learning experiences (Walters, 2014). These learning experiences should be evidencebased and focus on student engagement and the overall objectives of the student learning outcomes. There is much in the literature about ways in which to interact with students. However, some faculty appear to be more resistant to change than others. As a new faculty member entering academic practice, it is important to embrace innovative approaches to engage learners in the material. Walters

(2014) suggests that problem-solving based activities, learning groups, and evolving case studies provide students with dynamic learning experiences that are engaging and help students to learn the material.

Adult learners need to see the value in their learning experiences and require direct application of the subject matter to make learning stick. Weimer (2002) speaks about the importance of learning activities in which the learner is engaged and takes responsibility for the learning by becoming an active participant. Of course, for this to happen, the faculty member must plan learning activities that foster this type of education. Planning learning activities takes time, thought, and preparation to effectively align the activity to the learning outcomes and objectives of the course. The scholarship of teaching is about creating a rich environment with robust learning experiences in which the student feels accepted and engaged.

The scholarship of practice aligns well with teaching because the two rely on each other and often go hand in hand in nursing. The scholarship of practice is best defined as the transference of clinical knowledge that is acquired through clinical competency. Faculty must remain involved with practice standards as a means of evolving clinical practice with changing technology and evidence-based practice. The American Association of Colleges of Nursing (AACN) (1999) asserts the scholarship of practice is about focusing on providing care and services that address healthcare problems with the use of evidence to validate this level of practice. The scholarship of practice includes a number of strategies to stay relevant, including practice with direct or indirect care; research, teaching and scholarship; continuing education; writing; administrative approaches; and volunteering.

An argument can be made that nursing is largely a skill-driven profession. Within the framework of skills, critical thinking plays a large role in nursing practice. Congruent with critical thinking is the ability to recognize and respond to complex patient conditions with logical approaches to care. APN faculty with dated clinical skills may not translate cutting edge clinical care to students that require this information as a means of acquiring skills from their entry-level education. It is incumbent upon the faculty member to develop a competency plan that is driven by faculty development opportunities, practice opportunities, and other such experiences that help the APN faculty member remain relevant and engaged in practice. As faculty members enter the clinical environment with students, they must be prepared to address issues relating to the basic and advanced care of a population of patients. In addition, the faculty member needs to help students seek out opportunities for practical application of learning from class and simulation in the real clinical area as students engage in care for patients (Callen, Smith, Joyce, Brown-Schott, and Block, 2013). The scholarship of practice also focuses on methodologies for providing students with unique, student-centric learning opportunities within the clinical area that addresses the skill needs of the student. APN faculty are well suited to address these learning issues through approaches that meet the student's overall needs and address learning outcomes for the clinical course.

The scholarship of discovery is defined by the utilization of empirical findings that add to the scientific body of nursing knowledge and help to advance care standards to improve patient outcomes. Discovery is about learning new information that is derived from research or translating empirical research to change practice (American Association of Colleges of Nursing, 1999). APNs entering an initial academic assignment may discover the university requires some level of academic research as means to generate new knowledge or generate revenue for research from grants and other benefactors. The APN may be required to publish on a predefined schedule or generate new research studies; he or she may be asked to present at a scholarly conference or participate in peer-evaluations as a means of discovery. The scholarship of discovery is part of the faculty platform and may be required for the APN to earn tenure as an associate or full professor for the university.

The scholarship of service is focused on giving back to the community and taking part in services that benefit those in need. The APN may be required to participate in community work through volunteerism or to address a community health issue and present solutions for this issue within the college of nursing or for the university as a whole. Service can be incorporated as part of the clinical experiences with students and can focus on providing meals to the elderly on a predetermined schedule, helping in a community food pantry, or working with a vulnerable population to address healthcare needs or provide increased access to care in the community.

### Educating Nursing Students on Population Health

As mentioned earlier in this textbook, APNs are well positioned to teach population health because of the depth of knowledge that APNs possess in caring for populations, families, and individuals. The premise of dealing with population health is to look at the population as the patient and focus care and services based on the presenting needs of the population (National Advisory Council on Nurse Education and Practice, 2016). With the passage of the ACA in 2010 and with emerging global health issues that have impacted the population of the United States, now is the time to shift focus in nursing education. Nursing education has traditionally educated nursing students through an acute care model of learning experiences. Clinical faculty members bring students to the hospital on a pre-assigned floor, make random assignments, and hope students receive the skills they need to make the learning experience meaningful. Decreasing lengths of stay and limited clinical experiences make teaching clinical nursing more challenging than ever.

Nursing education today is under threat of having limited clinical sites in which to teach students the traditional models of nursing. Hospitals care for those with highly complex care needs and chronic illness. Moreover, patients are being discharged from hospitals to facilities with lower levels of care (e.g., subacute care, long-term care, or assisted living facilities) or to home and are recovering with community-based care at a more rapid pace than in the past. This change is driven mostly by reimbursement, but can also be attributed to evidence which suggests that the hospital is not always the safest place to recover. Despite this changing demographic, traditional nursing schools are still focused on providing clinical experiences in the hospital. Some nurse educators would argue that the laws and rules need to change to promote a more population health focus for nursing schools (Simpson & Richards, 2015). Others would argue nursing's origin is in the hospital and this is where nurses are best trained. Nursing schools today can re-envision population and community health curricula and make changes to course offerings to include more of the social and behavioral sciences. This change can help to promote models of care that are more focused on social policy and the way people respond to community-based healthcare (National Advisory Council on Nurse Education and Practice, 2016). These models can address the need for healthcare policy advocacy, promote nursing as a leader in population health initiatives, and place a focus on future trends in population health concerns and needs into the future.

## Strategies for Teaching Population and Community Health

It is clear there is a need to re-envision the way in which population and community health is taught in today's nursing school. However, APN faculty members can translate their education, experience, and knowledge of community and population health into valuable and meaningful learning experiences for nursing students. Weimer (2002) suggests that adult learners want to take responsibility for their own learning but look to faculty members as the holders of the knowledge. As educators, it is important to release the reins of control over the classroom learning environment and give up the traditional methods to convey information.

Nursing programs both at the community college level and the university level are beginning to see a new generation of students enter programs that have used technology for their entire lives. Individuals in this new millennial generation, in general, may have short attention spans, require constant engagement, and lose interests very rapidly. The notable strength of those in this population is their willingness to use technology as a significant part of learning, confidence, altruism, appreciation for innovated approaches to learning and their ability to foster and embrace change (Montenery et al., 2013). Montenery et al. (2013) asserts that the millennial generation is a cohort born between 1980 and 1992; others would expand this timeline up to the year 2003, but there is no current agreement on the timeline. The millennial generation, born to baby boomers, is viewed to have high self-esteem, lack a long attention span, have high levels of confidence, embrace team-work, and have a view of the world that is based on the impressions received from their use of multiple social media platforms. This generation uses social media and other forms of technology to document their everyday lives, selfies (a picture of one self), and time with friends. According to Montenery et al. (2013), "They [millennial generation] develop critical thinking through experimentation and active participation" (p. 405). This means educational platforms need to speak to these pressing characteristics if nurse educators hope to provide learning experiences that have meaning, are engaging, and help to convey important skills and information to millennial nursing students.

The millennial generation is entering nursing school during a time in which the student mix is quite diversified. One of the most significant challenges faculty members face today is how to design teaching and learning strategies that will promote and include the multigenerational makeup of the nursing class room. Nurse educators are often faced with a student mix that includes young adults, middle-aged adults, those in college for the first time, or those making a mid-life shift in careers to become a nurse. This multifocal aspect of teaching can present challenges and opportunities when defining learning experiences to meet the needs of each individual student. However, research supports the use of innovation and engaging learning platforms for all generations as adult learners.

### Case Vignette

Donita is a pediatric nurse practitioner (NP) that works fulltime in a pediatrician's office as one of the primary healthcare providers. This practice is very busy, but Donita enjoys the interaction she has with the children and families. She has recently agreed to work as an adjunct clinical professor for a local nursing program. She will be working with students taking a pediatric course in a prelicensure program and will be the supervising clinical professor for a group of eight students in a community-based pediatric clinical rotation two days per week. Donita understands the student population she will be working with this semester is highly diverse both in culture and age.

The learning objectives for the clinical experience this semester include prioritizing clinical care to a pediatric population through history and assessment and defining community needs through a windshield survey of the local community.

Describe how Donita can help the different generations represented in her class focus on the learning objectives. Will Donita need to have different planned clinical activities for each agegroup or can she define one learning activity for her clinical group?

Donita wants her students to understand clinical history, and assessment can provide information that may not always be spoken and may reflect a need in the community that is not being met. Describe the teaching strategies Donita may want to use to convey this message to her students. Provide at least two strategies that Donita might use as she teaches this important concept.

Donita's students will be working at multiple community agencies. What approach can Donita use to ensure her students are achieving the learning objectives for the clinical experience? Describe at least two different approaches.

Toward the end of the clinical rotation, Donita asks for feedback from the nurses on her students' performance overall during the clinical rotation. Describe why it is important to allow the nurses to provide feedback on the student performance overall. In addition, describe why clinical success should be measured by the professor and not the nurses.

Flipping the classroom is an approach that addresses the interactive needs of adult learners and can provide meaningful and active learning experiences to all students. The idea of flipping the classroom has become an important teaching strategy over the last decade and promotes the notion that students engage in learning the material on their own prior to coming to class. This means students complete required readings, watch videos, and learn the various concepts or central points of the lesson on their own. Class time is reserved for higher level learning in which the faculty member designs learning activities that promote the practical application of what was learned through the reading. In this environment, faculty members can be more effective in helping students apply concepts and skills and can provide direct and immediate feedback on the application. Brame (2013) asserts that engaged learning, such as those found with a flipped classroom experience, can help to promote active learning in adults and improve learning evaluations.

Designing innovative and unique learning experiences takes more time and preparation than the traditional lecture platform. Although students may prefer the passive learning environment, studies have demonstrated that adult learners learn more and prefer an active learning experience in which application of the concepts is at the core of the learning activity (Brame, 2013). This active learning environment requires the APN faculty members to employ strategies that move learning from passive to active. Approaches being used include the evolving case study, in which students are challenged to problem-solve as more information becomes available; the use of audience response systems that allow students to engage in responses anonymously; and highfidelity (HF) patient simulators that allow students to learn and practice highrisk procedures safely (Montenery et al., 2013). Each of these approaches provides an innovative and creative way to engage learners that helps to promote critical thinking and develop important clinical skills. Additional strategies, such as virtual learning platforms and podcasts, are being employed routinely by nursing faculty members to help students become active learners. The importance of using technology to create a strong learning environment that is active cannot be understated. However, these approaches require the nurse educator to do an inventory and reflect on his or her ability to meet the demands of nursing students today. The increasing use of technology may challenge some faculty members who have grown used to the traditional lecture method and may feel threatened or scared these new strategies may not work or students may fail examinations. Faculty development programs and continuing education need to be focused on helping faculty members gain the skills needed to be part of this brave new world of innovative technologies. This becomes especially important when faculty utilize HF patient simulation as a learning tool in the classroom and nursing laboratory.

*Case Vignette*

Mary Robinson, APN, MSN, RN, is a professor in a prelicensure bachelor's program that leads to eligibility upon graduation for students to sit for the National Council Licensure Examination—Registered Nurse (NCLEX-RN). She is teaching population health to a group of undergraduate nursing students. As she prepares for this next class on EcoMaps and GenoGrams, she wants to provide students with a flipped classroom experience in which the students read about EcoMaps and GenoGrams prior to class. Her preparations for the class will allow students to develop a deeper understanding of these two learning activities, which she hopes will promote the student's success.

As Ms. Robinson prepares for this class, how would she define the flipped classroom?

Ms. Robinson wants to better define the role of active and passive learning for her students. What steps can she take to better define the differences in active and passive learning and how can she translate this to her students?

As Ms. Robinson prepares for her class, what activities would she assign her students as homework and why?

Ms. Robinson is preparing for the classroom learning activities. What application activities can she plan that would promote engagement of her learners?

## High-Fidelity Simulation

HF patient simulation is a teaching and learning approach being used by many nursing programs to enhance active learning in both the classroom and nursing laboratory. HF simulation allows faculty members to define specific patient scenarios that are aligned with learning objectives to help nursing students develop critical thinking skills in a safe environment. According to Turner (2017), the use of high-fidelity simulators provides nursing students with clinical learning experiences on health conditions they may rarely see in nursing school. This is perfect for teaching population health, because faculty can create population-based health concerns or issues within the platform to help students with critical thinking on epidemiology, population, and community health issues that may be seen rarely in the population. HF simulation also provides faculty with the opportunity to develop scenarios specifically focused on population health issues that are present within the community of the students, which can promote active interest in learning. For example, an HF simulation scenario can be developed to address the issue of mumps in the population through assessment and taking a history. This experience can be coupled with an evolving case study to promote critical thought about the situation and require the student to devise a treatment plan that addresses the needs of the client and focuses on ways to improve the issue within the community. There are many options to employ this technology to educate on population health.

*Case Vignette*

Dr. Rah Linked, DNP, APRN, is a family nurse practitioner (FNP) and teaches in both the undergraduate and graduate nursing program for a large university in central Texas. He works closely with the HF simulation laboratory and often collaborates with the clinical director for HF on specific learning projects for his students. He has developed a growing concern about the increased prevalence of childhood diseases being seen in the community over the last few years and wants to address this issue with his students through HF simulation. He meets with the HF Clinical Director so they can develop some simulation scenarios that would promote an increased awareness of this issue with his students and wants to evaluate the students' critical thinking through these exercises.

Describe three approaches Dr. Linked might use with HF to evaluate each student's individual critical thinking?

Dr. Linked is clearly concerned about a community (population) health issue that is currently impacting the community. Why is it important for Dr. Linked to develop a specific simulation of an issue impacting health in his community?

Describe a simulation scenario you would develop for an issue of this nature impacting your community. Be specific about the learning objectives for this simulation.

Describe why learning objectives are an important part of simulation.

## Technology in the Learning Environment

Technology continues to emerge that has a very real and important impact on student learning. "Second Life" is an online virtual platform that promotes learning through interactive experiences in which the student is represented by an avatar. Within this virtual world, students can interact with learning experiences created by faculty designed to engage all aspects of the student's senses. The immediacy of the interaction is what defines this learning platform as something special. According to Reinsmith-Jones, Kibbe, Crayton, & Campbell (2015), the use of Second Life is a popular virtual platform that provides students with engaging learning experiences in which they can interact with peers and faculty in a collaborative manner. This technology is gaining popularity with many online schools to provide innovative and alternative teaching methods for student learning. Second Life has a great potential for population health students, because faculty members can define a virtual population, address prevailing community health issues within this population, and define specific learning experiences for students as they enter this reality and work virtually with a predefined population of clients.

There are many ways in which nursing faculty can engage learners. It takes the desire and willingness to step outside of the traditional approaches and design learning experiences that allow the student to interact, work collaboratively, and apply skills and concepts. Learning experiences for students should promote the understanding of theory and the scientific underpinnings of theory as it relates to nursing to practice.

*The APN Faculty Tool Kit*

As the APN begins to plan for clinical or academic practice, it is important to assemble all the tools learned from the APN's educational journey to support him or her in practice. With the amount of learning that takes place throughout the APN's education, it can be challenging to assemble a toolbox of skills that will help the APN teach population health to nursing students. The APN tool kit of skills should include a thorough and educated perspective on the needs of our aging population; focus on a holistic approach to care that is based in evidence and promotes wellness and disease prevention. Additional skills for the tool kit include recognizing that the demographic of the population is changing through aging and shifts in cultural norms, with the potential for new disease processes and illnesses that may not have been part of population care in the past. The APN must include skills about epidemiology, data collection, and the ways in which illness and disease impact the population. With a focus on the national health goals, the APN can provide immersive experiences for students that address prevailing healthcare concerns.

*Case Vignette*

Dr. Karen Lighting, DNP, APRN, is an Associate Professor of Nursing for a small BSN program in rural Idaho. She is teaching a population health course and wants her students to learn more about national health initiatives that would address some of the health issues impacting this small rural community. Dr. Lighting knows that, like most areas in Idaho and across the country, her small rural community is experiencing an increased prevalence of type 2 diabetes and CO and an increase in childhood diseases.

Describe three different websites Dr. Lighting could use to help students become more aware and familiar with national health initiatives.

Develop two learning activities she could use to help students develop a better understanding of the health needs within this community.

What approach can Dr. Lighting take to help students understand the importance of remaining aware of national health goals?

Define an educational activity students could develop to help promote awareness of prevailing health issues within this community.

## Summary

APNs who desire to teach need to include a thorough understanding of the mix in the nursing student population as multigenerational and one that requires patience and understanding of the learning needs of each generation. APN faculty need to reflect on teaching methods that can engage students and work to ensure the APN has the skills needed to develop and implement learning modalities that are technology based. APN faculty members need to understand and employ adult learning techniques that engage and foster a learning environment which is robust and rich with interactive and innovative approaches to help students engage in the development of critical thinking and the acquisition of skills.

The future of the health of our population in the United States and abroad can be positively impacted by nurses who understand the future of healthcare, future of population health initiatives, and needs of the next generation of nurses. Above all, the APN needs to remember, nursing is a life-long learning profession. What is learned in nursing school and APN education only establishes the base for this learning. The profession and healthcare are dynamic and are changing every day. Life-long learning addresses the need for APNs to remain current in practice and continue to learn throughout the life span of their careers. Professional development is an important and integral responsibility so that APNs can meet the needs of healthcare in their communities and for each of their students.

## Tool Kit and Resources

*Important Websites and Links*

American Association of Colleges of Nursing—DNP Essentials: www. aacn.nche.edu/publications/position/DNPEssentials.pdf

American Association of Colleges of Nursing—Masters in Advance Practice Essentials: www.aacn.nche.edu/education-resources/Mas-Essentials96.pdf

The Community Guide: https://www.thecommunityguide.org/

Public Health Grand Rounds: https://www.cdc.gov/cdcgrandrounds/

Healthy People 2020: https://www.healthypeople.gov/

Health Promotion—World Health Organization (WHO): http://www. who.int/healthpromotion/about/goals/en/

The Office of Disease Prevention and Health Promotion: https://health. gov/

APN Consensus Model: https://www.ncsbn.org/736.htm

National Organization for Nurse Practitioner Faculties (NONPF)

DNP NP tool kit: Process and approach to DNP competency based evaluation: http://c.ymcdn.com/sites/www.nonpf.org/resource/resmgr/imported/DNPNPToolkitFinal2013.pdf

*Discussion Questions*

1. Advance practice nurses have the education, experience, and knowledge to be effective teachers of population health. For this discussion, provide at least three evidence-based characteristics that qualifies a nurse practitioner to teach this course.

2. Today's nursing students are diverse in culture, age, and experience. Describe two student-centered learning experiences focused on population health that can be developed to help students understand the importance of national health goals.

3. Reflection: As you look to your own experience as a student, define a specific learning experience you had that was ineffective. How you would have changed that learning experience to be more engaging and focused on learning?

4. Describe how you would use a specific technology to enhance your teaching of a population health subject. For this discussion, define the technology you would use and how this technology would augment the content for this subject.

5. What are advantages and disadvantages for advanced practice nurses when it comes to licensure and certification? What key areas in education do the National League for Nursing (NLN) and AACN address in relation to advanced practice nursing education?

## Case Study 1

Jennifer is a family nurse practitioner (FNP) who has been active in clinical practice since graduating from APN school in 2003. She holds board certification through the American Nurses Credentials Center (ANCC) with a focus in family health. She has been working in a family practice office for the last five years and provides clinical support to the primary physician in the practice by making rounds to see patients in the hospital two days a week.

Prior to becoming an FNP, Jennifer worked as a registered nurse (RN) in the intensive care unit of a small rural hospital in North Carolina. Her entry-level education to nursing was through a baccalaureate (BSN) program that she completed in 1998.

Jennifer has recently been presented with an opportunity to teach population and community health in the local BSN program of the university from which she graduated. She has been teaching online in the RNtoBSN program for over a year and was invited by the dean to join the faculty in the prelicensure BSN program as an assistant professor.

Joining the university faculty would mean that Jennifer would need to leave her full-time position as an FNP. After many days of consideration, Jennifer agrees to accept the position with the university and leaves her FNP position. She agrees to stay connected with the practice will, as needed, manage patient rounding in the hospital on the weekends.

How can Jennifer meet the competency requirements for APNs if she is working parttime?

Jennifer has never taught prelicensure nursing students. What types of continuing education will Jennifer need to include in her development portfolio to teach a course in population health?

Jennifer will be teaching population health and community health. How can she prepare for these classes? What types of teaching and learning methods should Jennifer plan to use when teaching population and community health?

Jennifer is highly skilled in the use of technology. How can Jennifer translate these skills for successful use with HF simulation?

**Case Study 2**

Corey has been a registered nurse (RN) for six years. He started his nursing career as a licensed practical nurse and worked for 10 years before completing his associate degree in nursing and becoming an RN. After completing the associate degree, Corey worked for a few years in the emergency department for a very busy city hospital and gained a great deal of experience. The hospital began preparing for Magnet accreditation and started requiring existing nurses to go back to school to complete the bachelor's degree in nursing (BSN). After multiple requests, Corey decided he would finish the BSN and completed an RN-to-BSN program online.

Several years after completing the BSN, Corey decided to enter the local university to complete the education to become a clinical nurse specialist (CNS) with a focus on emergency care. He is scheduled to graduate with his masters of science in nursing as an advanced practice nurse (APN) in a few weeks and is thinking about his career trajectory. Upon graduation and board certification, Corey would like to work in the emergency department as a CNS, but he would also like to teach at the local university in the family nurse practitioner (FNP)/CNS program.

For Corey to practice as a CNS, what are the important steps he needs to accomplish before he can realize his goals?

The dean of the program determines that Corey is qualified to teach. What qualifies Corey to teach in an FNP/CNS program?

Corey has limited or no formal teaching experience. What continuing education would Corey need to include in his faculty development portfolio?

Describe the process for board certification and state licensing for APNs.

## Case Study 3

Casey is a nursing faculty member with the local community college. Most recently, the dean of the program revised the curricula (at the request of the faculty) to include a population health course. Casey understands the importance of this course, as more and more healthcare issues are being addressed within the community and students need to be aware of this prevailing healthcare dynamic. Casey is most concerned with cancer screening as a larger part of catching cancer prior to the spread of this disease systemically.

Casey recently had a conversation with her father about cancer screening; she learned during this conversation that he had not had a colonoscopy despite being 56 years of age. As a nurse practitioner, Casey knows the national health goal is for men and women to be screened for colorectal cancer after they turn 50 years old as a means of catching the disease early through colonoscopy. After encouraging her father to schedule an appointment for a colonoscopy, Casey decides to research this issue to help improve the number of people over age 50 receiving a colonoscopy screening. Much to her surprise, she is shocked to learn about the number of people who do not receive this screening. According to her research, some simply do not schedule the screening due to apathy; others do not schedule the screening because of limited or no health insurance; and a smaller population of people do not have this screening done because they do not believe they need it.

Casey believes this issue is important and decides to develop a learning activity out of the research she has done on colorectal screenings. She wants her students to develop an educational message for members of the community to help increase the number of people receiving this screening.

Describe the learning activity you believe Casey should develop, and share at least two approaches to this learning activity.

Define the research that students should do to confirm Casey's research. Should students work in groups or should they do their own research on the subject?

Casey wants to flip the classroom on this issue. Describe how Casey might go about flipping the classroom on colorectal screenings, and define two interactive learning experiences Casey would plan to engage student learning.

Provide two ways in which you would align the teaching to the learning objectives for this activity.

## Case Study 4

Michelle is a psychiatric mental health nurse practitioner (PMHNP) and works for a community mental health clinic. She also teaches the mental health and population health courses for a prelicensure nursing program. She has recently learned how to use podcasts to augment her classroom instruction. Michelle believes the use of podcasts allows students to revisit the material after reading the assigned chapter in the population health textbook assigned to the course.

In what ways does the use of a podcast help students grow their knowledge in population health?

Describe two strategies that a nursing professor can use to develop a podcast to engage students in learning activities.

Define one additional technologybased learning program that will enhance the learning experience for adult learners.

Describe how a nursing professor can align a podcast to meet the learning objectives for a course in population health.

## References

American Association of Colleges of Nursing. (1999). Defining scholarship for the discipline of nursing. Retrieved from http://www.aacn.nche.edu/publications/position/defining-scholarship

American Association of Colleges of Nursing. (2006). *The essentials of master's education for advanced practice nursing*. Washington, DC: Author. Retrieved from www.aacn.nche.edu/education-resources/MasEssentials96.pdf

American Association of Nurse Practitioners (AANP). (2013). Nurse practitioner state practice environment Retrieved from www.APRN.org

Brame, C., (2013). Flipping the classroom. *Vanderbilt University Center for Teaching*. Retrieved from http://cft.vanderbilt.edu/guides-sub-pages/flipping-the-classroom/

Callen, B., Smith, C. M., Joyce, B., Lutz, J., Brown-Schott, N., & Block, D. (2013). Teaching/learning strategies for the essentials of baccalaureate nursing education for entry-level community/public health nursing. *Public Health Nursing, 30*(6), 537–547. doi:10.1111/phn.12033

Colby, S., and Ortman, J. (2014). The baby boom cohort in the United States: 2012-2060. *United States Census Bureau*. Retrieved from https://www.census.gov/prod/2014pubs/p25-1141.pdf

Donley, R., Flaherty, M., Sarsfield, E., Burkhard, A., O'Brien, S., & Anderson, K. (2014). Graduate clinical nurse preceptors: Implications for improved intra-professional collaboration. *OJIN: The Online Journal of Issues in Nursing, 19*(3). doi: 10.3912/OJIN.Vol19No03PPT01

Fitzgerald, C., Kantrowitz-Gordon, I., Katz, J., & Hirsch, A. (2012). Advanced practice nursing education: Challenges and strategies. *Nursing Research and Practice*, vol. 2012, Article ID 854918, (8). doi:10.1155/2012/854918

Hain, D., & Fleck, L. M. (2014). Barriers to np practice that impact healthcare redesign. *Online Journal of Issues in Nursing, 19*(2), 5. doi:10.3912/OJIN.Vol19No-02Man02

Heller, B., Oros, M., and Durney-Crowley, J. (2000). The future of nursing education. Ten trends to watch. *Nursing Health Care Prospect, 21*(1), 9–13. Retrieved from http://www.nln.org/nlnjournal/infotrends.htm Google Scholar

Institute of Medicine (IOM). (2010). *The future of nursing: Leading the change, advancing health*. Washington, D.C.: The National Academies Press.

Montenery, S. M., Walker, M., Sorensen, E., Thompson, R., Kirklin, D., White, R., & Ross, C. (2013). Millennial generation student nurses' perceptions of the impact of multiple technologies on learning. *Nursing Education Perspectives (National League for Nursing), 34*(6), 405–409. doi:10.5480/10-451

Morin, K. H., & Bellack, J. P. (2015). Student learning outcomes. *Journal of Nursing Education, 54*(3-4). doi:10.3928/01484834-20150217-10

National Advisory Council on Nurse Education and Practice. (2016). *Preparing nurses for new roles in population health management*. Health Resource and Services Administration. Retrieved from https://www.hrsa.gov/advisorycommittees/bhpradvisory/nacnep/Reports/fourteenthreport.pdf

National Council for State Boards of Nursing. (2014). *Consensus model for aprn regulation*. Retrieved from https://www.ncsbn.org/Consensus_Model_for_APRN_Regulation_July_2008.pdf

Reinsmith-Jones, K., Kibbe, S., Crayton, T., & Campbell, E. (2015). Use of second life in social work education: Virtual world experiences and their effect on students. *Journal of Social Work Education, 51*(1), 90–108. doi:10.1080/10437797.2015.977167

Simpson, V., & Richards, E. (2015). Flipping the classroom to teach population health: Increasing the relevance. *Nurse Education in Practice, 15*(3), 162–167. doi:10.1016/j.nepr.2014.12.001

Turner, S. (2017). Using high-fidelity simulation scenarios in the classroom to engage learners. *Creative Nursing, 23*(1), 35–41. doi:10.1891/1078-4535.23.1.35

U.S. Department of Health and Human Services. (2016). Aging statistics. *Administration on Aging (AOA)*. Retrieved from https://aoa.acl.gov/Aging_Statistics/Index.aspx

U.S. Department of Health and Human Services. (2017) Center for Disease Control and Prevention. *Health, United States, 2015: With special features on racial and ethnic health disparities*. Retrieved from https://www.cdc.gov/nchs/data/hus/hus15.pdf

Van Vleet, A., and Paradise, J. (2015). Tapping nurse practitioners to meet the rising demand for primary care. *Kaiser Family Foundation*. Retrieved from http://kff.org/medicaid/issue-brief/tapping-nurse-practitioners-to-meet-rising-demand-for-primary-care/

Walters, K. (2014). Sharing classroom research and the scholarship of teaching: Student resistance to active learning may not be as pervasive as is commonly be-lieved. *Nursing Education Perspectives (National League for Nursing), 35*(5), 342–343. doi:10.5480/11-691.1

Weimer, M. (2002). Learner-centered teaching. San Francisco, CA: Jossey-Bass.

# Section 2

# Populations/Considerations/ Specific Areas

## CHAPTER 7

# Pediatric Issues

MARY LAWSON CARNEY, DNP, RNBC, CCRN, CNE

*An ounce of prevention is worth a pound of cure.*
—Benjamin Franklin—Poor Richard's Almanack

## Pediatrics Overview

**P**OPULATION HEALTH for pediatrics is, at its very foundation, future oriented. Although approaches employed for *all* populations are aimed at improving health and wellness through preventative strategies, the impact of these strategies in adults is limited when compared with those measures applied to pediatric populations.

Aside from the obvious health benefits that population health strategies can bring to the pediatric setting, one must also consider the impact on the potential of those children as citizens in our society. If we can at least partially reverse the conditions that lead to lifelong poor health/disability for even a small percentage of this population, the overall financial impact this could have on our nation would be tremendous.

Considering the idea that *present health equals future potential*, the life trajectory of individual children is threatened if we do not address these issues now (Chung, 2016). We also must consider the impact of these very real present issues on an individual's future quality of life.

The long-term impact of population health strategies has a ripple-like effect, and is felt as follows:

- *By individual families*—As child health improves, families can spend lesser proportions of their incomes on healthcare. Stopping this drain of dollars can potentially lead to a higher standard of living, better nutrition, improved and advanced education, and lifting the intergenerational cycle of poverty.

- *By our communities*—As the burden of funding care for individuals with chronic health conditions eases, more resources can be devoted to schools, infrastructure, community services, and public safety.
- *By the healthcare system*—Improvements in conditions such as obesity, inactivity, substance abuse, and nonaccidental trauma can have a decade long impact downstream. As healthier children become the norm, more attention and dollars can be devoted to improving quality of care and expanding research horizons.
- *By our nation*—An overall improvement in the health of our children translates into a potentially sustainable, generational improvement in the health of our nation.

When considering the population of children in our country, we must first define pediatrics as a distinct population. In doing so, one must give thought to the overall complexity of this population. Not only is there a tremendous continuum of developmental complexity from helpless newborn to adult, but also one must take other factors into account. For example, along this continuum lies tremendous variation in cognition, communication, mobility, and independence. A pediatric clinic might see newborns for well-baby checks, and their own teenage parents might also be patients as well. It behooves the practitioner to maintain awareness of this, as well as the ability of this diverse group to assent and consent to care and treatment. One must also consider that health-related lifestyle change in children is, unlike adults, almost wholly dependent upon the efforts of their caregivers. Therefore, the population defined includes acknowledgment of both an individual's dependency upon others and his or her movement upon the developmental continuum.

No introduction to pediatric population health would be complete without a discussion about transitioning these children to an eventual adult model of care. Some chronological adults are perhaps better served by remaining in a pediatric healthcare system. A striking example of this is those young adults with congenital heart defects, both repaired and unrepaired. Consider the case of children afflicted with single ventricle physiology. The caregivers (physicians, nurses, and others) in a traditional adult coronary care unit might have exceedingly limited knowledge and experience with the physiology of this condition, particularly after the multistage palliation resulting in Fontan circulation. For many of these patients, they continue to receive care specific to the heart defect in a pediatric setting, where it is not uncommon to encounter such individuals.

## Specific Dynamics for Advanced Practice Nurses

### Genomic Factors

One consideration in pediatric population health that presently occurs on a much more frequent basis than in the adult population is the survival of individuals afflicted with congenital conditions known to be caused by genetic anomaly. Historically, these individuals seldom survived early childhood. In past decades, those that did survive were relegated to live their lives in an institutional setting. Obviously, this is no longer the case, and rightfully so. We now encounter these individuals in the community setting on a regular basis.

The two leading factors influencing this phenomenon are intertwined. First, the treatments and technology that permit survival are continually evolving and improving. This includes the ability of perinatal teams to assess the genetic condition of parents (as carriers) as well as their unborn child. Additionally, as more individuals survive, more parents choose these life sustaining and prolonging therapies for their children who could not survive without it. What follows is a brief overview of four types of genetic variations that have impact on pediatric population health.

### Down Syndrome

The oldest known individuals with Down syndrome are currently entering their early 60s. This reflects several societal changes in the care and treatment of these individuals. The end of warehousing has had a substantial impact in the societal acceptance of these genetically atypical individuals. Additionally, they are now offered educational opportunities, as well as jobs and independent living situations. The advance of cardiac surgery for pediatric patients has also been a contributing factor to the survival of these individuals as a population.

### The Complexities of Congenital Heart Disease

As mentioned previously, individuals with formerly fatal congenital heart defects are now surviving to adulthood. This is the result of a number of factors, including advances in neonatal critical care, the development in the 1980s of prostaglandin infusion to buy time for these infants until surgical palliation/repairs can be made, advances in cardiac circulatory assistance including extracorporeal membrane oxygenation (ECMO), and prenatal ultrasound, which allows these individuals to be born into tertiary care centers where treatment is immediately available and planned.

The variety and complexities of cardiac malformation in children is truly stunning. As these children now begin to live to adulthood, the medical support team has grown to include school nurses/healthcare providers, who will need specific education regarding the anatomy and needs of individual children.

### Case Vignette: Monitoring the Hypoplastic Left Heart Syndrome Infant Interstage

Infants discharged home after first stage palliation of hypoplastic left heart syndrome (HLHS) (Norwood procedure) are at significant risk of death. Mortality estimates range from 10% to 18.9% (Cross, Harahsheh, & McCarter, 2014). Intense home surveillance programs have demonstrated improved survival of these children. Nieves *et al.* (2017) describe key components of the home surveillance program for these children in which advanced practice RNs play a substantial part. Key factors in this program are early recognition by parent/caregivers of seven key symptoms of decompensation—so-called "red flag" symptoms. They are as follows:

- poor feeding
- any weight loss for failure to gain weight for three days
- dyspnea or tachypnea
- oxygen saturation levels less than 75% or greater than 90%
- blue or pale appearance of the face, lips, or hands while at rest
- diarrhea, vomiting, and sweating
- irritability and fussiness

Another critical aspect of care for these fragile infants is continuity. Seeing the same provider at 50% or more of follow-up visits is linked to lowered mortality (Cross *et al.*, 2014). The nurse practitioner is well positioned to tie all factors of the infant's care (parent education, infant surveillance, and care follow-up) together into a cohesive whole.

### Sickle Cell Anemia

Sickle cell anemia afflicts 3.2 million persons worldwide. The prevalence in the United States (U.S.) is approximately 0.23% of the

African-American population. It is the single most common genetic disorder in Caribbean nations. Obviously, children with sickle cell anemia should be vigorously supported by a specialized team of hematology professionals. Advances in treatment and therapies now allow greater than 90% of these children to survive to adulthood in first world countries.

Sickle cell crises are triggered by three main factors: infection, dehydration, and acidosis. The biggest population health intervention for these individuals is infection prevention, particularly by means of vaccination. Additional preventative strategies include daily antibiotic doses during the preschool years, adequate hydration, and folic acid supplementation. Approximately 20% of children with sickle cell anemia demonstrate a degree of pulmonary hypertension, thus complicating their care and requiring the involvement of cardiology specialists. At present, bone marrow transplantation offers the only hope of cure.

*Cystic Fibrosis*

Cystic fibrosis is an autosomal recessive disease most often diagnosed during early childhood. It is one of the most widespread lifeshortening genetic diseases. The hallmark symptoms of failure to thrive and frequent chest infections place it high on the suspicion index for infants with poor weight gain and cough. Approximately 10% of diagnoses of cystic fibrosis are discovered through routine newborn testing. However, because of the high rate of false positive test results, many states and entire nations do not routinely test newborns for cystic fibrosis.

Approximately 30,000 individuals in the United States are afflicted with cystic fibrosis (O'Sullivan, 2009). Advanced treatments, such as mechanical percussion therapy, home means of mechanical ventilation, aggressive and prophylactic antibiotic administration, and bilateral lung transplantation have lengthened lifespan expectations from six months in 1960 to between 37 and 40 years in 2010. As with sickle cell anemia, an important population health strategy for this group of individuals is infection prevention by means of vaccines and other interventions. Particularly important for this group is the widespread protection via herd immunity gained by mass influenza vaccination programs, because respiratory infections are the leading cause of death in this group.

**Community Factors**

Any discussion of population health for pediatrics must include a frank discussion of environmental factors, specifically the communities in which American children live. The impact of these factors cannot be underestimated nor can the impact of public policy be separated from population health factors.

For example, 30 years ago, most of America's children walked to school, a distance of up to 2 miles each way daily. This is no longer the case. The real or perceived dangers of children walking themselves to school have all but eliminated this source of physical activity and, thus, calorie consumption for most children. The same can be said for unsupervised outdoor play. Coupled with the abundant availability of sedentary electronic forms of recreation and entertainment, obesity rates for all children, even the very young, have reached alarming levels (Ogden, 2014). Many public elementary schools are now lobbying for increased outdoor recess time for students to compensate for their sedentary lifestyles.

Many communities lack safe outdoor play spaces for children. Inner-city children are particularly impacted by this. Not only do cash poor cities fail to provide play space, but also what play space is available is often poorly maintained. The added burden of gang behavior and crime make these outdoor play spaces dangerous centers of violence by their very existence.

Overall, unsafe neighborhoods contribute negatively to pediatric population health in one of three ways. First, children who play outdoors unsupervised in these neighborhoods become targets for crime, youth violence, and gang behaviors. Secondly, some of these children will eventually participate in these activities. Finally, those children for whom protection from these unsafe neighborhoods means remaining indoors will most likely suffer from lack of physical activity and the results that accompany this lifestyle.

Air quality may also be a community factor impacting pediatric population health. Areas of high pollution have higher rates of asthma and associated respiratory conditions. Older homes in some communities can be sources of substantial numbers of allergens exacerbating this problem. Finally, communities in tropical climates may face challenges of their own with regards to vector borne illnesses such as Zika virus. As the world becomes a smaller place and international travel the norm, we can expect to see more of these mosquito borne illnesses in the United States. The emerging devastating threat that Zika virus poses to unborn children will require resources from public health, public sanitation, and the medical community at large (Lucey, 2016).

**Traditional Factors**

*Obesity*

The obesity epidemic in America is well documented. Pediatric population health interventions aimed at decreasing obesity can have a long-term impact on the health of our nation. Either these children become, through interventions, non-obese adults and do not allow their children to fall into the trap of obesity or they follow down the brutal path of life-long obesity and the long-term sequelae that accompany it. Additionally, obese children have an increased risk of other pediatric disorders, such as diabetes, hypertension, orthopedic problems, and sleep-related disordered breathing. Wang (2011) estimates medical expenditures on CO at $75 billion annually and project these costs to double every decade without the implementation of effective prevention programs.

These interventions must focus on the two key components in the development of obesity in children: (1) the overall lack of physical activity and fitness in children and (2) improving the nutritional state of these children. Both components must be addressed for any program to be successful and, both, like all interventions with this population group, are highly dependent upon the actions or inactions of the parents and/or caregivers.

*Mental Health*

Population health issues surrounding mental health treatment for pediatric patients is complex at best. A primary issue is the fact that children with serious mental health issues often find access to treatment limited because of the undue burden on an inadequate system of mental healthcare for pediatric patients. This is particularly troubling for children living outside of major urban areas. A child in the rural West, for example, may live hundreds of miles from the nearest provider of mental health services for children. The impact that telehealth services could have on this problem is self-evident.

Another issue is the impact of parental mental illness on the mental health of their children. A recent study found strong associations between parents who had a history of abusing marijuana, antisocial personality disorder, or a prior suicide attempt and the likelihood of children demonstrating suicidal behavior and violence as they age. When both parents exhibited these mental health issues, the risk was double (Akin, 2015). Early intervention for this group is crucial, and an interdisciplinary approach is required.

It bears repeating that early intervention and treatment of pediatric mental health disorders could have a profound impact not only on life-long costs associated with mental illness, but also on quality of life for decades to come for these individuals, their families, and their communities.

## Oral Health

Due in part to limited access to dental care, minority and poor children suffer disproportionately from dental caries and associated oral health conditions. According to the U.S. Department of Health and Human Services, a mere 20% of children under 21 years of age who were enrolled in Medicaid and eligible received preventative dental services (Lewis, 2000).

Although perhaps outside the purview and scope of the nurse practitioner, the impact of oral health on the overall health of children is substantial. Oral health is a significant contributor to overall health during childhood and into adulthood. During childhood, these impacts are most demonstrable in the areas of nutrition and selfesteem.

This is yet another area where an interdisciplinary approach can reap benefits. Although practitioners do not provide dental care, the importance of their advocacy for regular dental care and oral hygiene can make an impact. Adding questions about oral health and regular dental care to the screenings done at well-child visits impresses upon parents the importance of this oft-neglected aspect of pediatric care.

## Physical Activity

As previously discussed, physical activity in even very young children is in decline. Practitioners who treat adult populations are finding success with the "exercise as medicine" approach. Sedentary behavior is the single most positive predictor of future obesity in children (Herman, 2014). This is also an area in which practitioners should have a strong voice for the return of recess in elementary schools, as well as physical education courses up through and including all four years of high school. By making physical activity a normal part of a child's day, it may become a normal part of that person's adult day.

## Nutrition

No discussion of nutrition in the pediatric population would be complete without first mentioning the importance of breast-feeding during the first year of life. Support and encouragement for breast-feeding, of course, begins during the prenatal period. The benefits of breast-feeding past the neonatal period are well documented in the literature and will not be repeated here. Support resources offered in real time and available at the time of well-baby visits are ideal.

In no aspect of pediatric population health is the role of caring adults more important than in ensuring proper nutrition for children. Children's food preferences develop very early in life and once established are difficult to change. This should be a topic of constant ongoing discussion during well-child visits throughout childhood.

An Australian study recommended two simple changes to children's dietary habits that could have a profound impact (Doak, 2006). The simplicity of this would be easy to message to parents repeatedly. Those two changes are replacing sugary drinks with water and replacing most sugary desserts and snacks with fresh fruit. However, for families living in so-called "food deserts" (urban or rural areas without readily accessible, full service grocery stores), the fresh fruit part of the equation is easier said than accomplished. Again, an interdisciplinary approach involving care providers and dietitians/nutritionists is preferred.

### Immunizations

A discussion of the importance of routine vaccinations on pediatric population health in this chapter would be superfluous. Sadly, the most important discussion regarding vaccinations among care providers has now become how to combat the fringe antivaccine movement. Particularly onerous is the voice of celebrities who tout the nonexistent link between vaccines and such conditions as autism. These are important conversations to have with parents. An increasing number of practitioners now dismiss families from their practice who do not comply with vaccination guidelines.

Care must be exercised, however, in discussions with well-meaning parents (the "vaccine hesitant") who merely need to be guided to reliable information. The rise of social media and the parallel decline in discernment between real and falsified research has contributed to this problem. Although only education, often and repeated, can solve this problem, the importance cannot be overstated. Those children who cannot be vaccinated due to legitimate allergy or immunocompromised status must be given the benefit of herd immunity among their schoolmates and the general public. Providers must continue to point parents to reliable sources of information, show them how to recognize valid research versus anecdotal stories, and answer their legitimate questions with understanding (Shelby, 2013).

*Asthma*

Current estimates in the United States indicate that 9.5% of children have asthma (Trends in asthma morbidity and mortality, 2015) with a disproportionate number of these children being the poor and minorities. These children often lack access to subspecialty care, and it often falls to the primary care provider to direct and implement asthma care for these children.

One important contributing factor is poor air quality, both indoor and outdoor. Children living in urban areas are often exposed to both. Older housing is often a source of significant asthma triggers, such as mold, dust mites, cockroaches, and mildew. For low-income families, these triggers are nearly inescapable. Asthma education must encompass environmental factors as well.

Additionally, school-age children are estimated to be exposed to secondhand smoke. In other words, an estimated 24 million non-smoking children and youth are exposed to secondhand smoke largely because of their parents who smoke (Raghuveer, 2015). This is yet another area in which child health is almost entirely dependent on the actions of the adults who care for them. Pediatric care providers must provide a strong antismoking message, as well as offer tobacco cessation assistance, if these children are to maintain asthma control. Again, an interdisciplinary approach including the services of a pediatric respiratory therapist can take some burden off the primary provider. As with all pediatric population health interventions, aggressive tobacco cessation efforts directed toward parents will pay off downstream in healthier children and children who are much less likely to become smokers themselves.

*Sleep*

In 2013, the Centers for Disease Control and Prevention (CDC) declared insufficient sleep is a public health epidemic for both adults and children (CDC, 2013). Sleep deprivation impacts not only physical health, but also emotional health and normal growth and development. The causes of poor and insufficient sleep are many and beyond the scope of this chapter. However, one must recognize the dominant anti-sleep culture that exists in this country. "I'll sleep when I'm dead" and "Sleep is for sissies" are hallmarks of the American 24/7 culture. Pediatric care providers must consistently message the importance of sleep and recommend evidence-based sleep hygiene techniques. The essentials of sleep hygiene for children include the following:

- age-appropriate amounts of sleep, including naps for young children
- appropriate sleep environments: dark, cool, and devoid of electronic entertainment devices
- the importance of bedtime routines
- eliminating caffeine from the diets of children
- limiting screen time during pre-sleep hours

An additional consideration for those providers who care for infants is, of course, safe sleep for babies. The Back to Sleep campaign, an evidence-based bundle of safe sleep habits directed at parents and caregivers of newborns, has dramatically decreased the incidence of sleep-related deaths in newborns (Moon, 2011). Parents are instructed to not have the newborn lying in bed with them. The importance of having the infant in the bassinet or crib with proper swaddling and clothing is taught to parents during their hospitalization. However, co-sleeping and unsafe sleep environment deaths continue to happen. Again, consistent messaging of the dangers of these sleep environments cannot be overestimated.

*Nonaccidental Trauma*

The tragedy of nonaccidental trauma shakes pediatric care providers to the core. Even diligent care providers can miss subtle signs of abuse. Although conversations about shaken babies may occur prior to discharge after delivery, not every parent is equipped to deal with the demands of a newborn. Particularly troubling is when infants are left in the care of nonparents who have not received education on appropriate means of dealing with difficult newborn behavior. Pediatric care providers must continue to have these difficult, blunt, and unpleasant conversations during encounters with parents.

*Accident Prevention*

Accident prevention in the pediatric population is a continual and ever evolving source of concern. As children age, the types of accidents that might befall them change continually. Hot car deaths claim an average of 40 lives annually in this country, primarily among infants and young toddlers (MacLaren, 2005). Older toddlers, with their inquisitive nature, are at risk for laundry and dishwasher pod ingestion poisonings, as well as "purse poisonings" (Shah, 2016).

As children age and become more independent, education must occur regarding bicycle safety, including helmets. In addition, cultures in which learning to swim is not common see a disproportional number of their children succumb to accidental drowning. In China, where few children learn to swim, accidental drowning is the leading cause of death of children under age 14, topping both infectious disease and traffic accidents (Gardner, 2016).

Additionally, a recent study indicates that nearly one in five parents makes significant medication errors when dosing medication for their child (Phillips, 2016). This occurs even when parents are given appropriate dosing instruments, such as syringes. Fortunately, some pharmacies are now offering teach back/return demonstrations for parents who might be unsure about medication dosing.

*Diabetes*

As with all other conditions in childhood, a substantial contributing factor to treatment adherence in pediatric diabetes is the involvement of parents. The use of technology can be an important quality improvement tool, especially when used as a means of communication, follow-up, and feedback. Recent data suggest that children with type I diabetes who miss two or more appointments have a three-fold increased risk of diabetic ketoacidosis (DKA) and having a hemoglobin A1c level greater than 8.5 (Fortin, 2016). Missed appointments mean poor compliance and potentially loss to follow-up. Tele-practice models that incorporate appointments at a distance using Skype-like technologies could bridge the gap and improve compliance (Burke, 2015). Parents who could endanger their employment status by needing to attend in-person appointments with their child may now be able to attend regularly by means of technology—e.g., child in a school-based clinic and parent joining via online means

**Tools for Implementation and Quality**

*Screening Tools*

The University of Washington provides an extensive list of screening tools for pediatric care providers, covering a wide variety of physical, developmental, and psychological conditions. A link to this useful online resource is included in the references at the end of this chapter (Screening and Surveillance Tools, 2016).

The PedsQL is a useful tool that measures health-related quality of life in children and adolescents (Varni, 2016).

*Quality Considerations*

The Agency for Healthcare Research and Quality (AHRQ) website provides for nurse practitioners over 300 sortable, evidence-based practice guidelines specific to pediatric populations at www.guideline.gov.

*Discussion Questions*

1. Discuss how current social media platforms could be utilized to improve overall pediatric population health. Consider media platforms used by parents, children, schools, and communities.
2. What types of collaborative strategies could be implemented in at-risk communities?
   - Who are the stakeholders for health improvement in communities?
   - How could nonhealthcare stakeholders be brought into the discussion related to pediatric population health improvement?
3. How might an advanced practice registered nurse (APRN) implement Healthy People 2020 recommendations for children into a primary care clinic setting during well-child visits?
4. What factors would need to be considered in implementing group appointments for children with chronic health problems?

**Case Study 1**

*Targeted Obesity Prevention Strategies During Primary Care Visits*

The Agency for Healthcare Research and Quality (AHRQ) provides an excellent overview of approaches to integrate discussions about childhood obesity (CO) into every well-child visit (AHRQ, 2013). With the astonishing prevalence of obesity in pediatric populations, this education is crucial to improving the health of afflicted individuals.

The Guideline Summary provides the following three key goals for practices to work toward in order to embed routine discussions and interventions around obesity into every visit:

- To increase the percentage of patients ages 2 through 17 years who have an annual screening for obesity using body mass index (BMI) measured and whose BMI percentile status is determined
- To increase the percentage of patients ages 2 through 17 years with an annual BMI screening who have received education and counseling regarding weight management strategies, including nutrition and physical activity

- To increase the percentage of patients ages 2 through 17 years with a BMI screening percentile greater than 85 whose percentile decreased within 12 months of screening

## Case Study 2

*The APRN in School-Based Clinics*

The Massachusetts Department of Public Health funds 37 school-based health clinics in 17 communities in Massachusetts (Health, 2010). These clinics are located primarily within high schools and are staffed by pediatricians, pediatric and family practice nurse practitioners, registered nurses (RNs), physician assistants, dentists, dental hygienists, nutritionists, clinical social workers, mental health professionals, counselors, and health educators. They provide both primary care services and behavioral health services to the pediatric populations that attend those schools. This unique model of healthcare brings provider services to the students rather than expecting the students (as well as their parents) to travel to the provider.

These clinics are in areas with documented limited access to primary healthcare, high absenteeism and dropout rates, and high rates of eligibility for free or reduced cost school lunches. Parental consent is required for students to access these services; however, parents do not need to be present for a student to receive services. This favorably impacts the parents work absenteeism due to their child's health needs.

This unique partnership between school and health services is being copied and is expanding exponentially based on its success. The benefits are many:

- Parents do not need to leave their employment, travel to the child's school, transport the child to a provider's office, return the child to school, and then returned to work. This often results in missing an entire day of work for the parent and an entire day of school for the child.
- 94% of students seen at the school-based health center returned to class after being seen.
- Many chronic conditions can be managed by an interdisciplinary team available on-site during all hours that the child is at school. Management of these chronic conditions, such as asthma, by a school-based team results in better treatment adherence, fewer emergency room visits, and less frequent hospitalizations.

Primary care health services available to students include the following:

- physical examinations and immunizations
- school, sports, and employment physicals
- referrals to specialty providers
- care coordination for students with special health needs and chronic health needs
- treatment of acute injuries and illnesses
- laboratory testing and screening, including human immunodeficiency virus (HIV) counseling and testing
- reproductive health services
- oral health evaluations and treatments
- nutritional counseling
- health education
- health insurance enrollment
- prescriptions for medications

Behavioral health services include the following:

- assessments and screening for conditions such as depression
- individual and group counseling
- substance use and abuse screening, intervention, and referral to treatment

## References

AHRQ (2013). *Guideline summary: Prevention and management of obesity for children and adolescents.* (2013, July 1). Retrieved from Agency for Healthcare Research and Quality (AHRQ): https://www.guideline.gov

Akin, B. B. (2015). Co-occurence of Parental Substance Abuse and Child Serious Emotional Disturbance: Understanding Multiple Pathways to Improve Child and family Outcomes. *Child Welfare*, 71–96.

Burke, J. B. (2015). Telemedicine: Pediatric Applications. *Pediatrics*, 293–308.

Chung, P. (2016). Pediatric Population Health and Child Poverty. Mattel Children's Hospital at UCLA, Los Angeles.

Cross, R., Harahsheh, A., & McCarter, R. (2014). Identified mortality risk factors associated with presentation, initial hospitalization, and interstage period for the Norwood operation in a multi-center registry. *National Pediatric Cardiology- Quality Improvement Collaborative.*

Doak, C. V. (2006). The prevention of overweight and obesity in children and adolescents: A review of interventions and programmes. *Obesity Reviews*, 111–136.

Fortin, K. P. (2016). Missed Medical Appointments and Disease Control in Children with Type I Diabetes. *Journal of Pediatric Health Care*, 381–389.

Gardner, H. (2016, October 9). Forget those 18 Olympic medals. *Indianapolis Star*, p. 3B.

*Guideline summary: Prevention and management of obesity for children and adolescents.* (2013, July 1). Retrieved from Agency for Healthcare Research and Quality (AHRQ): https://www.guideline.gov

Health, M. D. (2010). *Here for the Kids: The School-Based Health Center Model at work in Massachusetts.* Boston: MDPH.

Herman, K. M.-t.-y.-o.-1. (2014). Sedentary behavior in a cohort of 8-to 10-year old children at elevated risk of obesity. *Preventative Medicine*, 115-120.

*Insufficient sleep is a public health epidemic.* (2013). Retrieved from Centers for Disease Control: www.cdc.gov/Features/dsSleep

Lewis, C. G. (2000). The Role of the Pediatrician in the Oral Health of Children: A National Survey. *Pediatrics*.

Lucey, D. G. (2016). The emerging Zika pandemic: Enhancing preparedness. *JAMA*, 865–866.

MacLaren, C. N. (2005). Heat Stress from Enclosed Vehicles. *Pediatrics*, 109–112.

Moon, R. (2011). SIDS and other sleep-related infant deaths: expansion of recommendations for a safe infant sleeping environment. *Pediatrics*, 1341–1367.

Nieves, J., Uzark, K., Rudd, N., Strawn, J., Schmelzer, A., & Dobrolet, N. (2017). Interstage Home Monitoring After First-Stage Palliation for Hypoplastic Left Heart Syndrome: Family Education Strategies. *Critical Care Nurse*, 72–88.

Ogden, C. C. (2014). Prevalence of Childhood and Adult Obesity in the United States, 2011-2012. *JAMA*, 806–814.

O'Sullivan, B. F. (2009). Cystic Fibrosis. *The Lancet*, 1891–1904.

Phillips, D. (2016, September 12). *One in five Parents Makes Major Dosing Errors.* Retrieved from Medscape: http://www.medscape.com/viewarticle/868707

Raghuveer, E. A. (2015, November 2). *Cardiovascular Consequences of Childhood Secondhand Tobacco Smoke Exposure. Retrieved from Circulation*: http://dx.doi.org/10.1161/CIR.0000000000000443

*Screening and Surveillance Tools.* (2016, November 5). Retrieved from University of Washington Developmental & Behavioral Pediatrics: https://depts.washington.edu/dbpeds/Screening%20Tools/ScreeningTools.html

Shah, L. (2016). Ingestion of Laundry Detergent Packets in Children. *Critical Care Nurse*, 70–75.

Shelby, A. E. (2013). Story and Science. *Human Vaccines & Immunotherapeutics*.

*Trends in asthma morbidity and mortality.* (2015, November 2). Retrieved from American Lung Association: www.lung.org

Varni, J. (2016, October 17). *The PEdsQL Measurement Model for the Pediatric Quality of Life Inventory.* Retrieved from PedsMetrics: Quantifying the Qualitative: http://www.pedsql.org

Wang, Y. M. (2011). Health and economic burden of the projected obesity trends in the USA and UK. *The Lancet*, 815–825.

## CHAPTER 8

# Gerontology and the Aging American

VERONICA LaPLANTE RANKIN, MSN, RN-BC, NP-C, CNL, CMSRN
KOTAYA GRIFFITH, MSN, RN, NP-C, CNL

## Aging Within the U.S. Population

THE future of America is certain to witness an accelerated rate of graying that can be defined "chronologically, physiologically, and functionally, (and) all of which might modify the phenotype of an individual, but might not affect the lifespan" (Azhar & Wei, 2015, p. 12). When considering population health as a topic of interest, the geriatric population is a very important topic of study. The most commonly used number to define entry into the geriatric population is 65 years of age (Besdine, 2016). Geriatrics denotes the medical provision of care to elderly patients, whereas gerontology is the study of aging and its biological, sociological and psychological impact on the patient (Besdine, 2016). This chapter will analyze aspects of the geriatric population to focus on and improve effective care provision within this population.

A major step in analyzing a population is to assess the quantity of that populace in relation to the entire population. According to the Administration on Aging (2016), in 2014, the geriatric population consisted of 46.2 million persons, which represented 14.5% of the United States (U.S.) population at that time. This number is expected to increase to 21.7% by the year 2040; by year 2060, the geriatric population is projected to more than double, totaling approximately 98 million persons (Administration on Aging, 2016). Data trends, as seen in Figure 8.1, project the greatest and fastest anticipated growth rate by the year 2050 to be in the 85 and older portion of the total population (U.S. Federal Interagency Forum on Aging Related Statistics, 2012). Furthermore, in 2012 the U.S. Federal Interagency Forum on Aging Related Statistics (USFIFARS) noted a significant increase of 65,000 people within the centenarian population aged 100 years or older. While exciting, care providers and clinicians must then consider the compounded issues related to living longer, which include chronic disease management, polypharmacy, additional need for resources and assistance, and additional social needs necessary to prevent cognitive decline. These issues will be discussed more in depth later in this chapter.

According to the Centers for Disease Control and Prevention (CDC) (2015), the life expectancy in the United States has increased within the last 20 years. The aggregate U.S. life expectancy for both sexes increased from 73.7 in 1980 to 78.8 in 2013. As seen in Figure 8.2, the life expectancy of the male has increased at a larger rate than that of the female (Centers for Disease Control and Prevention, 2015). For patients age 65 years at the time of the CDC's 2015 assessment, the life expectancy for females was 20.5 for females yielding an age of 86.5 years old and 19.3 for males yielding an age of 84.3 years old. This information is especially important when planning to care for sex-related chronic diseases and the future needs within a population.

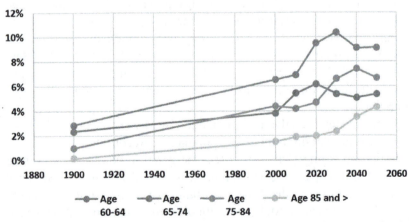

**FIGURE 8.1.** *Older Population Percentage of Total Population. Projected increases within the elderly population of the United States total population separated by age. Chart created from data provided by the U.S. Federal Interagency Forum on Aging Related Statistics, U.S. National Center for Health Statistics. (2012). Older Americans. Key indicators of well-being. Washington, DC.*

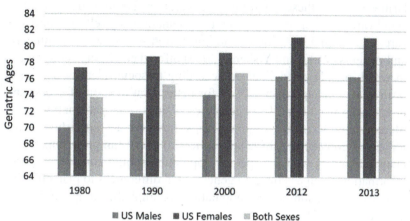

**FIGURE 8.2.** *U.S. Life Expectancy from 1980–2013, author created from CDC, 2015.*

## Generational Differences in Geriatrics

Leik (2014) provides the age classification of "young-old" ranging from 65 to 74 years of age, "middle-old" ranging from 75 to 84 years of age, and "oldest-old" as aged 85 years and older. Another way of evaluating the geriatric population is by categorizing cohorts by generations, which are based on birth years (Wang & Yisheng, 2015). Although no exact and agreed upon age range exists for generation delineation, the popular stereotypes within the geriatric population include Traditionalists (born before 1945) and Baby Boomers (born between 1945 and 1964) (Becton, Walker, & Jones-Farmer, 2014; Jiri, 2016). Information delineating the characteristic types of people born within these generations center on events and experiences of that time range. Traditionalists were born during the Great Depression and World Wars I and II. Some experienced the GI Bill and even the Korean War. Because of these events, the stereotypical characteristics of people born within this time are described as loyal, saver-mentality, and a high regard for authority, with a military influenced perspective of "top-down" (Jiri, 2016). Baby Boomers were born directly after World War II and into the mid-1960s. They grew up in the 1940s, 1950s, and 1960s and were influenced by the Great Depression, the attack on Pearl Harbor, the Cold War, protest movements, Vietnam, emergent rock music, drugs, and anti-segregation drives. The stereotypical characteristics of people born within this time are achievement-oriented, competitive, and independent minded (Becton *et al.*, 2014). Differences and similarities between these two different generations could be used to understand various perspectives within the population, as well as to augment care, educational techniques, and interaction styles between clinicians and patients. Wang and Yisheng (2015) offered an alternative approach in which people are delineated according to social identity instead of birth year. This approach allows for better stratification of everyone's uniqueness per their life experiences, values, and personality types. Stereotyping according to generations, however accomplished, is not fail-proof considering there are outliers to every sample group. Clinicians planning care for a specific population should consider valuable information, such as common generational differences to plan effective care and interactions within populations (Campbell, Campbell, Siedor, & Twenge, 2015).

## Causes of Mortality Within the United States

According to the CDC (2015), the top 10 causes of death within the U.S. population included heart disease, cancer, chronic lower respiratory disease, unintentional injuries, stroke, Alzheimer's disease, diabetes, influenza/pneumonia, kidney disease, and suicide. From 2013 to 2014, a decrease was noted in each of these rates, except for unintentional injuries, stroke, Alzheimer's disease, kidney disease, and suicide. In 2014, chronic lower respiratory disease and unintentional injuries tied in rates (CDC, 2015). Care directed by a population health focus should be well rooted in knowledge concerning mortality rates so that prioritized primary, secondary, and tertiary care can be structured to tackle known offenses within a population. Resources such as education, health programs, and preventative care initiatives can greatly impact health outcomes within a population by providing robust, effective modalities to change unhealthy habits and behaviors.

## Theoretical Concepts of Aging

Additional tactics to help evaluate and change health behaviors within a population include the use of theory and concepts models. Theories and conceptual models can be used to understand behavior and assess a patient's readiness for change. Examples of various theories and models related to behavior change are discussed below for care providers and clinicians to consider when caring for geriatric patients.

## Transtheoretical Model

Prochaska's (2008) Transtheoretical Model denotes five stages of behavior change, including precontemplation, contemplation, preparation, action, and maintenance. Although progression through these stages is often nonlinear with frequent repeated cycles, these stages can be used to assess and gauge an individual's readiness for change (Butts & Rich, 2015). Precontemplation describes the unconscious stage before an individual considers change, whereas contemplation denotes that consideration for change has begun (Prochaska, 2008). Prochaska (2008) described the preparation stage as that in which the individual identifies the problem and has created an action plan with the intention of acting on the plan. Prochaska describes the action stage as the stage in which behavior modification is occurring and the maintenance stage as the time in which sustainment of the behavior change is sought after to avoid relapse (Prochaska, 2008).

## Self-Efficacy

Another concept to consider when assessing behavior change is Bandura's concept of self-efficacy. Bandura (1977, 1989) described this as one's personal assessment of the ability to carry out a specific action or behavior that influences execution of that action. Bandura (1997) later noted that self-efficacy is especially vital for influencing change in healthy behavior efforts despite the opposing barriers or challenges experienced throughout the task. Romppel *et al.* (2013) noted that self-efficacy requires adaptive action on the part of the individual to control opposing demands within the environment. Mouloud, Fonseca, and Abdelkader (2015) posited that self-efficacy influenced the power of decisionmaking abilities, the strength of effort invested in the behavior change, the level of perseverance against hindrances, or the resilience to hardship. Butts and Rich (2015) noted that one vital goal of behavior change and wellness within the realm of healthcare is to promote high levels of selfefficacy in clients to try to halt unhealthy habits and/or deal with illness and an everchanging sense of self. Gandoy-Crego, Clemente, Gómez-Cantorna, González-Rodríguez, and Reig-Botella (2016) noted that the awareness of self-efficacy facilitates understanding concerning one's own abilities, including thoughts which act as motivators of action and then serve as determinants to be used to predict future behavior change. Gandoy-Crego *et al.* (2016) further highlighted that these determinants of behavior become changing conditions that are reworked and altered according to the information received and processed from different sources, such as past experiences, the observed behavior of others, verbal persuasion, and one's own perception of his or her physiological state. This work provides insight concerning ways in which healthcare providers can use personal experiences and contextual features to help promote successful and sustained behavior changes.

A study by Romppel *et al.* (2013) provided evidence that high levels of self-efficacy positively affects disease management and physical outcomes for patients. The concept of self-efficacy influencing the effort applied to behavior change is well supported in the literature by an overwhelming number of studies that applied the concept to explain outcomes. An article by Bandura (2012) shared the results of a study conducted on stock investors, which revealed that the investors with stronger levels of self-efficacy set higher goals for themselves, devoted more effort to their investment choices, and performed better than those with weaker levels of self-efficacy. This article also revealed that people with high levels of self-efficacy compared to those burdened with self-doubt were more open to new experiences, less disturbed by stressors, and potentially more outgoing within personal relationships. Another article also supported this finding and postulated that higher levels of self-efficacy positively influenced important coping behaviors necessary to successfully complete tasks (Bihlmaier & Schlarb, 2016).

Healthcare providers, as well as caretakers, can use the concept of self-efficacy to help predict readiness and the potential for success and sustainment of behavior changes. A strong understanding in self-efficacy is especially important to healthcare providers and caretakers simply because it provides the tools and assessment baseline to predict successful behavior change similar to that of coaches and athletes. The caretaker's or coach's ability to know what their patient or athlete feels or thinks about their own skills and abilities is important for goal setting purposes (Mouloud *et al.*, 2015). If deficiencies are identified, the caretaker or coach can then use tactics such as education and training, community resources, and even the assistance of the patient's family or support system to help create plans of care with reasonable and agreed upon goals that raise the level of self-efficacy.

### Health Belief Model

Glanz, Rimer, and Viswanath (2015) cited Gochman's definition of health behavior from earlier work completed in 1997 as "those personal attributes such as beliefs, expectations, motives, values, perceptions, and other cognitive elements; personality characteristics, including affective and emotional states and traits; and overt behavior patterns, actions, and habits that relate to health maintenance, to health restoration, and to health improvement" (p. 10). Using this definition, The Health Belief Model explains why people adopt healthy or unhealthy behaviors. Butts and Rich (2015) described the Health Belief Model as being a central concept regarding the prevention and management of disease. This model is made up of six concepts that assess readiness to prevent, detect, and manage disease. These six concepts include perceived susceptibility which reflects to vulnerability, perceived severity which considers the consequences, perceived benefits referring to the welfare, perceived barriers which are the obstacles, cues to action that prompt movement, and self-efficacy which is selfconfidence to successfully complete a task. Castonguay, Filer, and Pitts (2016) added a seventh concept, which is modifying variables to represent the individual characteristics that affect opinions and health behaviors. In order to promote and sustain positive behavior changes, a realistic plan of care must be tailored to the needs of the patient and the patient must possess a sufficient level of self-efficacy coupled with education, resources, and a support system of some type. Research supports tailoring interventions to target and include the patient's family or support system to help enhance and sustain positively outcomes.

## Psychosocial Development

Erik Erikson's theoretical stages of psychosocial development attempt to explain the impact that life experiences and influences have on human development from childbirth to adulthood. This theory elucidates the mechanisms by which one may deal with adversity or misfortune in life (Svetina, 2014). It also sheds light on the development of behaviors that may be healthy or unhealthy in nature, which ultimately affects the health of the geriatric population. This theory is made up of eight stages, but for the purposes of this chapter the final three stages, which are theoretically experienced during adulthood, will be discussed. Each stage is written in conflicting verbiage that presents the uncertainty that Erikson is portraying of each stage. These three stages include intimacy vs. isolation, which is experienced during the young adult years (ages 18 to 35); generativity vs. stagnation, which is experienced during the middle-aged adult years (ages 35 to 64); and integrity vs. despair, which is experienced in late adulthood (65 to death) (Leik, 2014). Intimacy vs. isolation centers on the uncertainty of seeking companionship or being alone. This stage can certainly be fulfilled later in life, completely skipping the age range of early adulthood, but Erikson's theory reflects that thoughts related to love are generally seriously considered during this time of life. Generativity vs. stagnation centers on career establishment and making a difference within a society. This is significantly driven by the fear of inactivity or being insignificant to others. In this stage, people devote significant energy and effort to careers and building relationships within their family, communities, churches, or other social networks. Integrity vs. despair centers on reflection, from which wisdom can be actualized. This reflection can inspire feelings of contentment and satisfaction for some and despair and sadness for others, depending on their perspective of success with having led a meaningful life. Many people within this stage may seek to find the purpose of their lives, reflecting on whether their lives were worth the struggle, whereas others will press harder to reaffirm their vitality and ability to contribute to society. Although age ranges are provided for each stage, the stages are interrelated, and the task at each stage is to resolve the uncertainty or threat experienced at the present stage to advance into the next stage (Svetina, 2014). According to Erikson's theory, the achievement of wisdom involves revisiting previous stages of uncertainty and "renewing psychosocial accomplishments" (Perry, Ruggiano, Shtompel, & Hassevoort, 2015, p. 253), similar to self-reflection. Perry *et al.* (2015) authored an article that evaluated two qualitative studies to investigate how older adults adapt to change and use wisdom in new situations. The findings from this article revealed that older adults reasserted independence and self-sufficiency by applying creative problem solving skills based on the knowledge and skills obtained from past experiences, to solve new issues from present day (Perry *et al.*, 2015). The findings from this article highlight the importance of engaging the geriatric population in creating plans of care that reassert their wisdom based on new education provided by healthcare providers (Perry *et al.*, 2015).

**Physiological Processes of Aging**

As the body ages, normal physical and metabolic changes can be expected. This section will focus on normal aging changes of the geriatric adult so that deviations can be actualized as abnormal changes.

*Skin*

As the human body ages, skin atrophies, meaning that the epidermis, dermis, and subdermal layers of the skin becomes thinner. This change results in fragile skin that is slower to heal and easier to damage. The skin becomes less elastic and develops hyperpigmentation and hypopigmentation issues because of changes in melanocyte production. With aging, hair becomes gray, and there are noted changes in the production of vitamin D in the skin (Gallagher, 2013). Sebaceous and sweat gland activity slows down significantly, which leads to drier skin and, in turn, potentiates skin cracking and infections. Nail growth slows and become thicker, more brittle, and yellow in color. Skin conditions, such as seborrheic keratosis, senile purpura, and lentigines (also known as "liver spots"), are common normal findings with the skin of the geriatric population (Leik, 2014).

*Eyes*

As the human body ages, the lenses of the eyes lose elasticity, resulting in presbyopia, which leads to close vision changes. The detrimental effects of aging are found not only within the lenses, but also in other vital areas of the eyes, including the cornea, ocular surface and adnexa, and the retina (Lin, Tsubota, & Apte, 2016). Additional common changes found with the eyes include cataracts, glaucoma, arcus senilis, age-related macular degeneration, and others that may require eye wear, eye drops, or surgical procedures for correction and restoration of visual abilities (Owsley, Huisingh, Clark, Jackson, & McGwin, 2015). Lin *et al.* (2016) noted that, although the significant impact of age-related visual changes is well supported in the literature, modern-day treatment modalities are somewhat inadequate, with infancy-staged strategies aimed at reversing or decelerating deterioration.

*Ears*

With aging, the most common sensorineural hearing loss experienced is high-frequency hearing. This is a result of degenerative ossicle changes, wasting away of hair cells, and less auditory neurons of the ear (Leik, 2014). According to Phillips (2016), special attention should be paid to the cognitive assessment of older adults with hearing loss due to the "potential for hearing loss to deplete cognitive reserve, contribute to communication difficulties and social isolation, the loss of input from environmental stimulation, or a combination of these factors" (p. 45S).

*Neurological System*

As the human body ages, neurological changes may be greatly apparent. Age-related changes within the nervous system may affect the function and cognition of the older adult. Changes such as reduced neurons and levels of neurotransmitters, coupled with alterations of dendrites and glial cells of the brain, contribute to such changes as slowed muscle coordination and reduced muscle strength, agility and coordination (Boltz, Capezuti, Fulmer, & Zwicker, 2012). Although these changes should be mild in normal aging, they can adversely affect the daily functioning of the geriatric patient. Additional changes commonly experienced within the elderly population include the change of febrile response to infection, reduced thermoregulation responses, an inability to differentiate colors, reduced reflexes, increased risk for sleep disorders, and reduced ability to multitask as performed at younger ages (Leik, 2014).

## Cognition

Aging affects the human cognition whether it is to a mild degree or more severe. Phillips (2016) noted that the changes occur within many domains, including learning and memory, the speed of processing, executive functioning, attention span, and reasoning abilities. Cognition assessments are extremely important for healthcare providers to identify declines and changes early on (Leik, 2014). Cognition changes vary from individual to individual so documentation is necessary to pinpoint and measure the degree of change.

## Heart

As the human body ages, the intimal layers of the arteries become thickened and tortuous in the physiological sense. This results in arteriosclerosis, which increases systolic blood pressure readings due to increased resistance on the vasculature system of the body. Baroreceptor response to position changes is reduced, which results in an increased risk of orthostatic hypotension, falls, or fainting. Cardiac reserve declines in the geriatric patient, resulting in a reduced ability to increase the heart rate and cardiac output, as related to an increase in cardiac demand. Additionally, an S4 sound may be heard upon cardiac auscultation (Boltz et al., 2012). Sclerosis of the atrial and mitral valves increases the risk of valve dysfunction, leading to aortic regurgitation and mitral stenosis among other changes. The loss of pacemaker and conduction cells within the heart also potentiates arrhythmias and electrocardiogram changes (Leik, 2014).

## Lungs

Respiratory function gradually deteriorates in the geriatric patient due to the anatomic and physiologic changes related to aging (Ito & Mercado, 2014). A reduction in respiratory muscle strength, as well as a loss of elastic fibers of the lung, may result in reduced response to hypoxia and air trapping within the small airways. Chest wall rigidity, which is also associated with normal body changes related to aging, results in an increased anterior-posterior chest wall diameter. A reduced number of cilia coupled with reduced efficiency of coughing results in mucus buildup, which increases the geriatric adult's risk for infection and insufficient oxygen exchange (Leik, 2014). Because of these changes, certain conditions develop, such as immunity impairment, pulmonary inflammation, and the enlargement of air spaces. Additional insult and acceleration of these changes is seen with exposure to noxious elements, such as gases, smoking, inhaled substances, etc. (Ito & Mercado, 2014).

## Liver

As the human body ages, the liver, which filters wastes from the body, atrophies in size and mass, resulting in reduced blood flow and functioning (Leik, 2014). Fatty depositions within the liver are common with age, as well as an increase in the volume of cholesterol levels. This coupled with the greatly reduced metabolism of low-density lipoproteins in the liver results in increased blood cholesterol levels, which can be life-threatening. Aging reduces the liver's regenerative abilities and, because the liver will repeatedly attempt to heal itself, progressive liver fibrosis develops with age (Kim, Kisseleva, & Brenner, 2015).

## Kidneys

As similarly seen with other organs, the kidneys atrophy in size and mass with age. This is especially important because renal clearance of drugs and other toxins of the body is greatly reduced with age. Research shows that the glomerular filtration rate (GFR) of the kidneys starts to decrease as early as age 40 (Leik, 2014). This is influenced by the decreased number of functional glomeruli secondary to sclerotic changes of the organ and the compensatory hyperactive actions of the remaining nephrons (Denic, Glassock, & Rule, 2016). Denic *et al.* (2016) noted a reduction every decade in the GFR of the kidneys by 6.3 mL/min/1.73 m$^2$. The risk of damage related to drugs that are primarily cleared by the kidneys is especially dangerous in the elderly, potentiating the risk of kidney injury.

## Musculoskeletal System

Deterioration of the skeletal system is common with aging. Articular cartilage deteriorates, giving way to compression fractures and kyphosis of the spine. Such changes are worsened by osteoporosis, osteopenia, rheumatoid arthritis, ankylosing spondylitis, and osteoarthritis, which are additional conditions commonly seen with aging. Decreased muscle mass and strength are noted, especially within the arms and legs. The rate of bone healing and growth is greatly reduced because of the decreased number of osteoblasts and bone resorption (Leik, 2014). Regional pain related to aging must be assessed thoroughly because of its ability to significantly impair mobility and the ability for older adults to work, resulting in chronic and sometimes excessive use of analgesics (Palmer & Goodson, 2015).

## Psyche

In an article by Allphin (2015), an important question is asked: "What happens to us when we are no longer in demand, when newer analysts become involved in our organizations and we need to step aside to make space for them, or we are not asked to take on roles we once filled with great interest and hard work?" (p. 50). This question is a serious concern for geriatric patients in that, for many older adults, their occupations or roles are central to their identity. Allphin (2015) noted that a patient described the realization of loss of career or primary role within society as a "phantom pain" (2015). This can also be related to the loss of fine motor skills; sensory abilities, such as hearing, seeing, and tasting; and phenotypical loss of youthful beauty. Allphin (2015) also noted that, although most older patients acknowledge the fact that they have led full lives, the majority are still plagued with thoughts questioning what they should do next for however long or short their time may be. Additionally, depending on the individual's perspective, which is influenced by factors such as experience and culture, wisdom can be positively or negatively impacted by age. A study by Gordon and Jordan (2016) revealed that age differences negatively influenced cognitive opinions of wisdom between people. This study revealed that people rated others as less knowledgeable and more sensitive as the age-gap between the two parties widened (Gordon & Jordan, 2016).

## Geriatric Challenges

Older adults may report some challenges related to the normal aging process from physiologic changes, such as declining vision and hearing, taste changes, and reduced sleep. However, there are additional challenges that older adults may face that are not necessarily due to the normal part of aging but are likely related to chronic disease processes, disabilities, and environment factors. These challenges include but are not limited to multiple comorbidities, polypharmacy, loss of independence, financial difficulties, advance care planning, ageism, substance abuse, and elder abuse.

Multiple comorbidities, or chronic conditions, are common among older adults and are defined as two or more chronic diseases that requires complex management and impact functional status and quality of life (National Quality Forum, 2012). The American Geriatrics Society expert panel on the care of older adults with multiple morbidities reported in 2012 that more than 50% of older adults have at least three or more chronic illnesses (American Geriatrics Society, 2012). The challenges associated with multiple comorbidities arise from the complex treatments, adverse effects, and increased burden of disease. Most older adults find that difficulty adhering to the treatment for a single disease and having two or more chronic conditions further increases the complexity. In addition, some older adults have cognitive, visual, and hearing impairment, which can have a huge impact on the ability to manage chronic diseases. For an individual to be effective in managing multiple chronic diseases, he or she needs to have the ability to perform complex tasks, such as medication administration. According to Sergi, De rui, Sarti, and Marizato (2011), one main challenge of the older adult's medication consumption is related to multiple comorbidities versus age. Therefore, older adults with multiple chronic diseases are at a high risk for polypharmacy and likely to have a higher incidence of adverse drug effects.

Polypharmacy is a term used to describe the regular routine of taking multiple medications that consist of five or more agents. In 2012, adults aged 65 and older in America accounted for 13% of the total population but had utilized a third of all prescription medications used at that time (Ham, Sloane, Warshaw, Potter, & Flaherty, 2014). The challenges associated with older adults consuming multiple medications include the increased risks for drug-to-drug interactions and adverse outcomes. In a study conducted by Ahmed, Nanji, Mujeeb, and Patel (2014), they found a 70% occurrence of polypharmacy and 10.5% incidence of adverse drug reactions among older adults aged 65 or older. According to Sergi *et al.* (2011), the evidence-based guidelines and longer life expectancy of today have caused increased issues related to polypharmacy. Thus, polypharmacy has caused many adverse effects, such as falls and hip fractures (Sergi *et al.*, 2011). Consequently, it is extremely critical that older adults are provided ongoing education about polypharmacy and its potential adverse effects. Sergi *et al.* (2011) stated that a comprehensive geriatric assessment has shown favorable outcomes, including improved functional status and lower mortality rates. Therefore, the implementation of a systematic process for a geriatric medication review would have considerable benefits in this vulnerable population and should be a top priority in any patient encounter or patient care setting that serves older adults.

Multiple comorbidities also increase disease burden, which is linked to time, high costs of treatment modalities, and information overload. Boyd *et al.* (2014) defined treatment burden "as a patient's perception of the aggregate weight of the actions and resources they devote to their healthcare, including difficulty, time and out of pocket costs" (p. 118). The high costs of multiple comorbidities are related to frequent doctor visits, resources, medications, and hospitalizations. For example, an older adult diagnosis list including diabetes mellitus type 1 or 2, chronic kidney disease, hypertension, hypothyroidism, and congestive heart failure will likely require frequent routine follow-ups by multiple healthcare professionals for effective disease management. A high risk for acute changes requiring hospitalization is extremely likely if this person is not closely monitored. Thus, ineffective management of chronic diseases leads to poor outcomes and reduced quality of life. Because of the negative outcomes associated with the complexity of multiple comorbidities, health professionals should be both knowledgeable and prepared to assist older adults in managing and coping with these chronic conditions.

Functional status is a main determinant in the older adult's health status, because it greatly affects quality of life. This should therefore be a major focus in any geriatric assessment. Functional status is a descriptor of an individual's activity level and his or her ability to complete activities of daily living (ADLs). ADLs include abilities such as bathing, dressing, toileting, continence, transferring, and feeding. The instrumental activities of daily living (IADLs) are meal preparation, ability to use the telephone, shopping, laundry, medication management, housekeeping, driving, and finance management. The loss of function in two or more ADLs will likely require additional support from a caregiver or placement in a skilled nursing facility, long-term care facility, or assisted living facility. The loss of independence is a common and significant fear within the older population. The loss of independence not only is a physical factor of consideration, but also can be a mental and emotional factor of consideration, oftentimes leading to depression. According to Ham *et al.* (2014), the loss of independence is often the indicator of disease progression and a forecaster of mortality. Therefore, maintaining a high functional status is vital for older adults, serving as an essential element for a high quality of life. As a healthcare professional, it is important to encourage older adults to participate in physical exercise and social activities to help maintain their functional abilities. The loss of independence can also have a significant financial impact and can become a burden to both the individual and the caregiver. Financial security is a major deciding factor in maintaining a person's current lifestyle and residence, securing caregivers and/or finding permanent placement in a nursing facility.

Financial difficulties are also widespread among older adults because of their limited resources. As a result, the lack of financial resources can interrupt care and hinder communication, which leads to poorer outcomes and higher healthcare costs. Mutchler, Li, and Xu (2016) published in their insecurity report that 34% of single older adults live above the poverty line but lack the income that is required for economic security. Mutchler *et al.* (2016) further reported that more than four out of 10 single older adults in America are at risk of being unable to take care of their basic needs. Therefore, one event or unexpected bill can have a significant financial impact and likely lead to poverty for many older adults. Limited resources are barriers for the older individual to access essentials such as food, medications, and shelter. Ziliak and Gunderson (2016) stated that over 10 million older adults in America faced the risk of hunger. Proper nutrition of the older adult is a major factor in determining mortality rate. Ensuring that older adults have access to well-balanced meals is a critical step in providing adequate care within this population, also serving as a deciding factor concerning life or death. Sadly, some older adults experience financial abuse or neglect by caregivers, which predispose them to emotional and physical stress.

Unfortunately, older adults also confront discrimination because of their age, which is known as ageism. Discrimination in any form often causes misconceptions and interferes with right judgments. According to Ham *et al.* (2014), ageism can have negative impacts and can "lower self-esteem, reduce opportunities, and lead to isolation, loneliness, and depression" (p. 8). Ageism also leads to inappropriate conclusions that in some cases have caused misdiagnoses. It is imperative that complaints and concerns of the older adult are not minimized or disregarded as a normal part of aging but are validated. For these reasons, healthcare professionals should be aware of ageism and its negative impact and should examine their own biases toward the aging population.

Substance abuse is unfortunately another common problem among older adults. Substance abuse among the baby boomer population is expected to increase by 5.7 million in 2020 because of their history of illicit drug use (Blank, 2009). Alcohol is the most common substance that is abused among older adults, followed by misuse and abuse of prescription drugs (Gage & Melilo, 2011). According to Alpert (2014), one to two million older adults use alcohol to cope with grief or loneliness. The effects from substance abuse can have considerable health risks on chronic conditions and cognitive and functional statuses. There is an increased risk of falls with injury associated with alcohol use. Sadly, it often goes undetected in older adults until there is an adverse event. It is essential that older adults are screened for substance abuse and provided education concerning its adverse effects.

Moreover, elder abuse is another problem older adults face that often goes unnoticed. According to the National Council on Aging (n.d.), one in 10 older adults aged 60 years or older have encountered some form of elder abuse. Sadly, only one in 14 cases are reported to local authorities (National Council on Aging, n.d.). Bonnie and Wallace (2003) estimate between one and two million adults aged 65 years or older in the United States have experienced elder abuse or neglect by a caregiver. It is important to know that elder abuse includes physical abuse, emotional abuse, sexual abuse, neglect, exploitation, and abandonment (National Council on Aging, n.d.). It is mandated by most states that healthcare professionals report elder abuse to authorities. Special attention should be focused on the assessment and documentation of any suspected abuse.

**Advance Care Planning**

Advance care planning (ACP) involves making end-of-life (EOL) decisions based upon a person's preferences and the completion of advance directives (ADs) (National Institute on Aging, 2014). ADs are legal documents that communicate decisions about EOL care if a person is unable to communicate his or her own wishes (National Library of Medicine, 2016). The Patient Self-Determination Act of 1990 was enacted by the U.S. Congress to "safeguard the right of patients to participate in healthcare decisions and have those decisions heard through the execution of ADs" (Brothers, 2015, p. 1). The completion of ADs is a very important aspect of patient care, and its absence can have a significant impact upon the patient, family, and healthcare costs. According to CDC in 2014, 70% of Americans lacked an advanced care plan. In a study conducted by Rao, Anderson, Lin, and Laux (2014), there were approximately 75% of 7,946 participants surveyed in the United States who did not have an AD. They found that the top reason for not having ADs was due to a lack of awareness (Rao *et al.*, 2014).

Sadly, most older adults are often uninformed about ADs. They may be frequently faced with multiple challenges associated with managing complex chronic conditions that lead to multiple hospitalizations, poor outcomes, and reduced quality of life. These chronic conditions can also cause an increased burden of hospitalizations and can result into serious medical complications among this vulnerable population (Hickman *et al.*, 2016). Therefore, adherences to evidence based clinical guidelines are essential to providing quality care and improving outcomes within the older population. In 2012, the Centers for Medicare and Medicaid Services (CMS) launched an initiative to reduce avoidable hospitalizations among residents in long-term care facilities to combat poor outcomes and rising healthcare costs (Hickman *et al.*, 2016). Hickman *et al.* (2016) reported "evidence suggesting advance care planning and Physician orders for Life Sustaining Treatment (POLST) have the potential to reduce unnecessary and burdensome hospitalizations of nursing home residents" (para. 3). In addition, Taylor (2016) reported "Medicare is the largest insurer of medical care provided at the EOL accounting for 25% of total Medicare spending in the last year of life" (para. 1). The average healthcare spending for "Medicare recipients who died in 2014 was $34,529" (Taylor, 2016). Consequently, to address these concerns, there is a heightened focus on ACP for early identification of goals and preferences of these individuals (Hickman *et al.*, 2016).

According to Detering, Silveira, Arnold, and Savarese (2016), there are several benefits for completing advanced care plans and ADs that include ensuring care is aligned with patient wishes, improved communication among families and the healthcare team, reducing hospital costs, and "a higher satisfaction with the quality of care" (para. 10).

Brinkman-Stoppelenburg, Rietjens, and Van (2014) completed a systematic review on ACP's impact on EOL care. These authors found several studies that showed a reduction in hospitalization rates associated with having Do Not Hospitalize (DNH) orders. Brinkman-Stoppelenburg *et al.* (2014) also found that ACP was associated with an increased compliance with patient's wishes and an increased satisfaction with quality of care for the patients and their families. Having an advanced care plan was also found to reduce the risk of stress, depression and anxiety (Brinkman-Stoppelenburg, *et al.*, 2014). The identified benefits of AD completion in these studies have shown favorable outcomes for the patient and families by ensuring patient goals and preferences are the main driving force in their care.

Wholihan and Pace (2012) found several innovative programs for ACP planning in the community that were linked to the progression of EOL decision-making "earlier in the illness continuum" and that have shown a reduction in hospital admissions. Among the various programs identified, Respecting Choices® was highlighted because of the significant impact it had on the community and cost of EOL care (Wholihan & Pace, 2012). The Respecting Choices program was first implemented at Gundersen Lutheran Medical Center in La Crosse, Wisconsin. Findings showed "the cost of care per patient during the last 2 years of life in LaCrosse was estimated at $18,000, well below the national average of over $25,000, with only 13.6% of deaths associated with a stay in intensive care" (Wholihan & Pace, 2012, p. 174). The Respecting Choices program received national recognition for ACP initiatives that increased awareness of Ads in the community and a reduction in hospital costs (Wholihan & Pace, 2012).

ACP should be an ongoing discussion with each patient encounter to ensure that the patient's voice is heard and wishes are honored. Older adults have a higher incidence of multiple chronic diseases, polypharmacy, and adverse outcomes and, therefore, are at a higher risk for hospitalization. Because of these factors, having ADs will be beneficial for older adults and for the healthcare team by providing clear direction to guiding care. Palliative and hospice care are additional services that may be beneficial for adults by providing symptoms management or EOL care.

## Major Insurance Carriers

According to the Centers for Medicare and Medicaid Services

(CMS) (2015), on July 30, 1965, President Lyndon B. Johnson signed the bill that led to the creation of Medicare and Medicaid. Many changes have been made to the original Medicare and Medicaid programs over the years in that Medicare has more parts than it originally had, more citizens are eligible now than before, and the program offers more benefits than it did before. In 1966, approximately 19.1 million Americans were covered with Medicare insurance. As of 2015, approximately 55 million Americans were covered by Medicare (Centers for Medicare and Medicaid Services, 2015). Although no conclusive evidence exists proving that Medicare and Medicaid lower mortality and morbidity rates, improved medical coverage that reduces out-of-pocket medical costs for the elderly positively influences medical compliance and healthier lives (Centers for Medicare and Medicaid Services, 2015). The parts of Medicare and Medicaid that pertain to the geriatric population are summarized below according to CMS.

*Medicare*

Medicare is a health insurance program provided by the federal government for people aged 65 years and older, people of various ages with certain disabilities, and people with a diagnosis of end-stage kidney disease. Medicare consists of various parts that cover different services with various associated costs.

*Part A* is considered hospital insurance because it covers inpatient hospital stays, hospice care, skilled nursing facility stays, and some aspects of home healthcare that are approved (Leik, 2014). Medicare Part A does not carry a premium fee for individuals that qualify for Social Security benefits. Additionally, if the individual paid Medicare taxes while employed, the Medicare Part A monthly premium is usually waived; otherwise, a monthly premium may be required. Stipulations exist that require payment by the patient after 60 days of hospitalization. This payment gradually increases as the number of hospitalized days increase.

*Part B* is considered medical insurance because it covers out of hospital services with a goal to prevent, diagnose, and treat medical conditions for its members. It covers services charged for doctor's visits, outpatient procedures and care, medical equipment and supplies, and preventive care services (Leik, 2014). Part B has a premium that must be paid directly by the individual, or it can be deducted from Social Security or other benefits received by the individual.

*Part C* is called Medicare Advantage. This insurance is a voluntary health plan that requires individuals to enroll. This plan, provided through Medicare and offered by private companies, combines benefits from Part A and Part B; however, copays and premiums vary between companies (Leik, 2014). Although variability exists within each plan, it usually covers prescription drugs, hearing, vision, and dental care, as well as alternative care, such as chiropractic and acupuncture therapy, wellness, and gym memberships.

*Part D* covers prescription drugs but has limitations and drug criteria. This plan, just like Part C, is voluntary and requires monthly premiums; individuals must enroll after gaining prior approval (Leik, 2014).

## Medicaid

Medicaid is a federal and state funded program that pays for health-related services for federally mandated eligibility groups, which include low-income individuals, elderly patients, and disabled people who meet criteria set by each state (Leik, 2014), among others. Although federal requirements guide the basic guidelines of the program, Medicaid is administered by each individual state. This means that criteria change from state to state according to poverty levels and the citizens who make up the state's population (Medicaid.gov, The Official U.S. Government Site for Medicare, n.d.). Federal guidelines also allow each state to decide upon covering optional eligibility groups that do not fit within the mandated group. Mandatory benefits required by every state by the federal government include inpatient and outpatient hospital services, doctor's visits, laboratory and radiology services, home health services, and many more. Additional benefits that may be covered at the discretion of the state to include vision care, eye wear, chiropractic and alternative therapies, foot care, dental care, prosthetics, etc. Some states also cover mental health services. Income-related eligibility is based on each individual state's poverty level. Geriatric patients already receiving Supplemental Security Income benefits or other assistance usually find greater ease with acquiring Medicaid services.

## Disease Prevention and Health Promotion

Disease prevention and health promotion are key factors influencing the ability of older adults to live healthier, high quality lives. Heart disease and cancer are the two leading causes of death among older adults aged 65 and over (Centers for Disease Control and Prevention, 2015). According to the CDC (2013) for cardiovascular and stroke prevention, recommendations for the older adult include using daily aspirin, maintaining appropriate blood pressure control, maintaining proper cholesterol management, and stopping smoking (i.e., smoking cessation). Aspirin, although proven to be useful in cardiovascular and stroke prevention, must be taken under the supervision of a medical prescriber (Centers for Disease Control and Prevention, 2015). The CDC (2013) reported that a diet rich in fruits and vegetables reduces the risk of some cancer and chronic diseases among older adults. Therefore, the CDC (2013) also recommends that older adults consume five or more fruits and vegetables daily.

## Charity Meal Distribution Organizations

Meal distribution resources are available throughout the nation within communities, regions, and states. The exact resources available depend on location, federal funding, charitable contributions, and staffing resources. A few examples of these resources include the Red Cross, local Meals on Wheels organization, soup kitchens, etc. The common mission of these organizations is providing balanced meals to community members who need help, including geriatrics or disabled citizens due to illness or disease (Friendship Trays, n.d.). Acquiring many of these services cost little to no money at all. Additionally, local churches often provide food pantries and outreach ministries that also provide food and aid to those in need.

The CDC (2015) reported that the third leading cause of death among older adults aged 65 years and over was chronic lower respiratory diseases. For health promotion and to minimize bacterial respiratory illnesses, older adults should receive the influenza and pneumococcal vaccinations as indicated by their medical provider. Guidelines state that the influenza vaccine should be given annually and either forms of the pneumococcal vaccine, Pneumovax® 23 or Prevnar 13®, should be given once after age 65 years (Centers for Disease Control and Prevention, 2016).

Unintentional injuries were the fourth leading cause of death among older adults, with fallrelated injuries being the top cause for hospital admission due to trauma. The CDC (2013) estimated that one out of three geriatric adults fall annually. According to the CDC (2013), because physical activity has been proven to reduce the risk of falls, it is recommended that older adults exercise at least 3 days per week for fall prevention. Additionally, removing throw rugs, ensuring proper lighting, and wearing proper foot wear are also advised for safety. Health professionals should also perform fall risk assessments routinely on older adults and take necessary measures to educate patients, families, and caregivers regarding falls prevention.

*SilverSneakers®*

SilverSneakers® is an exercise program covered by many health insurance plans for Americans aged 65 years and older (SilverSneakers, 2017). This program, created more than two decades ago, provides fitness classes that have been tailored to the geriatric population to improve strength endurance and over 60 year old fitness training to maintain health and physical training for older adults. Classes are performed to tunes favored by geriatric patients to maintain engagement and participation. The SilverSneakers organization has created partnerships with many insurance plans and retiree groups to ensure nationwide access for its members. This resource provides unlimited gym access at thousands of gyms nationwide, community fitness classes held at locations outside of the gym, and diverse group classes that provide various fitness techniques such as yoga, cardio-fit, etc. This resource also provides a great opportunity for socialization and relationship building for older adults.

Additionally, older adults with chronic diseases should adhere to their treatment plan and medications as prescribed, as well as to their follow up with a primary provider on a regular basis, to prevent acute exacerbations of chronic diseases. Tactics such as sending reminders for routine appointments and medication refills are advised for effective disease management (Leik, 2014). Lastly, patient education should always be a part of every encounter to ensure that older adults understand the disease trajectory, options of treatment, and complications related to noncompliance.

## Resources for the Geriatric Population

There are many resources within the community and world designed specifically for use within the geriatric population. These resources range from national organizations to online educational resources, community resources, and charity groups. A few of these resources will be discussed within this chapter.

*NICHE*

NICHE stands for Nurses Improving Care for Health-system Elders. According to Boltz *et al.* (2012), NICHE is a national program aimed at improving outcomes for geriatric patients by improving care quality and nursing competence within the practice setting. This is being accomplished by changing the culture of healthcare organizations to reflect consideration of the geriatric population within the mission statement, to acquire evidence-based resources and supplies for optimal care, and to create protocols and practices that require interprofessional collaboration towards geriatric care (Santamaria, 2016). To become NICHE designated, nursing leaders of the proposed NICHE leadership team within the facility must complete the NICHE Leadership Training Program (LTP). The LTP is a six-week affordable web-based program that provides online educational sessions and a guide to help leaders gain support and implement the program successfully within their organization (NICHE, n.d.). During the six weeks, leaders will engage in online webinar training sessions and interactive calls, complete practicebased assignments such as creating a steering committee for the system, conduct a SWOT (strengths, weaknesses, opportunities, and threats) analysis of the organization, and create a sustainable action plan based on findings from the SWOT analysis. Throughout this training, NICHE faculty members provide ongoing feedback for success; facility leaders network and learn from other facilities also completing the LTP; and participants receive more than 30 hours of continuing education. At the conclusion of the LTP, facilities are prepared to officially launch the practice of NICHE with scheduled interprofessional meetings, a plan for future practice, and resources for success, such as free access to the online NICHE Knowledge center for evidence-based resources provided within the "Try This" series, free webinars that provide continuing education credit for attendees, and other networking opportunities to contact other NICHE facilities to learn best practice ideas and tips (NICHE, n.d.). NICHE also provides free training curricula for nursing assistants and nurses to gain extra knowledge and serve as geriatric resources within their workplaces. At the completion of the specified modules, the clinicians receive a continuing education certificate that provides continuing education credit and serves as proof to their completed training in "geriatric friendly care." Annual benchmarking and program evaluation efforts involve assessing nursing competence in geriatric care through online Geriatric Institutional Assessment Profiles (GIAP) surveys provided by NICHE (NICHE, n.d.). These surveys with other quality assessment outcomes are used to measure success of each facility's NICHE program. Furthermore, levels exist to provide a competitive culture between the facilities to serve as a top-level NICHE facility within the program. The levels assess for older adult patient and caregiver representation on NICHE steering committees within the system, expansion of NICHE across service lines, geriatric resource nurse expansion to specialty units, and involvement with NICHE at the national level, among other criteria (NICHE, n.d.). Discounts are also provided to employees from NICHE-designated facilities to attend the annual NICHE conference. New York University's Rory Meyers College of Nursing has been designating appropriate healthcare facilities for more than two decades totaling more than 750 facilities to date, including acute care and long-term care facilities (Santamaria, 2016). Evaluations of NICHE-designated hospitals reveal improve clinical and cost-related outcomes, as well as improved nursing knowledge levels (Allen & Close, 2010; Boltz *et al.*, 2012; Guthrie, Schumacher, & Edinger, 2006; Pfaff, 2002).

### Organizations for the Geriatric Population

Many organizations exist with a primary focus of improving care and outcomes for geriatric patients. These organizations include, but are not limited to, the Administration on Aging (AoA), the American Association of Retired Persons (AARP), and the American Geriatrics Society (AGS). Each of these organizations are summarized below.

- AoA—The AoA is the principal sector of the U.S. Department of Health and Human Services created to implement the provisions included in the Older Americans Act of 1965 (OAA). This Act provides services and programs for geriatric patients to promote well-being and independent living within their homes and communities (Leik, 2014). The Act also permits the federal government to provide funds to states that provide services to support members of the population older than age 60 years. Under this administration includes offices such as the Office of Supportive and Caregiver Service, which provides funding for adult day care, caregiver support services, and services that promote health and wellbeing. Other offices included under this administration are the Office of Nutrition and Health Promotion Programs; Office of Elder Justice and Adult Protective Services; Office for American Indian, Alaska Natives and Native Hawaiian Programs; and Office of Long-term Care Ombudsman Programs (Administration for Community Living, 2015).

- AARP—AARP is a nonfederal, nonprofit organization made up of more than 37 million retired U.S. citizens aged 50 years or older. This organization is one of the most powerful lobbying and advocacy groups that has secured service and discounts for older Americans. AARP lobbies for issues related to medical care, employment, income security, and financial abuse prevention for its members. Additional perks of membership include discounts for medical and life insurance, medications, travel, glasses, groceries, car rental, etc. (AAPR Real Possibilities, n.d.).
- AGS—The American Geriatrics Society is a nonprofit organization for nearly 6,000 healthcare professionals who are devoted to improving the health, quality of life, and self-sufficiency of older people (Leik, 2014; American Geriatrics Society, 2017). This organization provides leadership to its members by implementing and advocating for programs that provide education, research, elder patient care, and public policy devoted to improving care quality and outcomes of the elderly. The organization's leadership is participating in numerous funded projects that affect elder care. A few of these projects include the Geriatric Emergency Department Collaborative, The Geriatrics Workforce Enhancement Program (GWEP), and the Geriatrics-Orthopedics Co-Management Planning Project (GOCo). The Geriatric Emergency Department Collaborative is designed to expand emergency medicine in the arena of eldercare through a collaborative that includes nine healthcare systems across the country. This collaborative has been funded with a two-year grant to implement evidence-based engagement between the nine systems included and create a plan for long-term sustainability and national expansion. The GWEP is a national system that provides technical support to 44 designated GWEP sites as needed through a coordinating center. This coordinating center provide resources, sessions, mentoring, and consultation services, as well as advocacy for funding purposes for its sites. The GOCo project seeks to market and spread nationally a model that will afford structured comanagement of geriatric orthopedic related care between interdisciplinary team members (American Geriatrics Society, 2017).

## PACE Program

PACE stands for Programs of All-inclusive Care for the elderly (Medicare.gov – PACE, n.d.). This program is a Medicare and Medicaid program designed to help older patients meet their care needs within the community to avoid admittance into a nursing home or care facility. PACE provides and coordinates collaboration between an interprofessional team to provide the comprehensive healthcare needs of an elderly patient. Services are provided within the home, the community, and PACE centers, as needed and directed by the team. For a patient to be eligible for PACE, he or she must be 55 years of age or older, must live in an area in which PACE services are available, must have documented proof certified by the state of residence that the patient requires skilled nursing care, and must be able to safely remain in the community with help from PACE services (Medicare.gov – PACE, n.d.). PACE programs include all the services covered by Medicare and Medicaid, essentially taking over the primary care of the patient and absorbing additional costs related to hospital readmissions, misdiagnoses, and lapses in healing. If services outside of that which is covered by Medicare and Medicaid are ordered, PACE will cover those expenses for its patients. Services provided by PACE include the following:

- adult day primary care (including doctor and recreational therapy nursing services)
- dentistry
- emergency services
- home care
- hospital care
- laboratory/X-ray services
- meals
- medical specialty services
- nursing home care
- nutritional counseling
- occupational therapy
- physical therapy
- prescription drugs
- preventative care
- social services, including caregiver training, support groups, and respite care
- social work counseling
- transportation to the PACE center for activities or medical appointments, if medically necessary

The PACE program has proven improvement in outcomes and is therefore spreading throughout the nation. Resources such as this program, which aims to keep patients within their homes instead of nursing facilities, are extremely popular within the geriatric population. Additionally, respite care opportunities provided to care takers of geriatric patients help to avoid burnout and compassion fatigue for those who are willing and able to provide assistance to PACE patients.

## Tool Kit and Resources

*Hartford Institute for Geriatric Nursing*: https://hign.org/
- The Hartford Institute is the geriatric sector of the New York University Rory Meyers College of Nursing program. For many decades, it has served as a robust resource for individuals interested in advanced care of the elderly through leadership and interprofessional collaboration.
- Features *ConsultGeri*, which is a resource bank that includes evidence-based geriatric protocols, device apps, team building tool kits, a "Try This" series with nationally recommended instruments for use within the geriatric population, hospital competencies for nursing orientation and ongoing evaluation, and online education modules.

*NICHE*: http://www.nicheprogram.org/

*PACE*: http://www.npaonline.org/pace-you
- *PACE Medicare resources*: https://www.medicare.gov/your-medi-care-costs/help-paying-costs/pace/pace.htm
- *PACE Medicaid resources*: https://www.medicaid.gov/medicaid/ltss/pace/index.html

*Respecting Choices*: http://www.gundersenhealth.org/respecting-choices/
- Respecting Choices® is an evidence-based model of advanced care planning (ACP) that offers a certification for ACP facilitators in First Steps, Next Steps and Last Steps (Respecting Choices Person-Centered Care, 2017). To become a facilitator, a specialized Respecting Choices training program must be completed.

*Definitions*
*Ageism*—discrimination based on age

*Geriatrics*—the medical provision of care to older adults

*Gerontology*—the study of aging and the biological, sociological, and psychological impact on the older patient

*Health Belief Model*—a theory that attempts to explain the internal

make-up and external influencing factors that relate to the health behaviors and choices made by an individual. This theory consists of
six concepts: perceived susceptibility, perceived severity, perceived
benefits, perceived barriers, cues to action, and self-efficacy.

*Medicaid*—a federal and state funded program that pays for health-
related services for qualified individuals that meet certain criteria,
such as low-income status, disabled, elderly, and pregnant women
and children, as set by each individual state.

*Medicare*—a health insurance program provided by the federal government for qualified people aged 65 years or older, the disabled, and
individuals diagnosed with end-stage kidney disease.

*NICHE*—an acronym an organization called Nurses Improving Care
for Health-system Elders. This national program provides resources
and training to improve outcomes for elderly patients by enhanced
care quality and nursing competence.

*Polypharmacy*—the routine of taking multiple medications that consist
of five or more agents.

*Self-efficacy*—an individual's personal assessment of his or her ability
to successfully carry out a specific action or behavior, which then
influences the execution of that action or behavior.

*Transtheoretical Model*—a theory that denotes five stages of behavior change that can be used to gauge an individual's readiness for
change. The five stages include precontemplation, contemplation,
preparation, action, and maintenance.

*Discussion Questions*

1. What are differences healthcare providers should consider between
   the baby boomer and traditionalist generations? Name ways in
   which education and goal planning can be altered to be more effective when considering these differences.

2. What are the developmental stages of the geriatric population?
   When considering the concept of self-efficacy and the challenges
   outlined in this chapter, how should a caregiver or healthcare
   provider's approach to care provision and recommended lifestyle
   changes be best accomplished?

3. What are common barriers associated with advanced care planning? Are these issues amplified within the geriatric population?

4. What are some measures providers can take to address some of the

top mortality issues and challenges outlined in this chapter? Name at least one example you have participated in that could address one of these issues.

5. What is the PACE program? What are some disadvantages to this program?

6. Explain the stages of the Health Belief Model and what perceived barriers a geriatric patient may be experiencing in applying lifestyle changes prescribed by a physician that include changes in diet, smoking, and exercise.

## Case Study 1

*Fall Incident*

Ms. Smith, a 79-year-old African-American female, presents to the hospital due to a fall at home, with multiple bruises and a left humerus fracture. She is unaccompanied by family but gives the numbers of her family to call and inform them of her incident. Ms. Smith reports that she was sitting on her porch talking with neighbors and, upon entering her house, she fell when her foot got caught in the door. Her baseline status received via telephone from a daughter who lives out of town informs us that she is normally an alert and oriented independent patient who lives at home alone with family assistance. Ms. Smith's daughter reports that if someone doesn't physically check on her daily, they at least call her, plus her close friend lives next door to her. We are also told by the daughter that the patient's son will be arriving soon. Ms. Smith reports a previous fall at home resulting in a rib fracture but adamantly refuses rehabilitation placement. The physician, case manager, and social worker attempt numerous times to talk her into going to a rehabilitation facility for a short-term stay. Every time this option is broached by the healthcare team, Ms. Smith immediately refuses and changes the subject. Upon assessing Ms. Smith's home medication list, the nurse informs the physician that Ms. Smith takes Neurontin 1800 mg at bedtime (QHS), along with a long list of other medications. The nurse informs the physician that Ms. Smith reported the highdose Neurontin due to gout. The physician, immediately thinking the fall could have been caused by the high doses of Neurontin, orders to hold the medication and prescribes Ms. Smith Ultram orally as needed (PO PRN) for pain. He also holds Ms. Smith's anticoagulant until the results of the computed tomography

(CT) scan performed in the emergency department (ED) are obtained. The physician places an order to consult physical therapy and orders an activity level of out of bed with assistance and close supervision for safety.

*Review of Pertinent History*: Falls, Gout, Polyneuropathy, Hypothyroid, Afib without anticoagulation management, Diabetes mellitus, Rib Fracture s/p previous fall, HTN, and Anxiety.

*Pertinent Physical Assessment*: Alert and oriented breath sounds clear in all fields, NSR without audible murmur, bowel sounds present in all quadrants, trace edema to lower extremities, scattered bruises over the body, brace in place to left upper extremity, PRN adapter in place to right arm, voids (no indwelling urinary catheter).

*VTE*: heparin SQ injection Q8
*Vitals*: WNL, cardiac assessment WNL

*Reflection Questions:*
- What are your top concerns for this case?
- What are potential plans of care?
- What are some differentials you can think of that are related to this patient's fall?

*Case Study Continued . . .*

Ms. Smith's adult son arrives with a few bags in hand prepared to stay in the hospital with his mother. Upon further assessment, the son leaves the room with the nurse and shares in the hallway of the unit that Ms. Smith's spouse died last month in a rehabilitation facility. He shared that, although his mother was too private to tell the team, she is extremely emotional about rehabilitation facilities. The son reports that Ms. Smith's home meds are correct and that her highdose Neurontin is being closely monitored and managed by her neurologist. The nurse obtains the name and number of the neurologist and gives the report and information to Ms. Smith's attending. The attending resumes her Neurontin after confirming the therapy with the neurologist. Throughout the night, the nurse recognizes that Ms. Smith exhibits signs of pain but refuses pain medications. Ms. Smith's blood pressure is elevated and she appears very restless.

*Additional Questions:*
What should the nurse do?

*Case Study Continued . . .*

While Ms. Smith is in the bathroom with the nurse's aide, the night shift nurse asks the son to see if his mother would take something for pain. Upon returning to her bed, the son assesses his mother, urging her to take something for pain although he knows she hates taking extra medications. Ms. Smith concedes, takes the medication, and is found resting within an hour. The next morning, physical therapy and occupational therapy work with the patient to find that she is still very independent and able to perform her ADLs despite her new injury. Ms. Smith reports to having a cane and wheelchair at home. As the physician enters the room, Ms. Smith's son informs the team that he will go home and live with Ms. Smith for a month to help provide assistance and 24/7 supervision to avoid rehabilitation. The physician updates Ms. Smith and her son that her scan and all her repeat laboratory tests and X-rays are normal other than the fractured humerus. He updates Ms. Smith and her son concerning the plan to follow up with the orthopedic specialist that assessed her in the ED after discharge, once the swelling has gone down. Physical therapy and occupational therapy assess Ms. Smith for additional needs and confirm that she is safe to return home with 24/7 supervision and assistance from her son. At discharge, the case manager arranges for home health physical therapy and occupational therapy. Teaching is provided to Ms. Smith and her son regarding fall prevention, constipation prevention, and safety due to pain medication use. Ms. Smith is given a followup appointment with the orthopedic specialist within 2 weeks after discharge. All members of the team are updated on the plan of care, including Ms. Smith and her son.

## Case Study 2

*Advanced Care Planning*

Mrs. Jones is currently being seen by Jane, a nurse practitioner (NP), for a routine followup. Her medical history includes diabetes mellitus type 2, hypertension, hypothyroidism, stress urinary incontinence, atrial fibrillation, congestive heart failure (CHF), and breast cancer in 2012. Over the past three months, she has been in and out of the hospital due to CHF exacerbations. During her hospitalization, palliative care was consulted to discuss goals of care and ADs, but Mrs. Jones declined to complete ADs at that time. During her visit with Jane, today, she asks about ADs and requests to complete one today. Jane asks her to explain what she understands about ADs. Mrs. Jones states that

ADs are written instructions detailing her wishes in the event she is unable to speak for herself. She further explains that after her recent experiences in the hospital, she is especially ready to complete the AD today. She further states that she does not want to be resuscitated or put on a ventilator and does not want a feeding tube. She also states that she has one daughter and would like for her to make her medical decisions if she is unable to speak for herself. Jane commends Mrs. Jones on her preparedness, stating that she clearly knows what she does and does not want done if her heart stops or she becomes unresponsive. Mrs. Jones shares that she desires to be comfortable and that she feels that "the good Lord" has blessed her with a good life. Jane informs Mrs. Jones that ADs are legal forms that include a living will and durable power of attorney for healthcare. She also shows her a copy of a Medical Orders for Scope of Treatment (MOST) form. Jane explains that the MOST form is a legal form for the state of North Carolina and is considered a doctor's order, which communicates an individual's medical care at the end of life (EOL). The MOST form addresses cardiopulmonary resuscitation (CPR) and medical interventions such as intubation, advanced airway management, mechanical ventilation, IV fluids, antibiotics, and feeding tube and specifies the defined timeframe if applicable. Mrs. Jones states that she would like to complete the forms today so that she can share them with her family and have them available the next time she is admitted back into the hospital. Jane explains each category of the MOST form and Mrs. Jones selects such options as do not attempt CPR (DNR), comfort measures, no antibiotics, no IV fluids, and no feeding tube. Mrs. Jones and Jane both sign the MOST form, and the original form is given to Mrs. Jones. A copy is scanned to her medical record, and Mrs. Jones is thoroughly educated and updated concerning her plan. Jane also has the clinic's social worker to assist with completion of the healthcare durable power of attorney so that Mrs. Jones can provide her daughter with a copy. Mrs. Jones states that since she has completed the MOST form and healthcare durable power of attorney, she does not think a living will is necessary.

- What are some reasons you might think Mrs. Jones would think of if she decided to decline completion of an AD?
- What are some of the determining factors for Mrs. Jones' participation in advanced care planning?
- When is the right time for advance care planning?

## Case Study 3

*Chronic Conditions and Polypharmacy*

Mr. James is an 85-year-old African-American male who was admitted into the hospital for a sustained fall with right hip pain for 2 days. His past medical history includes dementia, atrial fibrillation, hypertension, diabetes mellitus type 2, hypothyroidism, osteoporosis, degenerative joint disease, chronic pain, macular degeneration, depression, and history of recurrent falls.

*Hospital course*: Underwent right total hip arthroplasty, transfer to orthopedic unit for post op care. He developed increased confusion and was given Xanax 0.5 mg × 2 doses. He had increased pain and was placed on a Dilaudid Patient Controlled Analgesia (PCA). A sitter was placed at the bedside because of Mr. James' increased confusion. He was unable to urinate, and a urinary catheter was placed.

*Medications*: Coumadin 2 mg PO daily, Lipitor 40 mg PO QHS, Flomax 0.4 mg PO daily, Aspirin 81 mg PO daily, Lasix 40 mg PO daily, potassium chloride 20 mEq PO daily, Sertraline 20 mg PO daily, Donepezil 10 mg PO daily, Synthroid 75 mcg PO daily, Tylenol 650 mg PO Q6hrs prn pain, Metformin 500 mg PO BID, Zolpidem 10 mg PO QHS, Flexeril 5 mg TID, and Hydrocodone 5/325 mg 1 tabs PO Q6hrs.

*Labs*: Complete blood count with white blood count 10.1, hemoglobin 7.9, hematocrit 30, and platelets 225. Basic metabolic panel with sodium 130, potassium 3.0, glucose 150, BUN 35, and creatinine 1.65.

*Functional status*: During post-op course, he required moderate to maximal assistance with bathing, dressing, and transfers. He ambulated 10 to 15 feet with a physical therapist.

*Discharge course*: He improved slightly but unfortunately did not return to cognitive baseline and was discharged to skilled nursing facility for subacute rehabilitation care.

Identify the falls risk factors.

- What are some of the contributing factors of delirium?
- Identify medications that are high risk for geriatric patients.
- Why was Mr. James discharged to a skilled nursing facility?

## Case Study 4

*Elder Abuse*

Mr. Pate presents to the emergency department (ED) with a burn on his upper arm. Mr. Pate provides details related to how the burn occurred, stating that it was an accident but at times becomes foggy on certain details when further assessed by various healthcare providers. Mr. Pate appears disheveled and malnourished with a BMI of 16.7. His hair is uncombed, he hasn't shaven in days, and he is wearing dirty clothes with a soiled brief. His son remains by his side throughout the examination, oftentimes answering for his father and becoming annoyed by the number of questions the staff is asking of them. When Mr. Jones' son steps out of the room to use the restroom, the patient shares that he would like to go to a nursing facility instead of return back home with his son. He will not provide any other information but repeats his wishes. Upon the skin assessment, scattered bruises are noted over both the boney and non-boney prominences of Mr. Jones' body. He refuses to answer questions about abuse or neglect. Mr. Jones is alert and oriented and outside of the bruises is completely independent in taking care of himself.

- What are your concerns in this situation?
- What can you as a health provider do in this case?
- Is this patient appropriate for nursing home placement?
- What forms of abuse is this patient most likely enduring at home?

## References

AARP Real Possibilities (n.d.). About AARP. Retrieved from www.aarp.org/about-aarp/

Administration on Aging, U.S. Department of Health and Human Services. (2016). *Aging Statistics*. Retrieved from https://aoa.acl.gov/Aging_Statistics/index.aspx & https://aoa.acl.gov/Aging_Statistics/future_growth/future_growth.aspx#age

Administration for Community Living. (2015). Administration on Aging (AoA). Retrieved from https://aoa.acl.gov/

Ahmed, B., Nanji, K., Mujeeb, R., & Patel, M. J. (2014). Effects of polypharmacy on adverse drug reactions among geriatric outpatients at a tertiary care hospital in karachi: A prospective cohort study. *PloS One, 9*, 112–133. Retrieved from http://dx.doi.org/10.1371/journal.pone.0112133

Allen, J., & Close, J. (2010). The NICHE geriatric resource nurse model: Improving the care of older adults with Alzheimer's disease and other dementias. *Geriatric Nursing, 31*(2), 128–132.

Alpert, P. T. (2014). Alcohol abuse in older adults: An invisible population. *Home Health Care Management & Practice, 26*(4), 269–272. Retrieved from http://dx.doi.org/10.1177/1084822314527765

Allphin, C. (2015). Whither analytic identity when aging interferes? *Jung Journal, 9*(2), 50-57. Retrieved from http://dx.doi.org/10.1080/19342039.2015.1021232

American Geriatric Society. (2017). Who we are. Retrieved from www.americangeriatrics.org/about_us/who_we_are/

American Geriatrics Society Expert Panel on the Care of Older Adults with Multimorbidity (2012). Guiding principles for the care of older adults with multimorbidity: An approach for clinicians. *Journal of the American Geriatrics Society, 60*(10), E1–E25. Retrieved from http://dx.doi.org/10.1111/j.1532-5415.2012.04188.x

Azhar, G, & Wei, J. (2015). The demographics of aging and its impact on the cardiovascular health. *Current Cardiovascular Risk Reports, 9*(13), 1–6. doi: 10.1007/s12170-015-0441-x

Bandura A. (1977). Self-efficacy: Toward a unifying theory of behavioural change. *Psychol Rev, 84*, 191–215.

Bandura A. (1989). Human agency in social cognitive theory. *Am Psychol, 44*, 1175–1184.

Bandura A. (1997). *Self-efficacy: The exercise of control.* New York, NY: W.H. Freeman and Company.

Bandura, A. (2012). On the functional properties of perceived self-efficacy revisited. *Journal of Management, 38*(1), 9–44.

Becton, J., Walker, H., & Jones-Farmer, A. (2014). Generational differences in workplace behavior. *Journal of Applied Social Psychology, 44*, 175–189.

Besdine, R. (2016). Introduction to geriatrics. Merck Manuals. Retrieved from www.merckmanuals.com/professional/geriatrics/approach-to-the-geriatric-patient/introduction-to-geriatrics

Bihlmaier, I., & Schlarb, A. (2016). Self-efficacy and sleep patterns: A pilot study comparing sleep-disordered and healthy school-age children. *Somnologie, 20*(4), 275–280. doi:10.1007/s11818-016-0085-1.

Blank, K. (2009). Older adults and substance abuse: New data highlight concerns. *SAMHSA News, 17*(1). Retrieved from http://www.samhsa.gov/samhsanewletter/Volume_17_Number_1/OlderAdults.aspx

Boltz, M., Capezuti, E., Fulmer, T., & Zwicker, D. (2012). *Evidence-based geriatric nursing protocols for best practice.* (4th Ed). New York, NY: Springer Publishing.

Bonnie, R., & Wallace, R. (2003). *Elder mistreatment: Abuse, neglect and exploitation in an aging America.* Washington, D.C: National Academies Press.

Boyd, C. M., Wolff, J., Giovannetti, E., Reider, L., Weiss, C., Xue, Q, . . . Rand, C. (2014). *Healthcare task difficulty among older adults with multimorbidity. Medical Care, 52* Suppl 3 Suppl 2, ADVANCING THE FIELD: Results from the AHRQ Multiple Chronic Conditions Research Network (3), S118–S125. Retrieved from http://dx.doi.org/10.1097/MLR.0b013e3182a977da

Brinkman-Stoppelenburg, A., Rietjens, J. A., & Van, D. H. (2014). The effects of advance care planning on the end of life care: A systematic review. *Palliative Medicine, 28*(8), 1000–1025. Retrieved from http://dx.doi.org/10.1177/0269216314526272

Brothers, D. (2015). *Evidence-based advance directives: A guide for nurses.* [Adobe Digital Editions version]. Retrieved from http://search.proquest.com.jproxy.lib.ecu.edu/publication/50653

Butts, J., & Rich, K. (2015). *Philosophies and theories for advanced nursing practice* (2nd Ed). Burlington, MA: Jones & Bartlett Learning.

Campbell, K., Campbell, S., Siedor, L., & Twenge, J. (2015). Generational differences are real and useful. *Industrial and Organized Psychology, 8*(3), 324–408. doi:10.1017/iop.2015.43.

Castonguay, J., Filer, C., & Pitts, M. (2016). Seeking help for depression: Applying the health belief model to illness narratives. *Southern Communication Journal, 81*(5), 289–303. doi:10.1080/1041794X.2016.1165729.

Centers for Disease Control and Prevention (2013). The state of aging and health in America. Retrieved from https://www.cdc.gov/aging/agingdata/data-portal/state-aging-health.html

Centers for Disease Control and Prevention. (2014). Advance care planning and chronic disease management. Retrieved from https://www.cdc.gov/aging/advancecareplanning/

Centers for Disease Control and Prevention. (2015). National Center for Health Statistics, Mortality in the United States, 2014. Retrieved from www.cdc.gov/nchs/data/databriefs/db229.htm, www.cdc.gov/nchs/fastats

Center for Disease Control and Prevention (2016). Adult: Protect yourself with pneumococcal vaccines. Retrieved from https://www.cdc.gov/features/adult-pneumococcal/index.html

Centers for Medicare and Medicaid Services. (2015). On its 50th anniversary, more than 55 million Americans covered by Medicare. Retrieved from www.cms.gov/newsroom/mediareleasedatabase/press-releases/2015-press-releases-items/2015-07-28.html

Denic, A., Glassock, R., & Rule, A. (2016). Structural and functional changes with the aging kidney. *Advances in Chronic Kidney Disease, 23*(1), 19–28. Retrieved from http://dx.doi.org/10.1053/j.ackd.2015.08.004

Detering, K., Silveira, M., Arnold, R., & Savarese, D. (2016). Advance care planning and advance directives. *Up To Date*. Retrieved from http://www.uptodate.com/contents/advance-care-planning-and-advance-directives

Friendship Trays. (n.d.). Friendship Trays, Meals on Wheels in Charlotte-Mecklenburg. Retrieved from http://friendshiptrays.org/

Gage, S., & Melilo, D. K. (2011). Substance abuse in older adults: Policy issues. *Journal of Gerontological Nursing, 37*(12), 8–11. Retrieved from http://dx.doi.org/10.3928/00989134-20111104-01

Gallagher, J. (2013). Vitamin d and aging. *Endocrinology and Metabolism Clinics of North America, 42*(2), 319–332. doi:10.1016/j.ecl.2013.02.004.

Gandoy-Crego, M., Clemente, M., Gómez-Cantorna, C., González-Rodríguez, R., & Reig-Botella, A. (2016). Self-efficacy and health: The sehscale. *American Journal of Health Behavior, 40*(3), 389–395. doi:http://dx.doi.org/10.5993/AJHB.40.3.11

Glanz, K., Rimer, B., & Viswanath, K. (2015). *Health behavior: Theory, Research and Practice*. (5th Ed). San Francisco, CA: Jossey-Bass.

Gordon, J. & Jordan, L. (2016). Older is wiser? It depends who you ask…and how you ask. Aging, neuropsychology, and cognition, 24(1), 94–111. Retrieved from http://dx.doi.org/10.1080/13825585.2016.1171292

Guthrie, P., Schumacher, S., & Edinger, G. (2006). A NICHE delirium prevention project for hospitalized elders. In N. M. Silverstein & K. Maslow (Eds.), *Improving hospital care for persons with dementia* (pp. 139-157). New York, NY: Springer Publishing.

Ham, R. J., Sloane, P. D., Warshaw, G. A., Potter, J. F., & Flaherty, E. (2014). *Ham's primary care geriatrics a case approach* (6th Ed). Philadelphia, PA: Elsevier Saunders.

Hickman, S. E., Unroe, K. T., Ersek, M. T., Buente, B., Nazir, A., & Sachs, G. (2016). An interim analysis of an advance care planning intervention in the nursing home setting. *Journal of the American Geriatrics Society.* Retrieved from http://dx.doi.org/10.1111/jgs.14463

Ito, K. & Mercado, N. (2014). Stop accelerating lung aging for the treatment of COPD. *Experimental Gerontology, 59*, p. 21–27. doi: 10.1016/j.exger.2014.03.014

Jiri, B. (2016). The employees of baby boomers generation, generation X, generation Y and generation Z in selected Czech corporations as conceivers of development and competitiveness in their corporation. *Journal of Competitiveness, 8*(4), p. 104–123. doi:10.7441/joc.2016.04.07.

Leik, M. (2014). *Adult-gerontology nurse practitioner certification intensive review: fast facts and practice questions.* New York, NY: Springer Publishing Company.

Lin, J., Tsubota, K., & Apte, R. (2016). A glimpse at the aging eye. *Nature Partner Journals Aging and Mechanisms of Disease, 2.* doi:10.1038/npjamd.20163

Kim, H., Kisseleva, T., & Brenner, D. (2015). Ageing and liver disease. *Current Opinion in Gastroenterology, 31*(3), 184–191. doi:10.1097/MOG.0000000000000176

The Official U.S. Government Site for Medicare. (n.d.). PACE. Retrieved from www.medicare.gov/your-medicare-costs/help-paying-costs/pace/pace.html

Medicare.gov, The Official U.S. Government Site for Medicare. (n.d.). Your Medicare Costs. Retrieved from www.medicare.gov/your-medicare-costs/

Mouloud, K., Fonseca, A., & Abdelkader, B. (2015). Self-efficacy among the collective games players. *Journal of Physical Education and Sport, 15*(4), 805–808. doi:10.7752/jpes.2015.04123

Mutchler, J. E., Li, Y., & Xu, P. (2016). Living below the line: Economic insecurity and older Americans insecurity in the states 2016. *Center for Social and Demographic Research on Aging Publications.* Retrieved from http://scholarworks.umb.edu/demographyofaging/13

National Council on Aging (n.d.). Elder abuse fact. Retrieved from https://www.ncoa.org/public-policy-action/elder-justice/elder-abuse-facts/

National Institute on Aging. (2014). Advance care planning. Retrieved from https://www.nia.nih.gov/health/publication/advance-care-planning

National Library of Medicine (2016). Advanced directives. Retrieved from https://medlineplus.gov/advancedirectives.html

National Quality Forum (2012). Multiple chronic conditions measurement framework. Retrieved from http://www.qualityforum.org/Publications/2012/05/MCC_Measurement_Framework_Final_Report_document.aspx

Nursing Improving Care for Healthsystem Elders (NICHE). (n.d.). New York University, Rory Meyers College of Nursing. Retrieved from www.nicheprogram.org/program-overview/

Owsley, C., Huisingh, C., Clark, M., Jackson, G., & McGwin, G. (2015). Comparison of visual function in older eyes in the earliest stages of age-related macular degeneration to those in normal macular health. *Current Eye Research, 41*(2). Retrieved from http://dx.doi.org/10.3109/02713683.2015.1011282

Palmer, K. & Goodson, N. (2015). Ageing, musculoskeletal health and work. *Best Practice & Research Clinical Rheumatology, 29*(3), 391–404. doi:10/1016/j. berh.2015.03.004

Perry, T., Ruggiano, N., Shtompel, N., & Hassevoort, L. (2015). Applying Erikson's wisdom to self-management practices of older adults: Findings from two field studies. *Research on Aging, 37*(3), 253–274. Doi:10.1177/0164027514527974

Pfaff, J. (2002). The geriatric resource nurse model: A culture change. *Geriatric Nursing, 23*(3), 140–144.

Phillips, N. (2016). The implications of cognitive aging for listening and the framework for understanding effortful listening (fuel). *Ear and Hearing, 37*(1), 44S–51S. doi:10.1097/AUD.0000000000000309

Prochaska, J. (2008). Decision making in the transtheoretical model of behavior change. *Medical Decision Making, 28*(6), 845–849. doi:10.1177/0272989X08327068

Rao, J. K., Anderson, L. A., Lin, F. C., & Laux, J. (2014). Completion of advance directives among U.S. consumers. *American Journal of Preventive Medicine, 46*(1), 65-70. Retrieved from http://dx.doi.org/

Respecting Choices Person-Centered Care. (2017). Retrieved from http://www.gundersenhealth.org/respecting-choices/

Romppel, M., Herrmann-Lingen, C., Wachter, R., Edelmann, F., Düngen, H., Pieske, B., & Grande, G. (2013). A short form of the General Self-Efficacy Scale (GSE-6): Development, psychometric properties and validity in an intercultural non-clinical sample and a sample of patients at risk for heart failure. *GMS Psycho-Social-Medicine, 10*, 1–7. doi:10.3205/psm000091

Santamaria, J. (2016). The nurses improving care for healthsystem elders (NICHE) long-term care designation program. *Geriatric Nursing, 37*, 507. doi:10.1016/j.gerinurse.2016.10.004

Sergi, G., De rui, M., Sarti, S., & Marizato, E. (2011). Polypharmacy in the elderly: Can comprehensive geriatric assessment reduce inappropriate medication use? *Drugs & Aging, 28*(7), 509–511. Retrieved from http://dx.doi.org/10.2165/11592010-000000000-00000

SilverSneakers. (2017). Fitness for boomers and beyond. Retrieved from www.silversneakers.com

Svetina, M. (2014). Resilience in the context of Eriksons' theory of human development. *Current Psychology, 33*(3), p. 393–404. doi:10.1007/s12144-014-9218-5

Taylor, T. (2016, July 21). An update on costs of end-of-life care [Blog post]. Retrieved from http://conversableeconomist.blogspot.com/2016/07/an-update-on-costs-of-end-of-life-care.html

U.S. Federal Interagency Forum on Aging Related Statistics, U.S. National Center for Health Statistics. (2012). Older Americans 2012, Key indicators of well-being. Retrieved from https://agingstats.gov/docs/PastReports/2012/OA2012.pdf.

Wang, Y., & Yisheng, P. (2015). An alternative approach to understanding generational differences. *Industrial and Organized Psychology, 8*(3), 390–395.

Wholihan, D. J., & Pace, J. C. (2012). Community discussions: A vision for cutting the costs of end-of-life care. *Nursing Economics, 30*(3), 170–176. Retrieved from http://go.galegroup.com.jproxy.lib.ecu.edu/ps/i.do?p=HRCA&u=gree96177&id=G ALE|A291496702&v=2.1&it=r&sid=summon

Ziliak, J. P., & Gunderson, C. G. (2016). The state of senior hunger in America 2014: An annual report, 1-17. Retrieved from http://www.nfesh.org/research/

## CHAPTER 9

# Military and Care for Veterans*

## CAROL ANN KING, DNP, MSN, APRN, FNP-BC

*"I only regret that I have but one life to give for my country."*
—Captain Nathan Hale (Hale, 1776)

## The Military Culture and Healthcare

### Introduction: Why We Serve

SERVING in the military is considered an honor for many living and working in local communities. Military service members (SMs) live by a code of loyalty, integrity, and selfless service. Men and women join the Armed Forces for many different reasons, but they all share the same commitment to protecting and defending the United States (U.S.) with significant sacrifices, including their own lives. The SM's identity and sense of self surrounds the military system, including rank, position, and uniform. SMs can learn a lot about each other just by looking at the uniform, which reflects the military career. The SM is not alone in his or her selfless sacrifice, as the families also share in every assignment, every *deployment*, every injury, and every promotion. Military communities have a unique culture and challenges that healthcare providers should understand to be able to effectively unite with the military SM and family as they strive to meet their healthcare goals (Westphal & Convoy, 2015). As healthcare providers, we must also consider the person under the uniform and how the sense of identity is transformed once the uniform is no longer worn.

*The information contained in this chapter does not reflect the views of the Department of Defense (DoD) and was not completed in the line of the author's official Army duty.

215

The military healthcare system is robust and complex, but it cannot provide all the required care to all the active duty SMs, retired SMs, and their dependents. The military healthcare system's primary aim is to promote and maintain the active duty force for wartime readiness (Mundell, Friedberg, Eibner, & Mundell, 2013). Thus, the retired SMs, dependents, and even active duty SMs may be referred to civilian providers for specialty and primary healthcare. Whether the advanced practice nurse (APN) is a contract or civil service employee of a military healthcare system, or a civilian provider working with active and retired military SMs and dependents, knowledge of the unique cultural consideration and population risks are imperative for positive health outcomes.

## Understanding the Military System

The modern military system is very complex with multiple layers and distinct organizations, making up the protection branch of the U.S. DoD. Service departments include the Army, Marines, Air Force, Navy, and Coast Guard. Within the main branches of service, there are levels of service with different duty requirements, including *active duty* and *reserves*. Active duty is full-time military service, whereas Reserves, including the *National Guard*, is typically part-time service responsibilities. However, all SMs have the same responsibility—to remain physically and mentally ready to protect and defend the constitution of the United States against all enemies, foreign and domestic (United States Code, 2012).

The value of National Guard and Reserve SMs should never be minimized, noting that these part-time soldiers provide an estimated 38% of the total fighting force in the United States (Reserve Force Policy Board, 2016). The main service branches have reserve branches, such as the Army National Guard and Reserves and Air Force Reserves. Although many active duty SMs subsequently transition to reserve status, thousands join the service directly into reserve status without ever serving first as active duty. Most service commitments require one weekend of training a month and two weeks of service during the years, and SMs stay prepared for mobilization and deployments. These reservists are typically called "weekend warriors"; however, these SMs are much more than weekend employees of the U.S. federal government. Many are called to active duty for war and peace-keeping missions both in the continental United States and abroad. Some Reservists/National Guard

SMs have had multiple deployments in support of the U.S. missions, spending years separated from their families and full-time civilian jobs, balancing both worlds to fulfill their commitment to serve and protect.

## Have You Served?

Service is the key foundation of the military culture. When completing initial patient assessments, part of the interview should include a review of military service or affiliation. Based on the age of the patient, simply start the conversation by asking, "Have you served or has a family member served in the military?" Affirmative answers can be explored further and can provide a broad understanding important to the healthcare team. Some questions that may be asked include the following: Are you/family member currently serving? In what branch did you serve? How long did they serve? When did you serve? What were your jobs in service? Were you involved in military conflicts? Are you a qualified Veteran? Are you currently receiving any healthcare services through the Veterans Administration (VA)? Do you have a VA disability rating? What type of *discharge* did you receive (if no longer serving)? The APN must also be aware that the SM or family member may not be willing or able to disclose much information because of several issues, including lack of trust, stress evoked by the questions, and a desire to separate themselves from the military completely as a means of coping.

Once the general assessment is complete, more detailed information will prove to be vital in development of the plan of care. However, this initial visit may not be the appropriate time for diving deep into the military service. Allowing time for rapport and trust to build is an important strategy, fostering a therapeutic relationship over time. Mistrust of healthcare providers is common among SMs and their families, especially in the civilian sector. Make sure that you end the time with the patient with a plan in mind to prepare the patient for further discussion. For example: "Thank you for your (or your family member's) service. At the next visit, we will talk a bit more about your military history, if you are agreeable to that."

Asking permission to discuss military service in more detail is essential, because the SM may not be ready, willing, or able to endure additional inquiry. Sensitivity to past experiences is critical in fostering a positive working relationship. An insensitive response would be, "Have you killed anyone?" Having to take a life in defense of the mission is an experience that is not glamourous, and this question can be a trigger for a significant post-traumatic stress reaction. The SM or family member may not have a positive military experience and may appear very bitter and angry toward a complex system of bureaucracy and denial of services or a less than honorable discharge. For example, an SM may be prematurely discharged and denied Veterans' benefits or expected compensation, because they developed diabetes or another medical condition that does not meet service retention standards. Family members may be disillusioned with the military system, because the SM is deployed or returned from deployment so different that the family system is negatively impacted. And the harsh reality is that some SMs give the ultimate sacrifice of their lives while serving in both training and combat situations. The APN must be prepared for the expression of feelings and beliefs contrary to one's own and remain objective, supportive, and focused on a mutual progress toward healthcare goal attainment.

### Watch Your Six

A common term used in the military is "watch your six." This phrase refers to the SMs' blind spots or the areas behind them where they cannot see. This is a term used to remind SMs to stay alert and on guard to stay alive. Additionally, SMs have a deep commitment to each other, guarding each other's "six." The SMs may mention their "battle" or "*battle buddy*," and these terms refer to a very close fellow SM who worked with the SM, and how they protected and supported each other through the challenges and celebrations of military service. The bond between battle buddies is strong, and the loss can be devastating, comparing the grief to be like a close family member's death (Pivar, 2004). Being in the service provides a sense belonging beyond what most people will ever experience. SMs train together, eat together, house together in close quarters, fight together, celebrate promotions and awards together, share family issues together, recover from injuries together, and die together. SMs trust each other with their lives and must depend on each other, because the group is truly depending on each member staying focused and completing the mission as ordered (Junger, 2016).

The APN needs to be aware that the SM's loss of a battle buddy is a major traumatic event and can lead to intense grieving and *survivor's guilt*. The SM may ask questions such as the following: "Why did I survive and my buddy didn't?" or statements like "He/she was a much better person than I am. I should have saved him. I couldn't save him. I wish it was me instead of him." The APN will not have the answers.

The key point to remember is that the SM suffered a loss and must progress through the stages of grief to promote future healthy adjustment. A spirituality assessment may be beneficial to help the SM accept the loss and reconcile himself or herself to a higher plan in life and death (Kick & McNitt, 2016). The military services have faith-based chaplains of different religions readily available for both active duty SMs and reservists. Referral to community services may also be beneficial. Faith and belief in something beyond what one can see and touch can provide comfort to the weary SM who has been shaken to their core by life-shattering events. Moody and Trogdon (2016) present a faith-based approach to many of the issues facing our military SMs, including survivor's guilt, and serves as a possible template to discuss spirituality with the SM and family.

### Shut Up and Color

*". . . Theirs not to make reply, Theirs not to reason why,*
*Theirs but to do and die..."*
—Tennyson (1854)

SMs live in an environment of discipline, structure, and order, being told when to eat, sleep, run, relax, train, and fight. Military systems have a very clear hierarchy of rank and authority. SMs receive orders and follow them and, when they do not, serious consequences can result, including the loss of troops. At times, SMs may not agree with or understand orders received by a higher-ranking SM, but the order is acknowledged and executed. SMs use the term "shut up and color" in a jovial manner to reflect the need to just do what has been ordered. The SM clearly understands that the order is to be carried out as long as there is no violation of the Code of Military Justice, rules of engagement, or international law (Junger, 2016). This lived sense of structure and obedience can prove challenging for SMs transitioning back to civilian work and home life. In civilian employment, where collaboration and negotiation is common, there is little place for the SMs' order to be carried out without debate or discussion. When the SMs' "order" is met with questioning or refusal to comply both in the home and in the workplace, confusion, impatience, and anger can follow. The APN can help the SM and family to balance the structure and order of the military with the flexibility and open communication needed for a positive home and work environment.

## Slick Sleeve

Not all SMs deploy to foreign countries and not all SMs are assigned to combat. Thousands of active duty and reserve SMs are required to be right here in the United States to support the war fighter. When a SM deploys to a combat zone for a minimum amount of time, usually 30 days, the SM earns a combat patch, which is worn on the uniform under the U.S. flag on the right arm. When SMs do not have a combat patch, they are called "slick sleeve." There is a sense of division among SM between those who have been deployed to combat and those who have not. However, not every SM has the opportunity to deploy and is given orders in a noncombat but equally critical role. Additionally, just because SMs have not served in a combat zone does not mean that they did not have experiences and deployments that could have affected their health. Training and humanitarian missions can be quite dangerous but still do not earn the SM a combat patch. Obtaining a clear understanding of military service will provide the APN with direction for exploration of potential healthcare needs. A SM can experience a significant injury or post-traumatic stress from many military related situations, not just war.

## Medical Readiness

The APN may be part of a military medical readiness program, as these requirements for medical readiness are transitioning to the civilian sector especially for National Guard and Reserve SMs. The services' medical readiness program requires regular health assessments and determination of fitness for deployment and specific assignments, considering both the physical and mental demands of the assignment. The services have clear standards for medical fitness that will guide the ANP in SMs' medical fitness considerations. The *Periodic Health Assessment* (PHA) is a screening tool to identify potential deployment-limiting conditions and facilitate appropriate referrals for additional evaluation and treatment if indicated. If the APN is part of the PHA process, it is imperative to document all conditions the SM reports regardless of how minor those conditions may seem at the time. What might appear to be minor to the APN or minimalized by the SM could be a potential deployment-limiting condition in the future.

The services also have a process to inform leaders of what the SM can and cannot physically or mentally do, called the medical profile. The profile explains specific limitations related to the SM's expected duties to ensure the SM has limited risk of further harm while allowing time for the SM to recover from the condition. The APN may be in a position that requires the completion of *medical profiles*, and this would require additional training and experience to understand the roles of the SM and how to effectively and correctly place limits on the SM. The APN must also understand that each SM has a job and when he or she cannot do his or her job due to an impairing medical condition, the fighting team now has a weakness to overcome.

## Physical Limitations: A Culture of Denial

For many SMs, physical strength and ability is part of a personal sense of identity. Disease, injury, or limitations are weaknesses that are difficult to accept. The Armed Forces have standards of physical fitness, and failure to meet these standards can result in limitations to deployment, poor performance evaluations, removal from certain jobs, and separation from service. For example, Army regulation 40-501 states that a diagnosis of diabetes mellitus that requires glycemic control does not meet retention standards and the SM can be discharged (Department of the Army, 2003). Consequently, SMs are notoriously known to avoid disclosure of health issues for fear of the health issue affecting their military careers. Even if the SM has never deployed, the required ongoing training contributes to many injuries. SMs have to train as they would fight, including carrying heavy loads, walking long distances, maneuvering through tough terrain, and living in harsh conditions.

SMs also tend to put pressure on other SMs who do report illnesses and injuries. For example, one branch's SMs have used the term "sick call ranger" to refer to a SM who goes to sick call instead of morning physical readiness training. The peer shaming is intended to make the SM stronger; however, it promotes a culture of denial towards actual maladies. This failure to disclose real health issues prevents timely evaluation and management, thus allowing minor issues to become more serious. This same cultural trend clearly affects the healthcare team and APNs, as many prior service members present with an extensive list of health issues that have been ignored while actively serving.

Orthopedic issues typically dominate the list of health concerns due to the strenuous physical demands of service. Shoulders, knees, feet, and spine injuries dominate the physical complaints of SMs, from either direct injury or overuse and gradual strain from repeated harsh physical demands. Advanced nurses need to complete thorough physical assessments, including subjective and objective evaluations. An SM may sit before the nurse and calmly reply with a stoic, "I'm fine," while suffering from chronic, daily pain due to unaddressed physical insults. A focused physical examination based on patient complaints may not be adequate to fully assess the SM's health insults. A comprehensive physical examination will frequently reveal health limitations and areas of insult due to deficits in range of motion, strength, and joint function (Rhon, Lentz, & George, 2016).

Other common health concerns that affect the general population also affect the military SMs, including hypertension, diabetes, cardiovascular disease, and cancers. Management of these health conditions is consistent with clinical practice guidelines used for all patients. The APN must consider how the chronic health condition will affect the SM if he or she is still serving. Preparations will need to be made prior to a deployment to ensure the SM has any necessary medications and receives the same level of care to prevent long-term complications.

*Case Vignette*

Major Mary, an Army Nurse Reservist, works as a neonatal nurse manager in her civilian job for 15 years at the same hospital. Major Mary received orders for deployment and has been deployed to Afghanistan for 9 months. During her deployment, she had a duty-related injury to her knee that required steroid injections and physical therapy with little progress. The healthcare team discussed surgery, but Major Mary decided against surgery while in theater and said she would manage until she could get home; she was prescribed celecoxib and tramadol to help manage her pain and permit her to continue with her military duties. Major Mary completed her deployment and post-deployment process and was released from active duty back to her civilian role as a nurse manager. The injury was duty-related; she is a qualified U.S. veteran and has been approved to use the VA healthcare system. The nearest VA system is 50 miles away. From your previous readings, consider the potential effects of a duty-related injury on Major Mary's quality of life. What are the potential implications and clinical considerations of the medications prescribed in Major Mary's treatment? What might be some complicating factors and challenges Major Mary could face with her transition back to her civilian job?

## I'm Being Deployed

When SMs are notified that they are receiving orders for mobilization or deployment, the SM enters a very focused "get ready" mode. They pack what is essential, wrap up any loose ends, and get their home lives in order. However, the response for the family being left behind is very different. Spouses must prepare to manage home responsibilities alone, and children must prepare to be separated from one of their parents. See Table 9.1.

The remaining parent assumes the responsibilities of both parents. The young son may be the "man of the house" or the young daughter may be expected to assume some of the duties of the deployed mother. Traditional lines of responsibility become blurred, and the remaining

TABLE 9.1. *Stages of Deployment Based on the Emotional Cycle of Deployment (Pincus, House, Christensen, & Adler, 2001).*

| Phase | Service Member | Family |
|---|---|---|
| Predeployment | "Ramping Up" mode, focused on the mission, bonding with unit instead of family, getting family matters in order, overwhelmed by all the tasks, beginning emotional detachment, arguments to distance self | Denial, anxiety, fear, sadness of pending separation, acting as if the SM is already gone, arguments/anger covering the sadness of being separated, busyness, "honey-do" lists |
| Deployment | Helpless to help the family, left out of family issues, loneliness, fear of loss of family relationships | Overwhelmed, worried, numb, disoriented, loss of sense of security, loneliness, helpless to help the SM |
| Sustainment-Settling In | Acceptance that direct support to the family is limited, focused on the mission, communication when possible, need to feel included in family still | More confidence, support from others/groups, home routines/norms established, remaining family members learn their roles, reluctant to tell SM about family issues |
| Redeployment | Anticipation, excitement, concern over completing the mission, decline in unit cohesion, "home" focused | Excitement, anticipation, nesting/preparing the home for the SMs return, difficulty making decisions, high expectations |
| Postdeployment | Satisfaction with mission accomplishment, reintegration back into home and family, awkward in the home, tension, emotional distance | Honeymoon phase, emotional, relief, loss of independence, back into traditional roles, tension, emotional distance |

family members face confusion and stress, especially during the beginning of the deployment (Padden & Posey, 2013).

The APN needs to be on alert for specific maladjustment behaviors in children, such as regression to an earlier stage of development, acting out at school and in the home and risk-taking behavior, including promiscuity, substance use, isolation, loss of interest in activities, and sleeping and eating disturbances. Early identification and integration of additional services to help children adjust to all phases of the deployment cycle can foster the children's resilience and integrate new positive coping skills for future challenges (Gewirtz, Erbes, Polusny, Forgatch, & DeGarmo, 2011).

### I'm Coming Home

When SMs transition back home after deployment, most families share great joy and excitement about being reunited. While the safe return of SMs is joyous, it can be the beginning of a stressful transition time for both the SM and those to whom he/she is returning. Helping the family, significant others, and the SM with this transition is an important role of the ANP, and care must be taken to maintain safety, open communication, and awareness for potential complications of transition. Family members had to assume different roles in the absence of the SM, and the reintegration can lead to feelings of not belonging, as if the home is no longer the SM's home. The SM may not feel needed any longer, because the family managed everything well during the deployment. Seemingly trivial matters, such as the living room furniture being rearranged, can be a source of tension in the home. APNs need to support the SM and family with encouragement to take the time to re-establish the marriage relationship slowly, listen to each other, discuss situations with the children including the house rules, support each other in front of the children, and remember to laugh. The positive emotional reattachment between the spouses is imperative for family adjustment after deployment.

### Adrenaline Junkie

Military service provides opportunities for SMs to challenge themselves physically and mentally, always ready to respond to threats. This constant state of readiness promotes a state of hypervigilance, with SMs living in a near constant state of flight or fight readiness. Especially when deployed in combat situations, SMs must remain mentally alert for threats from enemies, attacks from any direction, and threats they cannot readily identify. Explosive devices are hidden well and people, including women and children, are disguised as friendly civilians. As a result, SMs must remain highly suspicious and alert. Later, when SMs are no longer in that intense environment, they can find the transition difficult, unable to turn off that adrenalineinduced fight or flight response. When this need for the adrenaline response is coupled with a sense of invincibility that comes from surviving tours of duty, the SM is at serious risk of self-destruction. Some SMs will engage in risk-taking behaviors, such as highspeed driving, intense gambling, risky sexual behavior, substance abuse, interpersonal aggression, and suicide attempts (James, Strom, & Leskela, 2014). Driving at high speeds and riding motorcycles without helmets are some of the most common risk-taking behaviors that need to be recognized and discussed with the SM (Hoggatt *et al.*, 2015).

The SM may also seek adrenaline-evoking experiences in attempts to bury intense memories from combat. The numbness from the hyper-vigilance is a protective coping skill to avoid having to experience the raw emotions from past experiences. In *Ghost in the Ranks* by Dr. John J. Whelan, SMs discuss the hidden costs of military service, including the unreported daily battles in the minds of SMs struggling to make some type of sense of the horrors and loss suffered during war (Whelan, 2016).

## Case Vignette

Sam Smitty, a 36-year-old male, presents to your civilian primary care clinic, which is near a joint services (Army, Air Force, and Navy) military base with a military treatment center/hospital. He complains of severe lower back pain that began after he wrecked his 4-wheel all-terrain vehicle this past weekend. He says he is a resident of your state, is uninsured, and has not had any primary care for years. He says that he just needs to get checked out and get something for the pain. As you are completing your assessment, you notice a tattoo associated with military service and that his driver's license is from a different state. You ask him if he has served in the military, and he avoids the question by changing the topic. You suspect that he is an active duty SM, has been involved in a high-risk accident, and could possibly be fraudulently seeking pain medication or avoiding having to report the accident to his command. What are some of the warning signals in Sam Smitty's case?

How might you determine if Sam Smitty was in the military without violating patient confidentiality policies and laws? How can the APN work effectively and professionally with Sam Smitty to help him with his healthcare concerns?

## Mental Health Considerations

Military SMs are affected in some way, both positive and negative, during their course of service. SMs and their family members may be reluctant to disclose true stress and coping problems for many reasons, including the military culture of stoicism, stigma associated with mental illness, and the expectation that SMs and families manage life events and emotions alone to maintain proper appearances. SMs are expected to control their family members and keep the home life in order, and that expectation is passed to the spouse/significant other and children. Asking for help for issues beyond typical physical ailments and conditions is difficult, so the APN needs to develop a sensitive approach to addressing issues related to mental health. APNs need to be prepared for denial and withdrawal when mental health issues are discussed, because disclosure can be considered weakness in a world in which phrases such as "toughen up, buttercup" are mainstream.

## Post-Traumatic Stress

The American Psychiatric Association's *Diagnostic and Statistical Manual of Mental Disorders, Fifth Edition* (DSMV®) (2013) presents symptoms of post-traumatic stress disorder (PTSD) in four categories: intrusive thoughts, avoiding reminders, negative thoughts and feelings, and arousal and reactive symptoms, all of which last more than a month. PTSD is reported to be the third highest condition for veteran disability. Only tinnitus and hearing loss, both very common military health issues, have higher rates of disability compensation (Guina, Welton, Broderick, Correll, & Peirson, 2016). The actual prevalence of combat-related PTSD is difficult to determine but ranges from about 2% to 35% (Xue, Ge, Tang, Liu, Kang, Wang, & Zhang, 2015). Many are exposed to events that are traumatic, such as situations experienced in combat, personal assaults, motor vehicle accidents, and training accidents, but not all develop PTSD. We do not fully understand who will experience the reaction to stressful events to the point of creating dysfunction in one's life, but the most consistent predictor for PTSD is military combat (Bray *et al.,* 2016). However, there are risk factors and warning signs associated with post-traumatic stress reactions: female, minority, enlisted (not officer), prior trauma, pre-existing behavioral health conditions, duration of combat exposure, repeated combat exposures and deployments, lower education levels, and higher overall adverse life events (Xue *et al.*, 2015).

Post-traumatic stress reactions occur on a continuum, with an individual response in each person. Although some risk factors can be associated with PTSD, consider each person individually and avoid generalizations. Screening tools validated for primary care can be very useful to begin planning care for SMs and their families, such as the Primary Care PTSD Screen for DSM-5 (PC-PTSD-5) (Prins *et al.*, 2016). Screening tools provide a more objective screening for a condition and an avenue for the APN to being discussing the SM's response to traumatic events, opening dialogue to facilitate a positive therapeutic environment. For example, seemingly benign colors, smells, or sounds can trigger an extreme reaction in the SM. Many SMs are reluctant to talk about triggers for their stress, their experience of hypervigilance, or intrusive thoughts for fear of judgment and being considered weak and out of control. Positive screening results should be discussed with the SM and/or family member and an interprofessional plan for care developed in unity with the SM/family.

## Traumatic Brain Injury

The Centers for Disease Control and Prevention (CDC) (2017) defines traumatic brain injury (TBI) as an insult to the head by some type of bump, blow, or jolt significant enough to cause some disruption of normal brain function. The U.S. DoD (2017) reports that nearly 314,000 SMs have experienced a TBI during their service, both in training and in combat. For the SM, TBI is most likely to occur during noncombat situations, such as training exercises and recreational adventures, but the incidence of combat-related TBI has increased during the most recent Iraq and Afghanistan wars, primarily from explosive blast (McCulloch *et al.*, 2017). TBI is divided into mild, moderate, and severe ranges based on the physiological and psychological responses after the insult. The vast majority of all TBIs, estimated at approximately 85%, are in the mild category, followed by only 7.5% classified as moderate and 0.5% as severe. The remaining were either penetrating TBI or unable to classify based on estimates from 2014 (O'Neil, Carlson, Storzbach, Brenner, Freeman, Quinones, *et al.*, 2013).

The Glasgow Coma Scale (GCS), developed by Teasdale & Jennett in 1974, is still a key component of TBI assessment, and APNs need to understand how to complete the GCS and the clinical applications. Fortunately, as with many other assessment tools, smart phone applications exist for the GCS to provide the APN with the ability to quickly compute the score and move toward clinical interventions appropriate to the SMs level of compromise.

Symptoms of TBI depend on the severity, with the clear majority of all TBIs being mild. The SM with mild TBI may exhibit insomnia, memory changes, headache, sensitivity to light and sound, and dizziness. These symptoms generally resolve without complications, but a small number of SMs may suffer with chronic postconcussion symptoms. APNs should assess the SM for cognitive impairments, behavioral health symptoms including depression and anxiety, and somatic symptoms of headache and tinnitus (Summerall, 2017). When working with SMs, the APN must consider the whole person and review presenting complaints, symptoms, and results of assessments and examinations concurrently to help identify potential clusters of symptoms that could truly be related to one initial cause. The need for a holistic approach to the assessment and treatment of the SM is very evident in relation to TBI—one event can begin a cascade of many life-changing sequelae (Gregory, West, Cole, Bailie, McCulloch, Ettenhofer *et al.*, 2017).

### Substance Abuse

Alcohol, illicit drugs, and prescription drug misuse, abuse, and dependence are all of concern. Substance abuse and dependence by SMs has been associated with pre-existing substance use disorders or a result of trauma and life stressors associated with military service. In both situations, substance use disorders are a real threat to the SM and the family. The APN should include validated screening tools and evidencebased practice guidelines when working with the SM and family. Specific screening tools should be integrated into care, including the Alcohol Use Disorders Identification Test—Consumption (AUDIT-C), combined with appropriate clinical assessment and management, to include referral for additional services (U.S. Department of Veteran Affairs, 2015).

## Sexual Assault

Military sexual trauma (MST) is a term used to include sexual harassment and sexual assault experienced by an SM during service. Sexual harassment is defined as repeated unsolicited verbal or physical contact of a sexual nature that is threatening in character (U.S. Department of Veterans Affairs, 2017). Sexual assault is a sexual act on another person using threats or invoking fear or is committed when the person refuses consent or is unable to give consent due to some type of impairment or mental disease or defect (Uniform Code of Military Justice, n.d.). In the military, one cannot assume that women are the only victims of sexual harassment and/or assault. Both men and women are affected; however, harassment and assault have been under-reported, under-investigated, and under-estimated. Although estimates of sexual harassment and assault range from 22% to 84% in the military, SMs frequently withhold reporting of sexual misconduct for fear of repercussions, fear of damage to their military career, feeling the need to just "drive on," and fear of not being believed (Kintzle *et al.*, 2015). SMs live in environments in which they are in daily danger from nefarious sources, but assault risks from one of their own unit seems unthinkable. When a SM experiences sexual harassment or assault, he or she loses sense of security and trust, as one of the very group who is supposed to bond together in service against the enemy actually becomes the enemy (Creech & Borsari, 2014).

Seeking help after harassment and assault is hampered by fear, but the culture is changing. Military leadership has sent the message very clearly that sexual assault and harassment will not be tolerated and perpetrators will be held accountable. The service branches have programs specifically to prevent sexual harassment and assault and allow the affected SM clear courses of action should the SM experience these threats. The U.S. Department of Defense Sexual Assault Prevention and Response Office (2017) clearly presents the expectations for each service branch; provides resources for military leaders for awareness, prevention, and response; and provides victim advocacy support.

The SM who has experienced sexual harassment or assault can suffer long-term consequences seen long after separation from service, including depression, anger, irritability, feeling numb, trouble sleeping, attention difficulties, substance abuse, hypervigilance, isolation, relationship difficulties, and physical health problems. APNs need to consider these issues within the assessment and planning with the SM. Failure to seek counseling and support after the assault, minimizing the impact, is common among SMs, so APNs should offer additional counseling services, ideally with counselors who have specific sexual assault and post-traumatic stress expertise (U.S. Department of Veterans Affairs, 2017).

## Suicide

The VA estimates that an average of 20 U.S. military veterans commit suicide each day, comprising about 18% of suicides in the United States (U.S. Department of Veterans Affairs, 2016). In the active and reserve components of the service branches, there was an average of 480 suicides per year from 2012 through 2015, with a total report of suicides for the same period to equal 1,921 SMs (Franklin, 2016). Since 2012, suicide has surpassed death from combat and second only to accidents (Corr, 2014). Suicide is devastating, with the loss of a human life and extreme effect on the loved ones and the military. Although combat deployments may contribute to death by suicide, research supports that rates of suicide among SMs who have never deployed may exceed those who have deployed. The leading independent predictors of suicide include being male and having pre-existing mental health conditions prior to joining the military (LeardMann *et al.*, 2013).

The APN needs specific training on assessing for suicide, including the use of validated screening tools and developing an effective plan to protect the SM or family member from self-harm while respecting the rights of the individual. Key contributing factors that may precipitate may include recent transitioning back from deployment or mobilization, a limited support system, marital and financial stress, physical injuries, chronic pain, and substance use. However, the most important point for the APN to remember is that all patients are at risk for suicide at any given time and one cannot just look at a patient to determine suicidality. Understand that suicide is a real potential, do not be afraid to ask about suicidal ideations, and help the SM or family get the services needed to remain safe (Hall, 2016).

Beyond the red flags for a mental illness crisis in the general population, healthcare providers working with military service members and their families need to be alert for additional signs of potential harm to self or others. Those signs include isolation from typical support systems, trying to get back into the fight or similar civilian position that is dangerous, increased hypervigilance, changes in typical presentation at healthcare visits, or a sense of resolution with a calmness uncharacteristic for the person (Hall, 2016).

## Separation from Service

This tribal-type life builds a sense of belonging and identity so strong that some SMs have great difficulty transitioning to civilian life. Transitioning to life separate from the daily support from fellow SMs and outside of the structure and safety of the group is a high-risk period of potential maladjustment. The SM who does not have strong family support and who has also recently separated from service is at high risk for negative adjustment responses, including suicide (Martin, Houtsma, Green, & Anestis, 2016). APNs need to be aware of the SMs and family needs during this transition out of service and help the SM identify potential resources to ease the separation. The APN can provide the SM and family with a list of potential community groups, including the United Service Organization (USO) or the Veterans of Foreign Wars (VFW).

Retirement from service is a time of celebration, and SMs signify the end of a long, honorable service by proclaiming, "I'm going to the house!" This typically positive transition presents unique challenges for the SM, family, and healthcare team. The SMs are leaving their source of order, identity, and comprehensive healthcare and entering uncharted waters of becoming a civilian. Nurses can ease that transition by assessing the SM's support system and ongoing life plan. Key issues to consider include the following:

- Is the SM going to work outside the home?
- Who are the SM's main supports?
- Is the SM involved in a faith-based group?
- Is the SM returning to college or alternative skills training?
- Are there financial concerns?
- Is the SM enrolled in the Veterans Affairs system?

### Case Vignette

Marine Master Sergeant (MSG) John White has been diagnosed with diabetes and now requires medication to manage his condition. He has been deployed to Iraq and Afghanistan a total of four times and was preparing for a fifth deployment. But he has been told that he cannot deploy because his diabetes is not under control and his command questions his fitness for duty. MSG White is in your primary care clinic asking for documentation stating that his diabetes is under control and that he is medically ready to deploy. You review his medical records and complete an in-office hemoglobin A1c (HgA1c), which was 8.2. You know his diabetes is not controlled but fear that he will be discharged from the U.S. Marines, which would be devastating for him. Consider how you would present your clinical assessment and conclusion to MSG White. What nursing interventions would be appropriate to initiate for MSG White? Considering the potential for a medical discharge, what risks would you consider to be applicable to MSG White based on what you have read?

### Additional Considerations

SMs are faced with some unique situations that require discussion. APNs who have not experienced military life first-hand may find it difficult to understand why SMs or family members are struggling with readjustments. Military life involves frequent moves, generally every two to three years, in which the whole family must pull up stakes and reestablish themselves in a new state or even country. Without integration into a supportive community, the family can feel very isolated and some become reluctant to form friendship bonds or trusting relationships.

Another consideration for the APN is the unique issues faced by same sex couples and their challenges of acceptance and issues with military benefits. An unmarried same sex partner of a military SM is not afforded any of the rights and privileges of federal service, including healthcare and death benefits. But with the repeal of the Department of Defense's Don't Ask, Don't Tell, legislation in 2011, homosexual service members are no longer in fear of legal action and can marry. Not all states recognize same-sex marriages, but after the U.S. Supreme Court ruled to recognize same-sex marriage, military same-sex couples have equal benefits allotted to opposite-sex couples. To be eligible, the couple would need to be married in a jurisdiction that legally allows same-sex marriages (Military One Source, 2017).

Military benefits include healthcare at no cost for the active duty SM, spouse, and children, both biological and legally adopted. The military healthcare system provides a secure source of quality healthcare while the SM is on active duty. However, when the SM is no longer on active duty, the full military healthcare benefit ends. The family must find alternative health insurance that is typically not free, and this can be a source of significant stress and insecurity. This is especially true for families with members having complicated health conditions that require expensive interventions, such as cystic fibrosis or insulin-dependent diabetes.

Serving in the military can be rewarding, but it is not without risks and insults to the SM and the family, physically, mentally, and emotionally. Many have described the post-service changes as "the new normal." ANPs can help with this transition to a new and better state of being through building a trusting relationship and healthcare partnership with the SM and family. The ANP should expect that military SMs and families have been affected by military-related life experiences and may never the same. But they can be better, a better version of themselves.

**Take Care of Yourself!**

Working with the military SMs and family members can be very positive for the healthcare team as a means of supporting those who have sacrificed so much for freedom. Although we can never repay the SM and family for their service, we can show our gratitude by partnering with them to promote optimal health attainment. However, the complexity of the healthcare needs can be daunting. The APN must prioritize care concerns and develop an interprofessional plan with the patient, family, and necessary community and professional team members.

Potential integrated team members include both healthcare professionals, other professional groups, and the community. Healthcare team members may include behavioral health, physical therapy, occupational therapy, and specialty medical services, such as orthopedics, neurology, and cardiology. Other professional groups to consider include financial counselors and clergy. Community resources include recreational programs, local support groups, and family programs.

The experiences of the SM may influence healthcare providers, noting that sharing of the SM's lived experience may produce fear and anxiety in the provider. Before the APN begins asking SMs about their lived experiences, APNs must assess their own current level of coping and ensure they can handle what they might hear. For example, SMs may witness horrific human suffering and may have been in situations in which they were required to defend themselves and support their mission at the expense of others' lives. If the provider asks SMs to discuss what they experienced, the provider needs to be prepared for the accounts of war. Secondary post-traumatic stress (PTS) just from hearing the stories of SMs is possible, with the provider being negatively impacted with subsequent symptoms of PTS, including hypervigilance, anxiety, fear, and insomnia (Baum, 2016).

## Tool Kit and Resources

*Tools and Key Tips for APNs Working with Military-Connected Patients*

As a nurse, you are part of the most trusted profession based on public opinion for the past decade, and this places you in an important position to help SMs and their families manage the demands of military service and the challenges associated with the transition to civilian life. Here are some key points to remember as you move forward:

- Keep the promises you make
- Build rapport and trust over time
- Discuss the plan
- Assess for risky behaviors
- Engage the family when possible
- Have a list of referrals readily available
- Have a list of community integration options
- Set the stage for the visit and transition slowly with a distinct soft tone
- Coordinate with the VA/other healthcare team members
- Reconcile medications at every visit and check controlled drug state registries, if able
- Be prepared to hear the SM's stories, which could be difficult to understand. Be empathetic, but be honest. Avoid saying you understand when you probably have never experienced anything close unless you were a prior SM.
- Take care of yourself, recognizing that hearing stories of trauma and working with SMs who have sustained complex injuries can be difficult.

*Tool Kit/Resources*
*Veterans Crisis Line/National Suicide Prevention Lifeline*: 1-800-273-8255, https://health.mil/suicideprevention

*Military One Source even for Reservist*: http://www.militaryonesource.mil/

*Strong Bonds Program*: http://www.strongbonds.org/skins/strongbonds/home.aspx

*Family Readiness Groups*: Local to each unit/command. Look up the specific information in your area. Other resources include https://www.jointservicessupport.org/Default.aspx

*U.S. Department of Veterans Affairs* free training and free screening scales for use in primary care, including PHQ-9 and The Primary Care PTSD Screen for DSM-5 (PC-PTSD-5): https://www.mental-health.va.gov

*DoD Sexual Assault Prevention and Response Office*: www.sapr.mil

*Yellow Ribbon Reintegration Program*: https://www.jointservicessupport.org/YRRP/default.aspx

*Centers for Disease Control and Prevention*: Resources for Healthcare Providers on Traumatic Brain Injury & Concussion: https://www.cdc.gov/traumaticbraininjury/index.html

*United Service Organization (USO)*: https://www.uso.org/

*Veterans Administration/U.S. Department of Defense Clinical Practice Guidelines*: https://www.healthquality.va.gov/

*Veterans of Foreign Wars (VFW)*: https://www.vfw.org/

## Definitions

*Active Duty*—Full-time federal military service for a specific duration and opportunities to re-enlist or continue service based on satisfactory service

*Battle Buddy*—Close SMs serving together, forming bonds equal to strong family bonds

*Deployment*—Military orders requiring travel and service outside of the United States, typically overseas. CONUS orders mean the SM is assigned to a destination in the continental U.S. OCONUS means the SM has orders outside the continental United State.

*Discharge*—The official end of military service. Types of discharge include honorable, general, other than honorable, bad conduct, and dishonorable. Any discharge besides an honorable discharge will affect the SM's benefits after separation.

*Medical Profile*—A summary of a SM's physical limitations with an explanation of how the physical limitations affect the SM's ability to complete require Soldier actions

*National Guard*—National Guard component is the responsibility of the state and under the authority of the state's Governor. National Guard SMs are activated to respond to state emergencies and disasters.

*Periodic Health Assessment*—Annual physical history assessment required as part of military medical readiness, designed to identify actual and potential health issues or injuries that might affect ability to be deployed

*Reserves*—Part-time federal military commitment, typically requiring one weekend of duty a month and two weeks duty in the summer. However, the Reserve component of the military branches can be called up for active duty at any time.

*Survivor's Guilt/Grief*—Intense remorse and feelings of guilt for surviving after the loss of a close fellow SM. The SMs may state that they wish they had died instead of their battle buddy.

### Discussion Questions

1. Discuss the different stages of deployment and the potential facilitating actions the APN can take to promote healthy family transitions through the stages.

2. The SM's sense of identity is strongly associated with his or her military service. Discuss the implications for the SM when he or she is no longer in the military and the impact on the SM and family. How can the APN help the SM and family with this significant life transition?

3. Sexual harassment and assault incidents are under-reported in the military. Consider the implications of under-reporting and the effects/potential effects on the individual and the military as a whole. How can the APN promote health with SMs who may have experienced sexual harassment or assault?

4. SMs report mental health issues surrounding traumatic events related to combat situations, including what they saw, what happened to them within the course of their deployments, and what they had to do as part of the war mission. Consider the impact of the SM's stories of war on the civilian or military ANP who has never experienced combat. How can the APN protect himself or herself from psychological stress while allowing the SM to present his or her stories?

### Case Study

Byron is a 50-year-old decorated veteran of Operation Desert Storm and Operation Iraqi Freedom and an active duty Army Officer. He has had a successful career and all he knows is life in the military. He has a master's degree in computer science, is married, and has two grown children. He is traveling and has been in a car accident. He presents to your civilian emergency department minor care section because of a laceration on his forehead from hitting his head on the steering wheel during the accident. As you are completing his history, you ask him where he was going in his travels, and he replied that he did not have a firm destination, was on leave, and just decided to take a road trip without planning. He reports that his wife recently asked him for a divorce, because he would not retire from the military, and he just needed to get away to think. His blood pressure is elevated at 156/94, pulse is 98, respirations are 18, temperature is 98.3 oral, and pulse oximeter is at 98%. The focused physical examination was negative for any abnormal findings except for the 5 cm laceration on his forehead above his left eye. You examine the laceration, determine that sutures will be required, and proceed to clean the wound and suture it. Consider questions the APN would need to ask and further assessments that need to be done regarding safety of Byron and others.

- What would be some red flags that would warrant further evaluation?
- What additional information would you want to obtain before discharging Byron?
- What are some potential referral and/or support resources for Byron?

## References

American Psychiatric Association. (2013). *Diagnostic and statistical manual of mental disorders* (DSM-5®). Washington, DC: American Psychiatric Pub.

Baum, N. (2016). Secondary traumatization in mental health professionals: A systematic review of gender findings. *Trauma, Violence, and Abuse: A Review Journal, 17*(2), 221–235. doi:http://dx.doi.org.jproxy.lib.ecu.edu/10.1177/1524838015584357

Bray, R. M., Engel, C. C., Williams, J., Jaycox, L. H., Lane, M. E., Morgan, J. K., & Unützer, J. (2016). Posttraumatic stress disorder in U.S. military primary care: Trajectories and predictors of one-year prognosis: PTSD trajectories and prognosis predictors. *Journal of Traumatic Stress, 29*(4), 340–348. doi:10.1002/jts.22119

Centers for Disease Control and Prevention. (2017). Basic information about Traumatic brain injury and concussion. Retrieved from https://www.cdc.gov/traumaticbraininjury/basics.html

Corr, W. (2014). Surveillance snapshot: Manner and cause of death, active component, U.S. armed forces, 1998–2013. Medical Surveillance Monthly Report, 21, 21. Retrieved from https://www.afhsc.mil/documents/pubs/msmrs/2014/v21_n10.pdf

Creech, S. K., & Borsari, B. (2014). Alcohol use, military sexual trauma, expectancies, and coping skills in women veterans presenting to primary care. *Addictive Behaviors, 39*(2), 379–385. doi:10.1016/j.addbeh.2013.02.006

Department of the Army. (2003). AR 40-501: Standards of medical fitness. Retrieved from http://www.au.af.mil/au/awc/awcgate/army/r40_501.pdf

Franklin, K. (2016). Department of Defense quarterly suicide report. Retrieved from http://www.dspo.mil/Portals/113/Documents/DoD%20Quarterly%20Suicide%20 Report%20CY2016%20Q1.pdf

Gewirtz, A. H., Erbes, C. R., Polusny, M. A., Forgatch, M. S., & DeGarmo, D. S. (2011). Helping military families through the deployment process: Strategies to support parenting. *Professional Psychology, Research and Practice, 42*(1), 56–62. http://doi.org/10.1037/a0022345

Gregory, E., West, T. A., Cole, W. R., Bailie, J. M., McCulloch, K. L., Ettenhofer, M. L., Qashu, F. M. (2017). Use of a multi-level mixed methods approach to study the effectiveness of a primary care progressive return to activity protocol after acute mild traumatic brain injury/concussion in the military. *Contemporary Clinical Trials, 52*, 95–100. doi:10.1016/j.cct.2016.11.005

Guina, J., Welton, R., Broderick, P., Correll, T., & Peirson, R. (2016). DSM-5 criteria and its implications for diagnosing PTSD in military service members and veterans. *Current Psychiatry Reports, 18*(43). doi: 10.1007/s11920-016-0686-1

Hale, N. (1776). Retrieved from http://www.revolutionary-war.net/nathan-hale.html

Hall, L. (2016). Counseling military families: What mental health professionals need to know (2nd Ed.). New York: Routledge.

Hoggatt, K. J., Prescott, M. R., Goldmann, E., Tamburrino, M., Calabrese, J. R., Liberzon, I., & Galea, S. (2015). The prevalence and correlates of risky driving behavior among National Guard soldiers. *Traffic Injury Prevention, 16*(1), 17–23. doi:10.10 80/15389588.2014.896994

James, L. M., PhD., Strom, T. Q., PhD., & Leskela, J., PhD. (2014). Risk-taking behaviors and impulsivity among veterans with and without PTSD and mild TBI. *Military Medicine, 179*(4), 357–63. Retrieved from http://search.proquest.com.jproxy.lib. ecu.edu/docview/1522546540?accountid=10639

Junger, S. (2016). Tribe: On homecoming and belonging. New York: Hachette Book Group.

Kick, K. A., & McNitt, M. (2016). Trauma, spirituality, and mindfulness: Finding hope. *Social Work and Christianity, 43*(3), 97–108. Retrieved from http://search.proquest. com.jproxy.lib.ecu.edu/docview/1814147606?accountid=10639

Kintzle, S., Schuyler, A. C., Ray-Letourneau, D., Ozuna, S. M., Munch, C., Xintarianos, E., & Castro, C. A. (2015). Sexual trauma in the military: Exploring PTSD and mental health care utilization in female veterans. *Psychological Services, 12*(4), 394–401. doi: 10.1037/ser0000054

LeardMann, C. A., Powell, T. M., Smith, T. C., Bell, M. R., Smith, B., Boyko, E. J., Hoge, C. W. (2013). Risk factors associated with suicide in current and former US military personnel. *Jama, 310*(5), 496–506. doi:10.1001/jama.2013.65164

Martin, R. L., Houtsma, C., Green, B. A., & Anestis, M. D. (2016). Support systems: How post-deployment support impacts suicide risk factors in the United States army national guard. *Cognitive Therapy and Research, 40*(1), 14–21. doi:http://dx.doi.org.jproxy.lib.ecu.edu/10.1007/s10608-015-9719-z

McCulloch, K. L., Cecchini, A. S., Radomski, M. V., Scherer, M. R., Smith, L., Cleveland, C., ...Weightman, M. M. (2017). Military-civilian collaborations for MTBI rehabilitation research in an active duty population: Lessons learned from the assessment of military multitasking performance project. *The Journal of Head Trauma Rehabilitation, 32*(1), 70-78. doi:10.1097/HTR.0000000000000272

Military One Source. (2017). Understanding your benefits as a lesbian or gay couple in the military. Retrieved from http://www.militaryonesource.mil/health-wellness?content_id=271888

Moody, E.E., & Trogdon, D. (2016). First aid for your emotional hurts: Veterans. Nashville, TN: Randall House.

Mundell, B. F., Friedberg, M. W., Eibner, C., & Mundell, W. C. (2013). US military primary care: Problems, solutions, and implications for civilian medicine. *Health Affairs, 32*(11), 1949–55. Retrieved from http://search.proquest.com.jproxy.lib.ecu.edu/docview/1458312779?accountid=10639

O'Neil, M., Carlson, K., Storzbach, D., Brenner, L., Freeman, M., Quinones, A., ...Kansagara, D. (2013). Complications of Mild Traumatic Brain Injury in Veterans and Military Personnel: A Systematic Review [Internet]. Washington (DC): Department of Veterans Affairs (US); Appendix C, Definition of Mtbi from the Va/Dod Clinical Practice Guideline for Management of Concussion/Mild Traumatic Brain Injury (2009) Retrieved from https://www.ncbi.nlm.nih.gov/books/NBK189784/

Padden, D., & Posey, S. M. (2013). Caring for military spouses in primary care. *Journal of the American Association of Nurse Practitioners, 25*(3), 141.

Pincus, S.H., House, R., Christensen, J., & Adler, L.E. (2001). The emotional cycle of deployment: A military family perspective. *U.S. Army Medical Department Journal, 415*(6), 15–23.

Pivar, I. (2004). Traumatic grief: Symptomology and treatment for Iraq war veterans. Retrieved from https://www.ptsd.va.gov/professional/manuals/manual-pdf/iwcg/iraq_clinician_guide_ch_11.pdf

Prins, A., Bovin, M. J., Smolenski, D. J., Mark, B. P., Kimerling, R., Jenkins-Guarnieri, M. A., ... & Tiet, Q. Q. (2016). The Primary Care PTSD Screen for DSM-5 (PC-PTSD-5): Development and evaluation within a veteran primary care sample. *Journal of General Internal Medicine, 31*, 1206-1211. doi:10.1007/s11606-016-3703-5

Reserve Force Policy Board. (2016). Improving the total force by using the National Guard and Reserves. Retrieved from http://rfpb.defense.gov/Portals/67/Documents/Improving%20the%20Total%20Force%20using%20the%20National%20Guard%20and%20Reserves_1%20November%202016.pdf?ver=2016-11-17-142718-243

Rhon, D. I., Lentz, T. A., & George, S. Z. (2016). Unique contributions of body diagram scores and psychosocial factors to pain intensity and disability in patients with musculoskeletal pain in a military primary care clinic. *Journal of Orthopaedic & Sports Physical Therapy*, 1–24. doi:10.2519/jospt.2017.6778

Summerall, E.L. (2017). Traumatic brain injury and PTSD. Retrieved from https://www.ptsd.va.gov/professional/co-occurring/traumatic-brain-injury-ptsd.asp

Teasdale, G., & Jennett, B. (1974). Assessment of coma and impaired consciousness: A practical scale. *The Lancet, 304*(7872), 81–84.

Tennyson, A. (1854). Charge of the light brigade. Retrieved from https://www.poets.org/poetsorg/poem/charge-light-brigade

Uniform Code of Military Justice art. [120] (45b). Retrieved from http://www.ucmj.us/sub-chapter-10-punitive-articles/920-article-120-rape-and-carnal-knowledge

United States Department of Defense. (2017) Sexual Assault Prevention and Response Office. Retrieved from www.sapr.mil

United States Department of Defense (2017). Traumatic brain injury. Retrieved from https://www.defense.gov/News/Special-Reports/0315_tbi

U.S. Department of Veterans Affairs. (2015). Management of substance use disorders. Retrieved from https://www.healthquality.va.gov/guidelines/MH/sud/VADoDSUD-CPGPocketcardScreeningandTreatmentRevised12716.pdf

U.S. Department of Veterans Affairs. (2016). VA research on suicide. Retrieved from https://www.research.va.gov/pubs/docs/va_factsheets/SuicidePrevention.pdf

U.S. Department of Veterans Affairs. (2017). Military sexual trauma. Retrieved from https://www.mentalhealth.va.gov/msthome/asp

UNITED STATES CODE. (2012). 5 U.S.C. 3331 - OATH OF OFFICE. Retrieved from https://www.gpo.gov/fdsys/pkg/USCODE-2011-title5/pdf/USCODE-2011-title5-partIII-subpartB-chap33-subchapII-sec3331.pdf

Westphal, R. J., & Convoy, S. P. (2015). Military culture implications for mental health and nursing care. *Online Journal of Issues in Nursing, 20*(1), 47–54. Retrieved from http://search.proquest.com.jproxy.lib.ecu.edu/docview/1710044007?accountid=10639

Whelan, J. (2016). *Ghosts in the Ranks.* Victoria, BC: FriesenPress.

Xue, C., Ge, Y., Tang, B., Liu, Y., Kang, P., Wang, M., & Zhang, L. (2015). A meta-analysis of risk factors for combat-related PTSD among military personnel and veterans. *PloS One, 10*(3), e0120270. doi:10.1371/journal.pone.0120270

## CHAPTER 10

# Chronic Disease

SUSAN R. ALLEN, PhD, RN-BC

## Chronic Disease

CHRONIC DISEASE, also known as a chronic illness or chronic condition, is a health state that persists over a period of time. The condition may be treatable, leading to improved health in an individual with the disease, but it is typically not curable. The treatments for chronic disease can be simple to complex and relatively inexpensive to very costly. Chronic conditions may or may not impact quality of life. The number of people living with one or more chronic conditions in the United States (U.S.) and around the world continues to increase. In fact, as mortality rates among at risk populations drop, the number of people living with chronic conditions will increase.

## The Facts about Chronic Disease in the United States

According to the Centers for Disease Control and Prevention (CDC), the leading causes of disability and death in this country are chronic diseases (Centers for Disease Control and Prevention, 2017). In 2012, seven of the 10 top causes of death in the United States were chronic diseases. The term *chronic disease population* is actually an inclusive term that is used to broadly capture the many chronic diseases that exist in our society and markedly impact the overall health of our nation. Most chronic diseases are well known to both healthcare providers and the American public because of their high prevalence. These conditions include heart disease, stroke, cancer, type 2 diabetes, obesity, respiratory illness, and arthritis. Because many of these chronic diseases are preventable by reducing health risk behaviors, the potential impact of advanced practice nurses (APNs) in improving population health outcomes in this area may be limitless.

The CDC (2017) reported that nearly half of adults living in the United States in 2012 had at least one chronic disease, and 25% of adults had two or more chronic conditions. Heart disease and cancer together account for almost half of the deaths in the United States. The problem of obesity continues to increase; 78 million people, more than a third of American adults, are clinically defined as obese, with a body mass index [BMI] $\geq$ 30 kg/m$^2$. Obesity is also beginning at a younger age; nearly 20% of youth from 2 to 19 years of age are obese. The major consequences of obesity are two chronic conditions: cardiovascular disease and type 2 diabetes. Unfortunately, these two conditions frequently precipitate other chronic illnesses. For example, diabetes can lead to vascular disease, neuropathies, renal failure, and blindness. Another chronic condition, arthritis, causes more disability than any other chronic health problem by limiting the physical activities of individuals living with this condition (Centers for Disease Control and Prevention, 2017).

People with chronic diseases use healthcare resources to manage their conditions and prevent additional complications. The Centers for Medicare and Medicaid Services (CMS) noted that healthcare spending in the United States reached $3.2 trillion in 2015, or $9,990 per individual (Centers for Medicare and Medicaid Services, 2015). The costs of chronic disease management, and the health risk behaviors that may lead to these conditions, were reported to be 86% of the healthcare expenses in the United States in 2010 (Centers for Disease Control and Prevention, 2016). Health risk behaviors that can trigger chronic diseases are common in American society. These behaviors include poor nutrition, tobacco use, limited physical exercise, smoking and other tobacco uses, drug abuse, and heavy alcohol consumption. Health risk behaviors are preventable and, when present in an individual, may be reduced or eliminated through targeted counseling or treatment.

APNs, public health officials, and other healthcare providers must be knowledgeable about chronic diseases, their impact on those individuals with these conditions and on their caregivers, and their current and future impact on healthcare resources. More importantly, APNs must be well informed of the ways in which chronic diseases can be prevented or, when chronic conditions are present, how they can be successfully managed.

## The Impact of Chronic Conditions in the United States

The impact of chronic diseases on population health in the United States is staggering. The number of individuals living with chronic illnesses in the United States continues to grow and will do so for the foreseeable future. People are living longer because of improvements in medical treatment and other supportive therapies. For example, the number of children with chronic disease has increased significantly in the past four decades. From 1994 to 2006 alone, the number of children with chronic conditions more than doubled (Focus for Health, 2016). Many of these children are survivors of conditions that were fatal in the past but for which there are currently treatments, including cancer, heart disease, and the complications of prematurity. The number of children and youth with chronic disease continues to grow, and African American and Hispanic children are disproportionately impacted with these conditions (Van Cleave, J., Gortmaker, S. L., & Perrin, 2010).

The U.S. population is also aging, and the development of chronic conditions is often part of the natural aging process. The segment of the U.S. population known as the *baby boomers* comprise individuals born from 1945 to 1964 and is the largest population segment. This group is heavily influencing the rapid growth of those 65 years and older in the U.S. population. In 2016, the baby boomer generation was 52 to 70 years old (Mather, Jacobsen, & Pollard, 2015). In 2014, the U.S. Department of Human and Health Services Administration on Aging (U.S. Department of Health and Human Services Administration on Aging, 2016) reported that 46.2 million people were 65 years or older, or 14.5% of the population in this country. It is estimated that this number will double by 2060 to 98 million in this age group. In 2060, this group of older adults will be 21.7% of the population. In 2014, older consumers averaged out-of-pocket healthcare expenditures of $5,849, an increase of 50% since 2004. In contrast, the total population spent considerably less, averaging $4,290 in out-of-pocket costs. Older Americans spent 13.4% of their total expenditures on health compared with 8% among all consumers (U.S. Department of Health and Human Services Administration on Aging, 2016).

As stated earlier in this chapter, the most common chronic diseases and conditions in the United States in 2012 were heart disease, stroke, cancer, type 2 diabetes, obesity, respiratory illness, and arthritis (Centers for Disease Control and Prevention, 2016). Although the incidence of chronic disease increases as a person ages, chronic conditions do not impact only older people. There are individuals of all ages with chronic conditions, including infants, children, teenagers, and young adults. The rates of the major chronic diseases in the United States are not static, and the number of people with chronic conditions continue to increase. The death rates from these conditions also continue to change. For example, the death rate from dementia and its most common form, Alzheimer's disease, is increasing, whereas deaths from heart disease and cancer are declining (Centers for Disease Control and Prevention, 2016). A chronic disease affects not only the person with the condition, but also the family members, care providers, and communities in which the person lives. There is no aspect of the healthcare system in the United States that has not felt the impact of the growth of chronic disease. The social and financial burdens of chronic disease are significant and increasing. Care management across the continuum of care may assist in reducing the impact and burden of chronic disease and conditions and may lead to improvements in population health. Chronic disease impacts the entire family, whether grief over loss of health, impact on work capabilities, loss of income, or added cost for medical expenses.

## Chronic Care Management and the Continuum of Care

To manage chronic conditions effectively, the days of provider-centered, segmented care must end. Individuals with chronic conditions, especially those with comorbidities, access our healthcare systems for numerous reasons and in many ways. These systems include acute care hospitals, primary and specialty care office settings, urgent care and emergency departments, skilled nursing and rehabilitation facilities, and home care. The lack of coordination across these settings due to insufficient structures and ineffective processes for communication can be detrimental to any patient. A lack of well-coordinated care can be especially harmful to individuals with chronic conditions as they attempt to navigate the systems in which they receive care. The impact of the current and future incidences of chronic diseases is described in this chapter. Comprehensive health services must be available and accessible to treat individuals with these conditions, promote stabilization and remission, and prevent complications and the development of comorbidities.

The Institute of Medicine's (IOM's) report, *The Future of Nursing: Leading Change, Advancing Health* (2010), called for nurses to shape the future of healthcare by creating innovative patient-centered programs across the continuum of care. The IOM report asserted that no profession was better prepared to lead this critically important work. Nurses currently practice in settings throughout the healthcare continuum. Nurses are uniquely knowledgeable, not only about existing resources to manage care, but also about how to access and assist patients with using these resources. Nurses have long been the facilitators of patient transitions in care, and their experience in doing so has equipped them to meet the growing need for improved care management and a patient-centered continuum of care. However, the doctor of nursing practice–prepared (DNP-prepared) nurse cannot accomplish this without effective interprofessional partnerships across the continuum of care. If each discipline remains in its own silo without shared interprofessional decision making, very little will be accomplished to move patient care and the population health forward. The DNP-prepared nurse is poised to lead this challenging effort to improve healthcare delivery.

## Preventive Care in Chronic Conditions

Preventive care is typically directed toward reducing or eliminating the risk of an individual developing a disease or health condition. In patients with existing chronic conditions, the focus of preventive care is to reduce or eliminate the complications or comorbidities of the known disease. Preventive care of chronic disease requires the provider's knowledge of the early signs and symptoms of complications and of ongoing attentive screening to identify the development of any complications or comorbidities. Effective preventive care in chronic disease management requires a patient-provider partnership (Wiggins, 2008). Effective partnerships across the continuum of care are illustrated in the chronic care model.

## The Chronic Care Model

In their seminal article on improving chronic illness care, Wagner *et al.* (2001) proposed a care model that has been widely adopted by providers caring for individuals with chronic conditions. These authors identified that care delivery models at the beginning of the 21st century were primarily focused on *sick care*, or the care of acutely ill individuals. Healthcare systems were organized to respond to, and care for, any patient that came to their facility with an illness or injury that needed treatment by a care provider. Wagner and had his colleagues had an important insight. They noted that in an acute care model, patients are dependent on the care provider for diagnosis and treatment. In other words, patients are in a generally passive role in the acute care setting. Wagner et al. (2001) suggested care delivery systems must be redesigned to better meet the needs of chronically ill patients. They argued that the needs of chronic care patients were markedly different than those of acute care patients. In addition to the need for the actual treatment of their chronic condition's symptoms and disabilities, patients also require support for the following (Wagner et al., 2001):

- The emotional impact of having a chronic disease
- Dealing with complex medical regimens
- Lifestyle changes, some of which could be significant
- Accessing the resources they need to manage their disease

Additionally, patient dependence and passivity does not lead to effective management of a chronic disease. Minimally, the foundation of effective chronic disease management is a true partnership between the provider and patient, rather than a dependent relationship (Wiggins, 2008). The characteristics of this kind of partnership include support to create patient confidence and independence, mutual respect, and increased collaboration to manage the condition by decreasing provider control (Lawn, Delaney, Sweet, Battersby, & Skinner, 2013). Optimally, the patient with a chronic condition is a knowledgeable and actively engaged owner of his or her care, who partners with providers to access the resources and expertise needed to effectively manage his or her chronic condition (Improving Chronic Illness Care, 2017). How this can be achieved will be discussed in a later section of this chapter.

Chronic care models have been developed to illustrate the essential factors in chronic care management. An example of a chronic care model that was first published in 1998, and continues to be in widespread use today, is Wagner's Chronic Care Model (Wagner, 1998; Wagner et al., 2001). As was discussed in Chapter 2, the use of big data from clinical information systems and access to decision support resources are necessary to effectively care for individuals with chronic disease. Although individualized care remains vitally important for each patient, care providers must also be analyzing the effectiveness of specific treatment interventions for populations of patients with chronic conditions. Finally, sufficient community resources must be in place or developed, with the accompanying health policies and funding to support and sustain their existence. The model can be viewed at http://www.improving-chroniccare.org/index.php?p=The_Chronic_CareModel&s=2

## Chronic Care and the DNP-Prepared Advanced Practice Nurse

DNP-prepared nurses are uniquely well qualified to lead the care of individuals with chronic conditions. Fundamentally, the nursing perspective is broader and more inclusive than that of other care providers. The metaparadigm of nursing considers the person, their health, and the environment in relationship with the nurse, acknowledging the influences within and among each of these dimensions. Nurses care holistically for their patients and families, doing more than medically treating or providing technical skills. Nurses provide family-centered care and emotional support and coordinate of all aspects of care. Nurses acknowledge and respect that patients with chronic conditions are more than just their conditions. Nurses recognize that each patient is also a family member, a community member, and often an employee, student, or retiree. Nurses are aware of the influences of the social determinants of health and find and respect the strengths that each patient brings to providing their own self-care. When a patient is not able to care for his or her own needs, nurses identify and establish the supportive structures needed for effective care management. This holistic nursing perspective supports both the development of an effective provider-patient partnership and the coordination of care across the continuum. The DNP-prepared nurse leader must ensure these broader and inclusive perspective influences decisions made regarding the management of care for individuals with chronic conditions.

## Care Coordination and Care Management

In the Institute of Medicine's (IOM's) 2004 report, it was noted that nurses are the profession consistently responsible for the surveillance and "rescue" of patients regardless of the setting of care delivery and are accountable for the coordination and integration of patient care wherever healthcare is delivered (Institute of Medicine, 2004). Care coordination is the everyday work of a nurse; it is a basic competency of nursing practice. Care management, sometimes referred to as case management, is a term that is frequently used to describe care coordination for individuals with chronic conditions. Care management occurs across a continuum, not only across healthcare settings, but also into the community. Care management approaches for an individual patient are driven by the patient's healthcare needs because of the chronic condition; however, the patient's needs due to behavioral, social, and financial influences within his or her environment should also be considered. Care management occurs within an environment that is increasingly interprofessional, with members of different disciplines working together to meet the needs of the patient.

Within healthcare settings, patients with chronic conditions may be stratified, using tools designed for this purpose, to determine the level of care coordination and management that is needed for each patient. An example of a risk stratification tool is the LACE Index Scoring Tool for Risk Assessment of Death and Readmission (Van Walraven *et al.*, 2010), which can be used to predict a patient's risk for readmission following discharge from an acute care setting. Within the ambulatory setting, stratification levels are assigned to patients based on the complexity of the chronic condition, the number of comorbidities, the capacity of family or a social support network structure to support the patient in the community, and their financial means, including health insurance. Based on the risk stratification level, the patient is provided with additional care managers or other resource personnel to ensure all areas of the individual's needs can be supported.

### Nursing Leadership in Chronic Care

Nursing leadership is critical to creating improvements in healthcare (Institute of Medicine, 2010). The *Future of Nursing* report concludes that changes in nursing education, practice, and leadership must take place for there to be continued progress in healthcare. This report also states most nurses do not begin their careers with the thought of being a leader, but nursing leadership must be present for essential improvements in our healthcare systems to occur. The IOM argues that nursing leadership is needed at every level of an organization and across all healthcare settings (Institute of Medicine, 2010). As was stated earlier, care management is an interprofessional effort. Within any team, even those working toward a common goal, leadership is needed. Nurses can step up to fulfill this need. Because care coordination is a basic competency of nursing practice, and because of nursing's holistic perspective, nurses are well suited to be leaders of interprofessional teams caring for patients with chronic conditions.

The DNP-prepared advanced practice nurse (APN) has been academically prepared as a leader to create and oversee the chronic care health delivery systems and structures that must be in place for efficient and effective care management (American Association of Colleges of Nursing, 2006). This includes acquisition of the resources that are needed to accomplish the work of care management; that is, the workforce, physical space, information technology, and healthcare policies. The DNP has the knowledge and skills to ensure programmatic and structural quality and to lead improvement projects to advance programs to meet evolving needs. The DNP also has the background and ability to be a community leader in chronic care management through networking and advocacy to achieve and improve population health outcomes (American Association of Colleges of Nursing, 2006).

## Issues in Chronic Disease Management

### Social Determinants of Health

It is essential for individuals in advanced nursing practice roles to be aware of and consider the impact of the social determinants of health. Application of this knowledge is essential when caring for patients with chronic diseases. For individuals to achieve the highest level of health for whatever chronic conditions they may have, DNP-prepared nurses require a broader perspective beyond the actual health condition. They must recognize that the health system itself can no longer be viewed as capable of providing the entire solution for a patient's care needs. The patient with a chronic disease must be assessed within the context of the environment in which he or she lives. Social determinants of health include gender, race, income, economic stability, level of education, housing, and physical location. The World Health Organization (WHO) defines the social determinants of health as, "the conditions in which people are born, grow, live, work and age," and notes that they are primarily responsible for the health inequities that exist globally (WHO, 2012a; WHO, 2012b).

Chronic diseases disproportionately impact individuals who are socially disadvantaged. This is thought to be, at least in part, related to the stress-related biological processes that are present in people living in difficult circumstances (Lathrop, 2013). Lathrop also notes that people who are economically secure have better access to resources that assist them in managing their chronic conditions. The economically disadvantaged often have less access to care, lack the financial resources to afford their medications, have diminished availability of healthy foods, and live in an unsafe environment for physical activity, all of which are necessary to successfully manage a chronic condition. Whether directly caring for socially disadvantaged patients, or leading others in the care of these vulnerable populations, the DNP-prepared APN must be aware of these concerns and act to improve health equity (Lathrop, 2013).

*Access to Care*

Access to quality healthcare remains a major concern in the United States. After the implementation of the Patient Protection and Affordable Care Act (also referred to as the Affordable Care Act, or ACA), the number of uninsured adult Americans began to decline for the first time in more than a decade (Agency for Healthcare Research and Quality, 2014). Despite this fact, racial and ethnic disparities in the access to care continues (Caldwell, Ford, Wallace, Wang, & Takahashi, 2016). These authors report that African Americans and Hispanics overall have less access to care and poorer quality care than their white counterparts, and this is especially true for persons living in rural areas.

Access to healthcare is a multifactorial problem and is not caused only by a lack of health insurance coverage. Syed, Gerber, & Sharp (2013) conducted a systematic review of the literature, examining 61 peer-reviewed studies on transportation barriers to accessing care. Transportation was noted to be a basic but necessary factor in managing healthcare; it was found that patients with transportation barriers were often living in poverty. A lack of transportation resulted in the inability to receive appropriate healthcare services and delays in the treatment of chronic disease exacerbations which, in turn, led to worsening of existing chronic conditions, additional comorbidities and, ultimately, a decline in overall patient outcomes (Syed *et al.*, 2013). Transportation barriers led to late or missed clinic appointments and the inability to obtain the medications required for care of the chronic condition. Transportation barriers were found to more prevalent in the pediatric, elderly, and veteran populations (Syed, *et al.* 2013).

*Financial Resources*

The cost of managing a chronic disease can be staggering (Centers for Disease Control and Prevention, 2016). Patients with these conditions can quickly be overwhelmed with concerns about the costs and the overall impact on their financial security. Although nurses have a broad knowledge base and skillfully provide holistic care, there is opportunity to reach out to interprofessional team members who may be excellent partners in assisting patients to deal with the financial burden of having a chronic condition. Social workers have in-depth knowledge of available financial resources and the processes to access these resources that can assist a patient and his or her family to successfully cope with the costs of a chronic condition. Financial resources include governmental, foundation, and philanthropic support that may be accessed at the local, state and federal levels. Additionally, healthcare facilities may also have individuals in financial advising roles to assist patients with managing their healthcare insurance claims and establishing payment plans when needed.

## Community Resources and Support

The expression *It takes a village* is certainly applicable in the care of patients with chronic diseases. Resources in the community can be accessed to provide support to patients in the daily management of their chronic condition. Community health workers (CHWs) can have a meaningful role as frontline health workers at the most common place that care occurs, in the patient's home (Allen, Escoffery, Satsangi, & Brownstein, 2015). Efforts have been growing to legitimize the importance of CHWs as community partners to provide support to interprofessional teams and patients in the prevention, management, and control of chronic disease. This is most important for diverse populations and high-need individuals. Community health workers can bring real world insights to the interprofessional team. As members of the community, they can provide context needed to understand the concerns of the patient and the care team. They can be the bridge between healthcare and the community and are also able to provide culturally and linguistically meaningful health education, support adherence to self-care, and participate in case management and care coordination for people with chronic conditions (Allen, *et al.* 2015).

Numerous chronic disease-specific organizations are available in local and regional communities who have volunteers, often with the same chronic or family members with the conditions, to assist and encourage individuals in the care of their health. These organizations are also strong partners in the provision of education to patients and self-care management education materials for patients and professionals. Additional sources of community support for patients and their families is through patient to patient and family to family connections with the same chronic condition. These connections are generally facilitated by community disease-specific organizations or the family advisory boards of healthcare facilities. In pediatric chronic diseases, there may be healthcare provider staffed week-long summer camps that can be accessed for children and youth. These camps provide an opportunity for children with chronic conditions to have a true peer experience in how to manage their conditions and give the parents a week of respite from managing care at home. As a parent who had a child with diabetes said, *"It's the only week of the year that I can actually sleep without listening for a bed to shake indicating my son was having a hypoglycemic attack."*

## Health Literacy

According to the U.S. Department of Education, 32 million adults in the United States cannot read; of those who can read do so on average at a 7th to 8th grade level. This leads to a significant issue with health literacy in the United States. Health literacy is an individual's ability to find, read, and comprehend health information and obtain the services he or she needs to make informed decisions about his or her health. It is estimated that over 90 million adults in this country lack health literacy because they do not have sufficient understanding of human biology, how diseases impact the body, and how lifestyle behaviors impact health outcomes (Eadie, 2014). Individuals with low health literacy are frequently unable to comply with verbal or written healthcare instructions. Low health literacy can lead to poor management of a chronic disease, problems with medication adherence, and, consequently, an increased need for additional healthcare services (Eadie, 2014). Certain demographic groups, such as the elderly, lower socioeconomic status, and individuals for whom English is the second language, may be at higher risk for health literacy concerns (Tamura-Lis, 2013).

It is important for DNP-prepared APNs to ensure that nurses and care providers with whom they work understand and appreciate the impact low health literacy may have on all patients, but especially those with chronic conditions. Those caring for chronic disease patients must learn ways to identify these individuals, by familiarizing themselves with the behaviors they may see to detect health literacy concerns and by using the tools that are available to assess an individual's health literacy level (Lambert & Keogh, 2014). Teach-back is an educational method that can assist care providers in evaluating patients' understanding of how they should manage their care at home. The teach-back method will be described in the next section of this chapter.

## Innovations in Chronic Care Management

This chapter's section delineates promising innovative models and methods that have been successfully used in chronic disease management. The DNP-prepared APN can examine these models or methods for implementation in his or her practice when working with these populations.

### Interprofessional Care Model

Interprofessional care is essential in patients with chronic conditions. There is no single model for developing an interprofessional team or a procedure for successful implementation of an effective team. Actual multidisciplinary teams of individuals from a variety of disciplines have been in existence for quite some time; however, members of such teams frequently practiced in silos (Hurlock-Chorostecki, Forchuk, Orchard, Reeves, & van Soeren, 2013). Interprofessional team members practice in partnerships.

The actual process of interprofessional care is fluid, because each interprofessional care team is individually assembled to meet the physical, psychosocial, emotional, spiritual, financial, and/or community resource needs of a specific patient. Team members from various disciplines may enter the team as patient needs are discovered and leave as those needs are met. Some team members are continuous participants who are involved with managing the care of the patient as long as that patient is within a specific health system. In a constructivist, grounded theory research study, interprofessional teams led by a nurse practitioner were found to better understand the many aspects of a healthcare system, connect team members, and know and focus on the whole patient and family to provide better care (Hurlock-Chorostecki, *et al.* 2013).

### Patient- and Family-Centered Care Model

In patient- and family-centered care (PFCC), the relationships between healthcare providers and the patient and family are redefined (Institute for Patient- and Family-Centered Care, 2016; Institute for Patient- and Family-Centered Care, 2017). The patient and his or her family are viewed as allies in care. They become important and participatory members of the interprofessional team. Patients and families determine the members of their family and how each will participate in caring for the individual needing care. The collaborative partnerships that form in PFCC have been found to be mutually beneficial for everyone involved. In PFCC, there is an emphasis on care providers freely sharing information with the patient and family so decisions about care are made in partnership. This change in role relationships has led to increased ownership of care by the patient and his or her family and decreased dependence on the healthcare team.

The overall goal of PFCC is to promote the health and well-being of individuals and their families so they have increased autonomy and remain in control of their care. This perspective is based on recognition that patients and families are indispensable allies for all aspects of care. PFCC has been shown to lead to improved health outcomes, increased patient and family satisfaction with the experience of care, better care provider satisfaction, and cost savings due to better allocation of resources (Institute for Patient- and Family-Centered Care, 2017).

*Patient-Centered Medical Home Model*

As has been noted, no country in the world spends more dollars on healthcare for its citizens with too often poorer quality and worse outcomes than the United States (Agency for Healthcare Research and Quality, 2012). In recent years, the patient-centered medical home (PCMH) has been advanced as an effective approach to manage the care of patients with complex needs. As its name implies, a PCMH provides individualized care through partnerships with patients and their families to understand, value and, whenever possible, defer to each patient's unique needs, values, and culture (Agency for Healthcare Research and Quality, 2017). The five distinguishing characteristics of a PCMH are as follows (Agency for Healthcare Research and Quality, 2017):

- Comprehensive, relationship-based care provided by an interprofessional team that meets a large majority of the patient's needs.
- Patient-centered, holistic care with the goal of self-management at the level desired by the patient and family.
- Coordinated care across all elements of a healthcare system and into the community through clear and open communication.
- Accessible services with shorter care appointment wait times and 24-hour resource contact and communication availability through telephone and email.

- Quality and safety improvements using evidence-based care and clinical decision support tools.

Individuals with chronic conditions generally use more healthcare services than the average person, see a larger number and wider variety of healthcare providers, and receive care at multiple healthcare facilities (Agency for Healthcare Research and Quality, 2011). This often leads to fragmented care and an increased risk for missed communications between care providers. Although additional research and evaluation are needed, the PCMH model for care has shown promise to provide improved quality care at lower costs (Agency for Healthcare Research and Quality, 2013).

## The Motivational Interviewing Method

In the relatively recent past, there was increased recognition that the common practice of providing information and education on how to manage a chronic condition did not often achieve the health outcomes desired by the care provider. Simply telling an individual what they needed to do from the perspective of the expert care provider did not lead to the behavioral changes that were needed for a patient to effectively manage his or her condition (Linden, Butterworth, & Prochaska, 2010).

Motivational interviewing is a patient-centered process in which the care provider partners with the patient to determine the health goals the patient would like to achieve. Its focus is to assist the patient to explore and resolve the ambivalence he or she may have about adopting or changing behaviors to improve his or her health condition. Motivational interviewing is a health coaching technique in which the patient chooses the health behavior he or she would like to improve or the unhealthful behavior he or she could reduce or eliminate. Once identified, the patient and care provider work together to set short-term goals for behavioral change and clinical improvement. To learn how to use motivational interviewing when working with patients with chronic diseases, care providers need didactic education and simulated interviewing to gain competence and confidence in using this approach to selfmanagement goal setting. Research in motivational interviewing has shown positive clinical outcomes and healthcare utilization and costs (Linden *et al.* 2010).

## The Teach-Back Education Method

The widespread prevalence of low health literacy in the United

States was described in the previous section of this chapter. The teach-back approach has been used to evaluate the patient's understanding of the education content he or she has received to manage his or her care at home. During the teach-back method in the clinical setting, the care provider does the following (TamuraLis, 2013):

- Speaks slowly and uses plain language, communicating in short statements
- Supports verbal instructional content with illustrations
- Discusses only two or three key concepts
- Checks for understanding by requesting the patient ay what he or she just learned in his or her own words

Following the patient's expression of his or her learning, the care provider rephrases or provides additional information for the key areas that were not heard or only partially understood. If the patient repeats the content accurately, the care provider reinforces the self-management information. Teach-back methods are important to use in a variety of clinical settings, but especially in situations involving patients with chronic conditions and their families. In this case, these individuals will be managing their care at home away from the healthcare setting and for the remainder of their lifetimes.

**A Broader View**

The profession of nursing has emphasized the need for individualized patient care for several decades. As can be seen throughout this chapter, this approach continues to be of paramount importance when caring for patients with chronic conditions. However, a broader view is also needed when managing from the population health perspective. Care interventions can also be implemented across chronic disease populations.

Lail, Schoettker, White, Mehta, and Kotagal (2017) reported the results of a chronic conditions outcomes improvement initiative in a pediatric healthcare organization in the Midwest. In this initiative, over 27,000 patients with chronic diseases who were cared for by 18 interprofessional teams were followed over a three-year period. Their methods included review of the literature to determine evidence-based outcomes, the use of condition-specific patient registries within the electronic health record to evaluate population outcomes, patient stratification to provide the appropriate level of care management, inter-professional team huddles to plan and coordinate care before and after clinic visits, and self-management support. Over 13,600 of the patients in this quality improvement initiative had at least one improved outcome. The outcomes included clinical, functional, and patient-reported improvements (Lail, *et al.* 2017). This study illustrates the power of the broader view of population health management.

## Summary

In this chapter, the societal and financial impact of chronic disease in the United States was examined. The use of the chronic care model across the continuum of care was explored. Special issues in chronic disease management that should be recognized and attended to for successful management of chronic conditions were discussed. Finally, promising innovations to improve the management of chronic diseases were described. Nursing leadership in chronic disease management is essential. In 2016, a follow-up report to the Institute of Medicine's (2010) The Future of Nursing: Leading Change, Advancing Health recommends increased nursing leadership in the redesign of care delivery and payment systems; it was noted that nursing's unique perspective is essential for continued progress in healthcare (Altman, Butler & Shern, 2016). Once again, this new report stressed that additional nursing leadership is needed all levels of healthcare systems, from the bedside to the boardroom (Institute of Medicine, 2010). It was determined there has not been a sufficient increase in nursing leadership to influence health policy decision making (Altman, *et al.* 2016). Linda Burns Bolton, DrPH, RN, FAAN, the vice chair for the Committee on the Robert Woods Johnson Foundation Initiative on the Future of Nursing at the Institute of Medicine, stated this in 2011 at a keynote address presented at the annual convention of the National Nursing Staff Development Organization (Bolton, 2011):

> "If nurses would stand up and lead,
> and society would recognize nurses for what they are,
> we would improve the quality of, and transform healthcare . . .
> nurses must live up to being the most trusted profession,
> they must do more."

The DNP-prepared APN is poised to do just that and to stand up and lead to fill these needs.

## Tool Kit and Resources

*Chronic Diseases*: https://www.cdc.gov/chronicdisease/, https://www.
nih.gov/health-information

*Diabetes*: https://www.diabeteseducator.org/, http://www.diabetes.org/,
http://www.jdrf.org/t1d-resources/

*Hypertension, Congestive Heart Failure, Stroke*: http://www.heart.org/
HEARTORG/

*Cancer*: https://www.cancer.org/

*Kidney Diseases*: https://www.kidney.org/kidneydisease

*Alzheimer's Disease and Dementia*: http://www.alz.org/

*Pulmonary Diseases*: http://www.lung.org/

*Definitions*

*Care Management*—Care coordination for individuals with chronic
conditions that occurs across the continuum of care; also referred to
as case management.

*Chronic Disease*—A health state that persists over a period of time; also
known as a chronic illness or chronic condition.

*Continuum of Care*—The delivery of health services across an integrated system of healthcare facilities that provide all levels of healthcare;
i.e., primary care, acute care ambulatory follow-up care, rehabilitation services, and community services.

*Family-Centered Care*—A partnership approach to the provision of
healthcare decision making between the patient and his or her family
and the care provider.

*Health Literacy*—An individual's ability to find, read, and comprehend
health information and to obtain the services they need to make informed decisions about their health.

*Interprofessional Care Providers*—Licensed professional care providers (nursing, medicine, audiology, nutrition, child life therapy,
speech pathology, respiratory therapy, social work, pharmacy, physical therapy, occupational therapy, recreational therapy, and spiritual
and integrative therapies) working in partnership to care for patients
and their families, populations, and communities.

*Patient-Centered Medical Home*—Provision of individualized care
through partnerships with patients and their families to understand,
value and, whenever possible, defer to each patient's unique needs,

values, and culture. In a PCMH, comprehensive, relationship-based care is provided by an interprofessional team that meets a large majority of the patient's needs (Agency for Healthcare Research and Quality, 2017).

## Discussion Questions

1. What is the relationship between the social determinants of health and chronic disease outcomes? Choose a chronic disease and discuss an in-depth examination of these relationships.

2. The concept of a patient-centered medical home (PCMH) was described in this chapter. Discuss the ways in which the PCMH can improve management of a patient with multiple chronic conditions.

3. In this chapter, you learned chronic diseases are not limited to adult populations. They also impact children, and the number of children with chronic diseases is increasing. Consider and discuss the impact of chronic disease on the developmental needs of children.

4. Health literacy is a major factor in the successful self-management of chronic diseases. What are the implications of health illiteracy in managing chronic illnesses? Discuss how an individual's health literacy level should be determined and give interventions that are needed to support individuals with low health literacy.

## Assignments

- Design a community awareness plan for a chronic disease and target population of your choice. Include an implementation and evaluation plan.

- Develop a lobbying plan for a state legislative bill to increase funding for low-income communities with high rates of chronic diseases.

- Compare and contrast the rates and outcomes of chronic diseases in a minimum of five racial and ethnic groups in the United States and globally. Investigate and discuss reasons for these differences. Discuss the impact of access to healthcare on the chronic disease outcomes.

## Case Study 1

### Care Management in a Patient with Diabetes

Mr. D, a 62-year-old homeless male with lean body habitus, arrives at the hospital emergency department (ED). He states he is homeless and living in his car and has not seen his primary care provider for four years. He does not have a glucometer and says he has not taken his finger stick blood sugar for three years. Mr. D also mentions has not been eating because of his financial situation. He discontinued his metformin and all other medications four years ago. He states he has had type 2 diabetes for 15 years. Mr. D also reports he has a history of hypertension, hyperlipidemia, and a major depressive disorder. He indicates he smokes three packs of cigarettes daily.

Mr. D is admitted to the hospital with depression, suicidal ideation, and hyperglycemia with a glycated hemoglobin (A1c) of 13.0%. There was no evidence of retinopathy on physical examination. He has thickened toenails and a blister on his left plantar fifth toe. His anthropometric data are height 69 inches, weight 147 lb, and BMI 23.19 kg/m$^2$.

A consultation was immediately made to a primary care provider and a podiatrist. Diabetes socks were ordered. Mr. D received diabetes education from the inpatient nurse practitioner/diabetes educator (NPDE) before discharge to a shelter. A glucometer and glucometer supplies were ordered, and he was instructed on their use. Mr. D stopped smoking in the hospital and continued after discharge. He was discharged on basal/bolus insulin; Lantus 24 units once daily at the same time each evening; aspart insulin 6 units with meals, and metformin 500 mg twice a day.

Mr. D returned to for a follow-up appointment with the NPDE while waiting for his primary care appointment. He saw the podiatrist afterwards and received a consult for diabetes shoes. He was provided with nutrition education on how to eat healthy in the shelter.

A week later, Mr. D's blood glucose readings were 106 to 150 mg/dL. In three weeks, he was having low blood glucose readings in the 60s and 70s, and his insulin was reduced. A glutaminic acid decarboxy antibody test and an islet cell cytoplasm antibody test were ordered to check for type 1 diabetes. Mr. D tested positive on both laboratory tests. His metformin was discontinued after he was confirmed as a type 1 diabetes patient.

Mr. D's A1c reduced to 6.9% in 2.5 months and 5.7% in six months. The A1c goal range is under 7.0%. He transitioned to an apartment. Mr. D continues on basal/bolus insulin regimen and is now in good health.

Discuss the social determinants of health that influenced Mr. D's diabetes selfmanagement and need for hospitalization.

Mr. D received care from an interprofessional team while he was hospitalized. Considering his diagnoses on admission, what additional team members could have been involved in his care during his admission and as he transitioned back to the community? Why?

You are the care manager responsible for coordinating Mr. D's ongoing care after his return to the community. What support did he receive to assist him in managing his diabetes? What potential risk factors can you identify that may negatively affect his future health status? How will you mitigate these risk factors?

## Case Study 2

*Care Management in a Patient with Dementia*

Mrs. J, an 81-year-old woman with dementia and known hypertension, hyperlipidemia, and arthritis, was brought to her primary care physician's office by her daughter, who was accompanied by her elderly husband. Mrs. J and her husband lived independently in a retirement community. She was evaluated for vague symptoms of abdominal pain due to possible constipation. Neither Mrs. J nor her husband could remember the last time she had a bowel movement. After the physical examination was conducted, the primary physician ordered an abdominal x-ray. It revealed a possible mass in Mrs. J's lower right abdomen. She was immediately sent to the emergency department (ED) of a local hospital where the family had received care in the past.

In the ED, Mrs. J was referred to the oncall surgical and medical teams. Mrs. J did not understand her health condition, grew increasingly confused and frightened, and required sedation to complete the physical examinations. A computed tomography (CT) scan was ordered and showed a large mass wrapped around the distal end of the duodenum. The surgical team arrived soon after and recommended an immediate bowel resection of the distal duodenum and colon. They left quickly, saying they needed to get to the operating room to ensure a room was available for Mrs. J's surgery.

By this time, Mrs. J's three other children arrived at the ED. Her husband was upset, anxious, and said he was unable to make decisions about Mrs. J's care. The other family members were uncertain about how to move forward. The ED nurse caring for Mrs. J asked the medical doctor to come and speak with the family about treatment options to ensure their full understanding of the diagnosis, prognosis, and future care requirements. The nurse also invited the hospital chaplain to participate in the discussion. The care team had a frank discussion with the family about Mrs. J's potential outcomes so they could make informed decisions about the appropriate healthcare interventions for Mrs. J, also considering her age and dementia. After better understanding the probable outcomes of Mrs. J's healthcare needs and quality of life after the bowel resection, the family declined the surgery. Mrs. J was transferred to hospice care.

The receiving nurse and chaplain at the hospice facility had been fully informed of Mrs. J's history and the decisions made by the family, so they were able to immediately provide needed support and comfort to the family. The hospice care team partnered with the family to make decisions about palliative care measures that were in place to ensure Mrs. J's comfort during her remaining days. She had a peaceful death surrounded by the members of her family.

Think about dementia as a co-morbidity when other chronic diseases are present. Reflect on the family's decision, and discuss the pros and cons of their choice. What ethical issues did they need to consider?

What physical, psychosocial, and resources outcomes may have occurred if the family had chosen the surgical intervention?

Consider the three teams' behaviors. Which team(s) provided patient and family-centered care? Compare and contrast the team behaviors that led you to your conclusion.

## Case Study 3

*Care Management of a Patient with Congestive Heart Failure*

Mr. T, a 75-year-old man with a three-year history of congestive heart failure (CHF), is being prepared for discharge to home from a medical-surgical unit in an inner-city hospital. This was Mr. T's third admission for CHF this year. In addition to Mr. T's cardiac disease, he also has arthritis and an increasing visual impairment due to bilateral cataracts. Mr. T's wife of 50 years is physically healthy but has recently had increased problems with her memory.

Mr. and Mrs. T live independently on the second floor of a two-family home in a small town in a rural community with a population of 2,500. The town is located approximately 35 miles from the city where the hospital is located and where he had been admitted for CHF. The neighborhood in which Mr. and Mrs. T reside is in decline because of deteriorating local economic conditions. There is one family practice physician and two pharmacies in the town. The county health department employs a nurse practitioner, as well as public health and home health nurses. Mr. and Mrs. T have three adult children who no longer live in the town, but are within an hour's drive to their parents' home. Mrs. T has never worked outside the home and does not drive a car. There is no public transportation in the community.

Mr. T's cardiac status began improving on the second day of his admission, and planning began for his discharge. Two new medications were added to his current regimen of six medications, and dosages were adjusted on two of his current medications. Because of concerns raised by Mr. T's frequent hospital re-admissions for CHF, a doctor of nursing practice–prepared (DNP prepared) advanced practice nurse (APN) at the hospital invited several interprofessional team members to participate in the discharge planning for Mr. T. Interprofessional discharge planning was routine at the hospital, but in Mr. T's case, routine discharge care had not been effective. The team members at the initial meeting included the clinical nurses from the medical-surgical unit, the hospitalist caring for Mr. T, a pharmacist, a dietitian, a social worker and a case manager; the meeting was led by the DNP nurse. The DNP prepared APN proposed that members of the team consider innovative approaches that have been shown to be effective in managing the care of chronic disease populations. The team participated in a brainstorming session to generate ideas for improvements in the processes and structures to better support Mr. T in caring for his CHF after he returned home. A second meeting was scheduled two days later to continue the discharge planning.

- What innovative approaches in chronic disease management should the team have considered at their first meeting? Why?
- What access, environmental, and safety factors needed to be addressed? What were possible solutions for these issues?
- Were there key individuals missing at the first discharge planning meeting? Who should the team be certain to include in the second meeting? Why?

At the second meeting, decisions were made about Mr. T's follow-up care, and the discharge planning was finalized.

There were concerns about Mr. T's ability to adhere to his new medication administration schedule, as well as Mrs. T's ability to support him. What interventions could be used to increase the potential of their ability to correctly adhere to the medication schedule?

What are the community resources that should be accessed to support Mr. T's transition of care?

## Case Study 4

*Managing a Pediatric Sickle Cell Disease Population*

The complexity of disease management in chronic care populations has been discussed in this chapter. Chronic conditions like sickle cell disease require rigorous care management to prevent complications that can lead to disease progression and hospitalization. In the adolescent and young adult (AYA) population, care providers have found that peer-to-peer contact between adolescents and young adults who are diagnosed with the same chronic condition can lead to better health outcomes. Because of this, care management can be organized in a way that promotes contact between patients of similar ages and diagnoses. At pediatric healthcare facilities, outpatient AYA clinic days are established at regular intervals throughout the week for a number of chronic disease populations. Patients scheduled for these AYA clinic appointments are between 13 and 25 years of age. Depending on each patient's current health status, clinic visits can occur weekly, monthly, or bi-annually. An interprofessional team approach is used to manage the patients during these clinic visits. This is illustrated in a sickle cell population example at one facility below.

To provide individualized care in their population of patients, an interprofessional sickle cell team huddle occurs prior to the start of each AYA clinic day. A huddle is the term used to describe the gathering of the interprofessional team members who will be caring for the patients scheduled in clinic that day. At this huddle, each scheduled patient's plan of care is reviewed. It is determined which team they should be seen by that day, what blood work or other testing is needed, and if medications should be administered during their visit. Psychosocial issues are also reviewed. Pertinent care topics that need to be discussed with the patient are delineated. This plan of care is recorded at the time of huddle and is actively communicated to each of the care providers upon the patient's arrival to the clinic. For the sickle cell population, a visit typically consists of a clinical nurse and nurse practitioner assessment, a consultation with the physician care provider, and a follow up with the patient's care manager, social worker, and dietitian.

During the course of the clinic visit, any new pertinent information is disclosed to one or more of the patient's care providers. Frequent intentional communication among the care providers during the visit and detailed documentation of updates on the patient's status is critical. Following the AYA sickle cell patient's visit, any new information and changes to the plan of care are documented his or her electronic health record (EHR). This includes a synopsis of the patient's medical history, current health status, and future plan of care. Documentation in an EHR is essential for managing patients across the continuum of care, because it provides access to inpatient and community care providers who may also be involved in the care of each patient in the sickle cell population. At the conclusion of each clinic, a post-clinic huddle occurs during which the interprofessional team shares patient updates and any patterns that may have been identified within the population of patients seen in clinic that day.

- Discuss the strengths of the care management model presented in the sickle cell population case study.
- Describe any structural or process improvements that may strengthen the model.
- Explain the role of the DNP-prepared APN in establishing the structures and processes needed to provide care to chronic disease populations.
- How can the DNP influence the allocation of federal, state, and private insurer resources to care for populations of individuals with chronic diseases?

*Special Note*: Case Study 1 provided by Susan Brumm and Case Study 4 by Hannah Reed (Thank you).

## References

Agency for Healthcare Research and Quality (2011). Ensuring that patient-centered medical homes effectively serve patients with complex health needs. Retrieved from https://pcmh.ahrq.gov/page/ensuring-patient-centered-medical-homes-effectively-serve-patients-complex-health-needs

Agency for Healthcare Research and Quality (2012). Closing the quality gap series: The patient centered medical homes. Retrieved from http://effectivehealthcare.ahrq.gov/index.cfm/search-for-guides-reviews-and-reports/?productid=1177&pageaction=displayproduct

Agency for Healthcare Research and Quality (2014). The medical home: What do we know, what do we need to know? A review of the earliest evidence on the effectiveness of the patient-centered medical home model. AHRQ Pub. No. 12(14)-0020-1-E. Retrieved from https://pcmh.ahrq.gov/sites/default/files/attachments/the-medical-home-what-do-we-know.pdf

Agency for Healthcare Research and Quality (2017). *Defining the PCMH*. Retrieved from https://pcmh.ahrq.gov/page/defining-pcmh

Allen, C. G., Escoffery, C., Satsangi, A., & Brownstein, J. N. (2015). Strategies to improve the integration of community health workers into health care teams: "A little fish in a big pond." *Preventing Chronic Disease, 12*, 1–10.

Altman, S. H., Butler, A. S., & Shern, L. (Eds.) (2016). Assessing progress on the Institute of Medicine Report. *The Future of Nursing*. Washington, DC: The National Academies Press.

American Association of Colleges of Nursing. (2006). *The essentials of doctoral education for advanced nursing practice*. Washington, DC: American Association of Colleges of Nursing.

Bolton, L. B. (2011, July). *Nurse education leading change: Transforming staff development*. Keynote address presented at the annual convention of the National Nursing Staff Development Organization, Chicago, Illinois.

Centers for Medicare and Medicaid Services. (2015). *National health expenditures 2015 highlights*. Retrieved from https://www.cms.gov/research-statistics-data-and-systems/statistics-trends-and-reports/nationalhealthexpenddata/downloads/highlights.pdf

Centers for Disease Control and Prevention. (2017). *Chronic disease overview*. Retrieved from https://www.cdc.gov/chronicdisease/overview/

Caldwell, J. T., Ford, C. L., Wallace, S. P., Wang, M. C., & Takahashi, L. M. (2016). Intersection of living in a rural versus urban area and race/ethnicity in explaining access to health care in the United States. *American Journal of Public Health, 106*(8), 1463–1469. doi:10.2105/AJPH.2016.303212

Eadie, C. (2014). Health literacy: A conceptual review. *Academy of Medical-Surgical Nurses Newsletter, 23*(1), 1, 10–13.

Focus for Health. (2016). *Chronic illness and the state of our children's health*. Retrieved from https://www.focusforhealth.org/chronic-illnesses-and-the-state-of-our-childrens-health/

Hurlock-Chorostecki, C., Forchuk, C., Orchard, C., Reeves, S. & van Soeren, M. (2013). The value of the hospital-based nurse practitioner role: Development of a team perspective framework. *Journal of Interprofessional Care, 27*(6), 501–508.

Improving Chronic Illness Care. (2017). *The chronic care model: Model elements*. Retrieved from http://www.improvingchroniccare.org/index.php?p=Model_Elements&s=18

Institute for Patient- and Family-Centered Care. (2016). *Advancing the practice of patient- and family-centered care in hospitals: How to get started*. Retrieved from http://www.ipfcc.org/resources/getting_started.pdf

Institute for Patient- and Family-Centered Care. (2017). *Advancing the practice of patient- and family-centered care in primary care and other ambulatory settings: How to get started*. Retrieved from http://www.ipfcc.org/resources/GettingStarted-AmbulatoryCare.pdf

Institute of Medicine. (2004). *Keeping patients safe: Transforming the work environment of nurses*. Washington, DC: National Academies Press.

Institute of Medicine. (2010). *The future of nursing: Leading change, advancing health*. Washington, DC: National Academies Press.

Lail, J., Schoettker, P. J., White, D. L., Mehta, B., & Kotagal, U. R. (2017). Applying the chronic care model to improve care and outcomes at a pediatric medical center. *The Joint Commission Journal on Quality and Patient Safety, 43*, 101–112.

Lambert, V. & Keogh, D. (2014). Health literacy and its importance for effective communication. *Nursing Children and Young People, 26*(4), 32–36.

Lawn, S., Delaney, T., Sweet, L., Battersby, M., & Skinner, T. C. (2013). Control in chronic condition self-care management: How it occurs in the health worker-client relationship and implications for client empowerment. *Journal of Advanced Nursing, 70*(2), 383–394.

Lathrop, B. (2013). Nursing leadership in addressing the social determinants of health. *Policy, Politics & Nursing Practice, 14*(1), 41–47.

Linden, A., Butterworth, S. W., & Prochaska, J. O. (2010). Motivational interviewing-based health coaching as a chronic care intervention. *Journal of Evaluation in Clinical Practice, 16*, 166–174.

Mather, M., Jacobsen, L. A., & Pollard, K. M. (2015). Population bulletin: Aging in the United States. Retrieved from http://www.prb.org/pdf16/aging-us-population-bulletin.pdf

Syed, S., Gerber, B., & Sharp, L. (2013). Traveling towards disease: Transportation barriers to health care access. *Journal of Community Health, 38*(5), 976–993. doi:10.1007/s10900-013-9681-1

Tamura-Lis, T. (2013). Teach-back for quality education and patient safety. *Urologic Nursing, 33*(6), 267–271.

U.S. Department of Health and Human Services Administration on Aging. (2016). Aging statistics. Retrieved from https://aoa.acl.gov/Aging_Statistics/Index.aspx

Van Cleave, J., Gortmaker, S. L., & Perrin, J. M. (2010). Dynamics of obesity and chronic health conditions among children and youth. *Journal of the American Medical Association, 303*(7), 623–630.

Van Walraven, C., Dhalla, I. A., Bell, C., Etchells, E., Stiell, I. E., Zarnke, K., Forster, A. J. (2010). Derivation and validation of an index to predict early death or unplanned readmission after discharge from the hospital to the community. *Canadian Medical Association Journal, 182*(6), 551–557.

Wagner, E. H. (1998). Chronic disease management: What will it take to improve care for chronic illness? *Effective Clinical Practice, 1*, 2–4.

Wagner, E. H., Austin, B. T., Davis, C., Hindmarsh, M., Schaefer, J., & Bonomi, A. (2001). Improving chronic illness care: Translating evidence into action. *Health Affairs, 20*(6), 64–78.

Wiggins, M. S. (2008). The partnership care delivery model: An examination of the core concept and the need for a new model of care. *Journal of Nursing Management, 16*, 629-638. doi:10.1111/j.1365-2834.2008.00900.x

World Health Organization. (2012a). *What are the social determinants of health?* Retrieved from http://www.who.int/social_determinants/sdh_definition/en/

World Health Organization. (2012b). *Key concepts of the social determinants of health.* Retrieved from http://www.who.int/social_determinants/thecommission/finalreport/key_concepts/en/

## CHAPTER 11

# Obesity—Opportunities Across the Continuum

CHRISTINE RALYEA, DNP, MS-NP, MBA, NE-BC, CNL, OCN, CCRN
CECILIA ANNE RALYEA, BS

## Obesity Opportunities Across the Continuum

Population health issues and problems exist in all parts of the world and impact all ages. Hence, in 2000, the United Nations Millennium Declaration was signed, creating eight focal areas (goals). The United Nations (n.d.) identifies the eight goals areas as end poverty and hunger, universal education, gender equity, child health, maternal health, combat HIV/AIDS, environmental sustainability, and population partnership. One such population partnership that needs strengthening is the prevention and management of obesity. Obesity is defined as excess body fat and a body mass index (BMI) greater than the 95th percentile for age and sex on a growth chart (Centers for Disease Control and Prevention, 2017). Obesity is due to excess intake compared with calorie expenditure. According to the Centers for Disease Control and Prevention (CDC), if your BMI is less than 18.5 kg/m$^2$, it falls within the underweight range.

- If your BMI is 18.5 to < 25 kg/m$^2$, it falls within the normal range.
- If your BMI is 25.0 to < 30 kg/m$^2$, it falls within the overweight range.
- If your BMI is 30.0 kg/m$^2$or higher, it falls within the obese range.

Obesity is frequently subdivided into categories:

- Class 1: BMI of 30 to < 35 kg/m$^2$

- Class 2: BMI of 35 to < 40 kg/m$^2$
- Class 3: BMI of 40 kg/m$^2$ or higher.

Class 3 obesity is sometimes categorized as extreme or severe obesity (https://www.cdc.gov/obesity/adult/defining.html).

The APN can use a BMI calculator to make this calculation easy to compute. The necessary information for the patient is the height (feet and inches) and their weight (in pounds). Despite the span of almost two decades since the United Nations Millennium Declaration's conception in 2000, opportunities to impact and reduce obesity remain a focus due to serious health implications, such as diabetes and cardiovascular disease. Some of the many statistics found in the literature include "adult obesity prevalence increased drastically in the 1980s, 1990s, and early 2000s" (Eilerman *et al.*, 2014, p. 462); Finkelstein, Trogdon, Cohen, and Dietz (2012) predicted a 33% increase in obesity prevalence for individuals older than 18 years of age by the year 2030; and "worldwide obesity has doubled since 1980" (Seppala *et al.*, 2014, p. 349). According to Wang (2014), there are hazardous trends and correlations between obesity and mortality. This is alarming and takes a focus by all providers and advanced practice nurses (APNs) around the world. "Obesity has resulted in a significant impairment of health and longevity" (Ghouse, Barwal, & Wattamwar, 2016, p. 1). Obesity has created a patient safety dilemma by increasing surgical risks (Goode *et al.*, 2016) and exponential rise in healthcare costs. Obesity is a growing population health crisis that needs focus and attention from all healthcare providers.

## The Stigma of Obesity

Trotter (2016) acknowledges that obesity carries a visible stigma. When a patient is overweight, it is visible and *labels* him or her. However, compared with a patient with hypertension, for example, when this patient takes prescribed medications, the teammates at work (as an example) would not be able to label him or her as having a chronic illness, namely hypertension. Yet, when a patient is overweight, his or her size and potential limitations (e.g., on activities or pace of work) lend to discrimination. An obese individual may not be hired for a position he or she interviewed for or be assigned a project at work, and they may not be invited to participate on a team when compared with an individual of visibly healthier (normal) weight. Often, the obese patient also faces the societal stigma of thoughts of laziness. He or she is viewed as less active, unwilling to take responsibility for his or her personal health and wellness, and lacking control of his or her physical and mental health (Trotter, 2016). Often, these stigmas are inaccurate, and APNs are in a powerful role as healthcare authorities to change the way their obese patients are viewed. Hence, the APN role of advocacy is critical to addressing the population health issue of obesity.

## Obesity—A Crisis

Childhood obesity (CO) and obesity in adolescent and adult populations are complex problems. Obesity as a health issue is multifactorial and has been increasing in scope. In general, obesity has increased illness and diseases across the age spectrum, including (but not limited to) diabetes, cardiovascular disease, hypertension, and depression. CO also impacts the productivity of children and expands into later years. Because there is not an easy solution for treating obesity, prevention is the best strategy. Prevention begins with maintenance of ideal weights for parents who are their children's role models and should demonstrate healthy activity levels. Mothers can help prevent CO during infancy by breastfeeding. Exclusive breastfeeding for a minimum of six months can also reduce the occurrence of CO (U.S. Department of Health and Human Services, 2011).

CO is particularly prevalent in Hispanic populations; in fact, there is a rise in obesity prevalence rates by 34.6% (Wright, 2011). With over one third of Hispanic children facing OC, a call for action requiring a multifaceted approach for addressing this population health problem in the Hispanic community is proposed. A commitment needs to include both primary caregivers (parents, extended family members, school teachers, religious, and community leaders) and healthcare providers (multiple disciplines). The success can be seen only with full engagement of these stakeholders. The approach requires ongoing monitoring, reassessment, and behavioral changes. To be successful, a diverse and varied approach for interventions has been identified, such as formulating an action oriented public messaging campaign with associated verification for implementation processes. Additional cultural sensitivity and ethical considerations need to be considered when developing treatment plans for obesity prevention programs. Together, these interventions and strategies are proposed to improve health by reducing obesity.

Obesity is the most common childhood nutritional disorder in the world (World Health Organization, 2012). With the rise in CO, secondary diseases such as hypertension, cardiovascular disease (CVD), and type 2 diabetes are escalating (Wright, 2011). Phillips (2012) reported associations of CO with asthma, fatty liver disease, and joint pain. In addition, CO has psychological impacts. Specifically, depression, mood disorders, and low confidence are commonly secondary to CO (Sanderson, Patton, McKercher, Dwyer, & Venn, 2011). Childhood obesity is a population health issue that can be partially deescalated with regional public information campaigns. The campaigns should educate healthcare providers on intervention plans, early warning signs, prompt treatment plans, and ongoing assessment of CO.

### Case Vignette

A mother brings her three-year-old daughter TR in for her routine checkup and examination. Upon review of TR's trends in height, weight, and growth chart, TR had always been between the 80th and 90th percentiles for weight and at the 50th percentile for height. On this visit, you note that the weight is greater than the 99th percentile. As the APN, do you need to address TR's weight at this visit? If so, what will be your approach to elicit more information from TR's mother? What questions will you ask? How will you engage the mother in a wellness plan for TR?

### Obesity Impact on the Population in the United States

The direct impact on the population in the United States (U.S.) is an estimated $48 to $66 billion each year in direct medical costs associated with obesity and its comorbidities (Wang, McPherson, Marsh, Gortmaker, & Brown, 2011). Comorbidities and life impacts related to obesity include diabetes, cardiovascular disease, depression, stroke, issues with a decreased lifespan, an increase in time off work due to decreased mobility, an overall reduction in productive years of life, and many other chronic illnesses. Furthermore, secondary medical costs and healthcare related to obesity continues to rise annually. "The combination of rising obesity prevalence and increased spending on obese people has been estimated to account for 27% of the growth in US healthcare spending between 1987 and 2011" (Wang et al., 2011, p. 816). Wang et al. (2011) also reports that, if the current trends of CO continue, by 2020 three of every four (or 75%) of the American community will be diagnosed as obese. The cascading effects of obesity in the United States are serious and need attention. The awareness of this public health issue and call for action is essential. There is a strong need to reduce the immediate expenditures for medical care associated with obesity. Responsive actions would serve to reduce the resulting health concerns from obesity. Type 2 diabetes is one such health concern, to which poor weight management and obesity have contributed. Lee *et al.* (2017) shares that obesity in conjunction with diabetes has a higher mortality rate. This increases the cost of delivering care and contributes to the acceleration of chronic illness and declining quality of life.

According to Popkin, Adair, and Ng (2011), the rise in obesity has been associated with advances in transportation, leisure (television, computers), and home production (cooking, cleaning, and child care). Diets have suffered because of changes in the food supply. Production no longer focuses on hand raised/grown grains and legumes, so there has been a shift to mass food production with increased animal fats and refined sugars. This increase in mass produced food positively correlates with an increase in obesity. Can we become an advocate for health policies to reduce cost of healthy food such as fresh fruits and vegetables? When our patients are on a fixed income or have high medical expenses, the limited funds will be spent on the lower cost foods, which frequently have more carbohydrates with lower nutritional value. It becomes easier to go to a fast food restaurant and order off a *dollar menu* rather than prepare a chicken breast and broccoli at home. Perhaps, because obesity relates to these mealtime decisions, obesity is a family issue. Perryman (2011) completed a research project and has shown that a child has a 40% probability of obesity when one parent is overweight with an increase to an 80% probability of obesity when both parents are overweight. One can see that obesity of a familiar and cultural tendency needs strong attention and focus. This demonstrates the critical nature of engaging the entire family in lifestyle changes to reduce the obesity crisis in the nation.

## Case Vignette

In the same TR case, above, you hear from the mother that she is struggling between work and home. She drops TR off at daycare at 6:15 A.M., so she is eating two meals and a snack at daycare. Typically, she picks TR up after work around 5:30 P.M. and rushes home to get with the other children. When she comes home, dinners are often fast food or quick fix meals, including pasta, a sandwich with canned soup, or processed foods. TR's mother starts to cry and says all the children are gaining weight and she does not know what to do.

As the APN, what are several suggestions you can make to help TR's mother (and all the children)? What would be your recommendation for an appointment for the other children? When would you schedule the next follow up for TR? How can you best support mom?

## Scope of the Obesity Issue

The causes of obesity are attributed to many domains—environmental, socioeconomic, behavioral, genetic, metabolic, and cultural (Li & Hooker, 2010; Rooney, Mathiason, & Schauberger, 2011). Several examples of environmental factors have included the use of cars and public transportation instead of walking to school or work, which would increase steps and calories burned daily. The socioeconomic factors, such as high-income family, may include a high rate of eating out in restaurants, including food with higher calories, cream sauces, and alcohol consumptions adding to the total calorie count each day. The diversity of these contributing factors adds to the difficulty of addressing this population health problem. Resolving this issue requires addressing the causes and supporting lifelong nutritional changes to improve the health and well-being of the population.

Early assessment and diagnosis along with healthcare provider involvement is vital in the management of obesity. Healthcare providers can provide active involvement in many settings. The provider can use healthcare settings, schools, churches, and community groups as forums for education. Healthcare providers need to have a common understanding of reliable methods for effectively changing a population's behavior. These diverse providers must also focus on consistent and culturally sensitive communication for the family unit (Wright, 2011). This problem is massive in scope and requires a population response tailored to regional needs.

## Best Practice with Congruency

That prevention is the best plan for controlling obesity is supported and congruent in the literature as cited by Gill (2009); Faraz (2010); Han, Lawlor, & Kimm (2010); Kelly, Yang, Chen, Reynolds, and He (2008); and U.S. Department of Health and Human Services (USD-HHS) (2011). Prevention should be the focus at all levels of contact with youth, at home, in institutions (e.g., schools, employment), at community activities and functions, in the religious community, and during routine preventative care and clinic visits and within healthcare at all levels. In the home, this includes engagement of the entire family and extended family as able (Han *et al.*, 2010). Preventing obesity with programs such as Change4Life and Healthy Towns can help create awareness for healthier lifestyles, increase peer support, and support positive for behavior changes (Phillips, 2012). Employers have invested in monitoring teammate weights and offering incentives for healthy weights or weight loss. Church communities have sponsored health fairs with education on lifestyle choices, including increasing activity levels and nutritional counseling. Often this cannot be the healthcare provider alone. The APN must engage the patient's support systems for success.

## Multifaceted Intervention

Early comprehensive assessment of the entire family should include the parents' history of weight patterns, dietary habits, television time, activity level, and socioeconomic status and food insecurities. Next steps include acting upon information received to help support the family unit in early recognition of obesity concerns and early interventions to avoid the many associated health risks and concerns secondary to obesity (Kornides, Kitsantas, Yang, & Villarruel, 2011). Following detailed assessments, plans must include dietary, behavior modifications, exercise, support groups, health coaching, and other culturally sensitive measures to improve health perceptions.

Li and Hooker (2010) presented a strong case for modifying health policy. They suggested two components: advocacy and change. Advocacy includes modifying awareness, and the change component called for directed change in the food served and activity levels. When active engagement of the government to support healthy public policy focuses on prevention of obesity, the potential for improvements exist (Popkin *et al.*, 2011).

## Clinical Prevention and Population Health

Breastfeeding has been reported to have positive health effects (lower respiratory infections, lower leukemia, less diabetes, and CO), psychological effects (bonding between mother and newborn, less postpartum depression), economic impacts (savings in annual formula cost of approximately $1,500 per year, potentially lower cost from healthcare sick visits), and positive environmental effects (no package disposal from bottles and formula) (Stewart, 2012; U.S. Department of Health and Human Services, 2011). Healthy People 2010 established a goal of 75% exclusive breastfeeding initiation, 50% exclusive breastfeeding at six months, and 25% breastfeeding continuation for one year to help reap these benefits (U.S. Department of Health and Human Services, 2011). Because the Healthy People 2010 goal was not met, a call for action by the Surgeon General was announced. Following this call for action could give children the best start for a healthier future by preventing CO.

**Familiar Factors for Obesity**

Beyond breastfeeding, parental weight and role modeling activity levels also greatly impact CO. Perryman (2011) and Water (2011) identified engagement in parents to improve CO. As a correlation to the Millennium Development Goal for maternal health, a greater focus of prevention for CO could be supported by improving prenatal care. Improving prenatal care can be accomplished with prenatal education to support improved diets during pregnancy and, thus, healthier weight gains and with monitoring for gestational diabetes. Prenatal planning can also include improving pre-pregnancy weight and seeking an ideal weight preconception (U.S. Department of Health and Human Services, 2011). Prenatal nutrition effects on CO can be seen in studies of the Dutch Hunger Winter. The Dutch Hunger Winter is the period of famine during Nazi occupation of the Netherlands in 1944 and 1945. Evaluating health records from this era shows that mothers who are famished in their third trimester have babies with lower birth weights. Mothers who are famished in their first trimester, however, have babies with higher birth weights, and these children, as well as their children, are more likely to be obese into adulthood because of epigenetic patterns established in the womb (Carey, 2012).

Activity levels for parents, extended families, school leaders (teachers, physical education, nurses, administration), and community leaders (religious and others) need to role model healthier activity levels, such as taking stairs, walking short distances versus using public or personal transportation, and enhancing physical exercise commitments (Rooney et al., 2011). A personal motto used with my family is *when you can, sit instead of lie, stand instead of sit, and walk instead of stand.* An example includes if you are lying down watching television, change your position and sit up. This improves posture and breathing and exercises muscles that tend to get lazy. Engagement at home and the broader community to serve as role models and trigger greater activity levels can support prevention of the escalating CO trends.

## Cultural Sensitivity

An example of cultural sensitivity includes the Hispanic culture; family is their source of strength and extremely valued. They rely on each other and share their dreams within their family. Their Hispanic identity is a cultural point of. It will be essential to help them maintain their cultural identity and include their primary care providers across the family unit. Also, knowing the respect they have for their culture, trust must be developed and the messaging must be consistent with Hispanic values and must support family involvement.

The Hispanic community supports breastfeeding but often uses formula supplements in the early weeks of the newborn's life. This is a cultural concern for mothers' understanding of "no milk" during the first days of life. In the Hispanic population, early breastfeeding rates are higher than many cultures but fall off before the six-month period of benefit, per Healthy People 2010. Interventions aimed at encouraging and supporting women to maintain their cultural traditions, beliefs, and practices related to breastfeeding should be applied (Gill, 2009). Some of these culturally sensitive measures can be support for Le Leche community support groups and Bellas. Understand that the Hispanic cultural values first-day formula supplementation should be supported by healthcare providers. The focus on exclusive breastfeeding as soon as milk comes in and valuing the family engagement for breastfeeding success will yield greater results (Schlickau & Wilson, 2010; Faraz, 2010).

Translating the importance of family in the Hispanic culture will extend beyond the support for breastfeeding. The engagement of father in prenatal visits and prenatal education, understanding of role modeling healthy weight, and dietary choices will build potential commitment in implementation strategies for reduction of CO. This will include extended family as critical elements and involvement.

Cultural sensitivity across all ages must be considered when working with the obese patient population. For example, in Japan, cuisine is a major part of celebrations and their culture. In several parts of Japan, the slightly overweight women are more attractive and healthy. It will be important to support the value of food in these situations, but support optimal selections and portion intake.

He *et al.* (2016) mention that underweight women have concerns with infertility and difficulty carrying pregnancies to term. This has impacted the Chinese women of childbearing (ages 20 to 49 years), so young adolescents (ages 15 to 19 years) tend to maintain higher BMIs than in past years. Notably these age groups tend to increase their weight in the four to six months prior to conception as they were planning a pregnancy.

*Case Vignette*

Juan and Maria Hernandez are so excited to have their sixth child and finally have a baby girl. Juan always wanted a daughter; the extended family is frequently visiting and stays 24/7 with Maria in the room at the hospital. Maria did not go to any childbirth classes, because she only went the first time and she feels she knows everything about childbirth, childcare, and taking care of her new daughter Rosa. Maria starts to breastfeed in the hospital, but every four hours is additionally providing a bottle of formula. Maria shares with the APN, no leche. What would be your response to help Maria increase compliance with exclusive breastfeeding for six months?

## Ethical Considerations

The CDC respects the rights of parents to raise their children, but the CDC also needs to protect children from harm. The CDC sees CO as neglect because the parents are responsible for the indirect harm or negligence of their child. There have been cited cases when parents have criminal charges for neglect for their children's severe cases of obesity. It is extremely important to engage the parents and family unit in awareness, early assessment, and interventions for prevention and treatment of obesity. Providers must help parents understand their responsibilities and build accountability to minimize harm to the youth (Perryman, 2011). When caring for the Hispanic population, it is essential to get buyin from the family and extended family for the implementation plan for weight management (diet, nutrition, exercise, etc.) as a building block and foundation for successful lifestyle changes. Engagement and compliance with the plan will improve, and the outcomes will demonstrate greater obesity weight reductions.

Some obese patients will be candidates for a surgical intervention. There will be many severely obese patients who may consider a surgical intervention such as a gastric bypass as the only solution to their weight issues. As APNs, we make referrals to the specialist/surgeon. The ethical considerations may include the crucial conversations about the risks of the surgery (Goode *et al.*, 2016) and the need to be engaged in a weight loss program prior to surgery to demonstrate a commitment to the necessary lifestyle changes. Making a referral to the specialist without prior dialogue would be creating a conflict for expectations for the patient and potentially be a barrier for engagement of the patient for success.

As an ethical advocate, questions arise should government play a role in reducing obesity? What are the ethical considerations for the APN in managing obesity and reducing the rising rates of obesity? Can an APN who is significantly overweight be effective in education and developing an obesity reduction plan for a patient? These are important questions, and we need to challenge ourselves to be healthier. Can we afford to reduce our weight? What choices can we make for ourselves to be better role models and to reduce the rates of obesity? We can share successes and share personal stories with our patients for success.

## Obesity and Quality of Life

Often, we find that, in practice, patient education was completed to direct a decrease in intake and an increase in physical activity. Despite these efforts, the patient's weight either stays the same or often increases. True behavior modification does not get hardwired and become changes in practice. As an APN assessing a patient's health status related to his or her weight and obesity, your assessment must include how the patients weight (and size) impacts his or her quality of life. The use of the Health-Related Quality of Life (HRQoL) tool can be used (Seppala *et al.*, 2014). As a patient values health and more clearly understands the impact of their weight burdens, conscious efforts start to make correlations. Does an individual's weight impact their leisure activities, ability to complete a day's work, or daily chores including time spent with family? This supports a strong shift in focus, driving behavior modifications. Seppala *et al.* (2014) also comments on the critical nature of a provider's duty to help the patients avoid finding comfort in their poor health, being overweight, and obesity. This may include treating depression, aligning the patient with support groups, and offering a monthly weight check, group therapy for the patients with nutritionist, or low impact exercises. Information on dietary intake in obese people is divergent and often conflicting (Lovold-Mostad, Langaas, & Grill, 2014). This often makes dietary instruction complex and complicated. We have seen this with the variety of diet choices, such as high-protein, low-carbohydrate diets or simply counting calories, available online and offered by various programs. Often these choices host conflicting principles for success. Which diet do we recommend and which best supports the patients are important considerations. The low socioeconomic patient would not be successful on a high-protein, low-carbohydrate diet. The inability to purchase the higher percentages of lean meats and fresh vegetables would set him or her up for failure.

A best practice is to provide a food diary or journal for the patient to complete. Providing this as an exercise after completing the HRQoL questionnaire will lead to improved accuracy and documentation by the patient. The diary can be used to help the patient identify the triggers for eating and understand the concepts of portion control and overall choices made in a day or weeks' period. As the APN, it is important to take the time to understand through the eyes and perception of the patient. Weight reduction is not a simple task, so showing patients the possible rewards, such as improved quality of life, beyond the obvious physical change can help pique their interest in the journey.

Marteau (2011) explains the concept of nudging as a method to combat obesity. Nudging is the alteration of an environment to encourage a certain choice without the use of regulations. For example, placing the produce section at the front of a grocery store may encourage shoppers to purchase fruit and vegetables, whereas placing candy bars by the check-out encourages shoppers to purchase less healthy options at the last minute. Moving the candy to a center aisle or the back of the store could reduce this unhealthy shopping behavior by removing the convenience. In fact, replacing this candy with fruit increases the amount of fruit that teenagers purchase by 70% (Marteau, 2011). Another example of grocery store nudging is the placement of a designated area in the shopping cart for fruits and vegetables, which doubled the amount of fruit and vegetables that consumers bought (Marteau, 2011).

Nudging need not happen only in the grocery store to encourage healthy habits. Advertisements can also nudge. Beer commercials have been identified as a cause for the doubling of alcohol consumption in young people since 1960 (Marteau, 2011). Although this is a negative example of nudging, it shows the power advertising has in shaping consumer habits. Eliminating advertisements for unhealthy food options and increasing those for healthy options could perhaps change consumers' grocery lists. Advertisements for non-food items can also nudge viewers toward a healthier lifestyle. For example, seeing fitness trackers in the media may encourage people to buy a Fitbit™ or Jawbone™. As sales for the products increase, people will receive further encouragement to buy a fitness tracker of their own because their peers may have them, providing another nudge. Wearing a fitness tracker encourages physical activity (Cadmus-Bertram, Marcus, Patterson, Parker, & Marcy, 2016). Together, the APN and the patient can mutually agree on a daily goal for daily steps, setting the patient up for success. Ultimately the goal would be the recommended 10,000 steps per day, but initially a morbidly obese patient may have a goal of 1,000 steps a day. As goals are achieved, they can be advanced and build stamina and progress for the patient.

Thinking outside the box and utilizing technology to the fullest in today's world, the APN can monitor the obese patient's steps and activity level. Imagine the engagement if the patient did not meet his or her goal for three consecutive days and received a call from the APN as an advocate to assess what the barriers were and demonstrate a sense of care and commitment to the patient's wellness plan. Maybe the patient was ill and the APN can connect earlier for treatment to get the patient back on the wellness plan for the activity level goals set. The opportunity could truly build engagement for success. We know the phone call we receive after a procedure showing care and concern fosters outcomes and open communication between patient and provider. This is one example of a potential opportunity for the APN to advocate for a successful weight reduction plan for the growing obese population.

Another suggestion for the APN when he or she cannot offer obese patients a fitness tracker for monitoring and tracking their activity and steps daily would be to include activity monitoring with the food journal. Maybe this can be a patient that comes to a weekly support group. Maybe a group of obese patients and the APN together can meet weekly and schedule a reasonable walk/activity session and review journals. During this time, celebrate the successes and reconnect with all participants to build commitment and engagement.

### Case Vignette

Mr. Slow, 35 years old, is at church and you realize you haven't seen him in approximately four months. He is not well kept, is dressed in dirty clothes, appears slightly short of breath, and has gained about 20 pounds since your last encounter. Out of concern, you sit next to him, monitor his behavior during the service, and stay after church to speak with him. He acknowledges he is depressed and sad since his wife left him six months ago.

As a fellow church mate and APN, what can you do to help Mr. Slow? What would be your first recommendations? How can you engage the church community to help Mr. Slow?

## Additional Treatment/Management

ANPs have many considerations to make in the care and treatment plans of the obese patient. The plan must be individualized for each patient and address the following:

1. Establishing weight-loss goals
2. Lifestyle counseling
3. Increased physical activity
4. Dietary interventions
5. Ensuring adequate sleep
6. Medications
   —Identification of medications that can contribute to weight gain
   —U.S. Food and Drug Administration (FDA) approved medications for obesity
7. Bariatric surgery
8. Managing comorbid conditions
9. Follow-up and monitoring
10. Referrals for comorbidities, dietitian, multidisciplinary weight-loss clinic, and bariatric surgery
11. Considerations for weight gain in pregnancy
12. Patient education and resources. (www.clinicalpracticeguidelines. gov)

## APN as an Advocate for Reducing Obesity

Eyler, Nguyen, Kong, Yan, and Brownson (2012) studied the legislative proposals during the years of 2006 to 2009, finding 27 related to CO. The proposed recommendations included physical education, nutrition (including school dietary monitoring), and community topics. Nutrition included education on portion control, fat intake, and use of farm and home grown local products as examples. Several of the community topics included soda and snack taxes, breastfeeding, community food access, public transportation, trails for bikes and walking paths, menu labeling, and outdoor activity playgrounds. Despite these efforts, the United States continues to see a rise in CO.

Looking to the causes of obesity is essential when developing an intervention and program to effectively reduce the overweight and obesity crisis. Effective responses to obesity include dietary choice and activity levels (Boddy, Hackett, & Stratton, 2010; Bucha-Torre, Akre, & Suris, 2010; Darweish, 2012). Additional factors associated with obesity included genetics and environment, and a lesser correlation can be made with acculturation (Kornides *et al.*, 2011). Findings suggested that the parental BMI was consistently found to be a factor in CO rates (Wright, 2011). The socioeconomic status and parental income also play a strong role and impact the family member's BMI (Kornides *et al.*, 2011).

Opportunities exist for APNs to be a political advocate to drive policy changes addressing societal, environmental, and community changes for reducing obesity. Trotter (2016) suggests taxing sugar sweetened beverages (SSB) and using the tax revenue to lower costs of healthier food and support exercise programs. At the grade school level, one can advocate for healthier food choices on the school menu, no sale of SSBs, mandating physical activity each day as part of lunch periods, adding to the activity level with bus drop off at a greater distance on the school property, support of outside playground funding, weight management monitoring quarterly by the school nurse with nutrition counseling, and other such activities.

In your community, you can advocate for starting a walking group in your neighborhood, meet a group of people at 7:30 pm and walk for an hour as an example. Another thought is to advocate for developing a new walking trail. You can reach out to the local Boy Scout Troop that has scouts working on their Eagle Project and build support to develop such programs. At your church, you can offer a nutrition class and do a weekly weighin for a group of the congregation. In this group, encourage the maintenance of a diet journal that can be reviewed each week. You can reach out to your interdisciplinary team and have guest lecturers on various topics to improve health and improve the quality of life for the people.

## Summary

Obesity is a population health problem. The escalating rates of chronic illnesses secondary to obesity are well documented. Thus, there is higher medical cost expenditure and costs incurred by this population and their families. It requires engagement of the families as primary care providers to improve the health status of their patients. Prevention is the greatest opportunity for obesity reduction. Prevention starts with engaging the patients and family to establish and maintain a healthy BMI and increase their own personal activity levels. The family must engage in an understanding of the energy balance (energy-out with physical activity and energy-in from dietary intake) (Stewart, 2012). Optimizing care, including education on exercise, nutrition, managing weight gain during all aspects of life (pregnancy, stressors of life, school including college years as examples), and the importance of exclusive breastfeeding for a minimum of six months are essential. Additionally, engaging the entire family unit can add to the commitment for change and sense of pride in family and culture.

Obesity is multifactorial, and education alone cannot support lifelong and lifestyle changes. Actionable items must be embedded in the education using teach back for understanding, principles of health literacy, followed with monitoring, and rewards for success. Every APN, primary care provider, and healthcare worker needs to take accountability for this population health problem and understand his or her impact. Each person must model and embrace lifestyle changes to improve healthcare spending on obesity related illnesses.

## Tool Kit and Resources

www.clinicalpracticeguidelines.gov

To calculate BMI, see the Adult BMI Calculator: (https://www.cdc.gov/healthyweight/assessing/bmi/adult_bmi/english_bmi_calculator/bmi_calculator.html) or determine BMI by finding your height and weight in this BMI Index Chart

HealthPartners—Health Care Reform Series: Pediatric Dental: https://www.healthpartners.com/ucm/groups/public/@hp/.../cntrb_039418.pdf

CDC—Obesity: https://www.cdc.gov/obesity/adult/defining.html

Healthy Eating: www.healthyeating.com

Healthy Recipes: https://www.popsugar.com/Healthy-Recipes

Michelle Obama Let's Move Initiatives: https://letsmove.obamawhite-house.archives.gov/

National School Lunch Program (NSLP)—Food and Nutrition Service: https://www.fns.usda.gov/nslp/national-school-lunch-program-nslp

Obesity Help: www.obesityhelp.org

Obesity Definition—Obesity Prevention Source—Harvard T.H. Chan: https://www.hsph.harvard.edu/obesity-prevention-source/obesity-definition

## Definitions

*Obesity*—excess body fat, a body mass index (BMI) greater than the 95th percentile for age and sex on a growth chart (Centers for Disease Control and Prevention, 2010).

*Childhood Obesity (CO)*—obesity, excess body fat in the agegroup 0 to age 18.

*HRQoL Survey*—Health Related Quality of Life survey tool to determine a patient's view of health and the quality of life associated with their physical health.

*Nudging*—the alteration of an environment to encourage a certain choice without the use of regulations.

## Discussion Questions

- Beyond your professional work in the pediatrician's office, what are some political advocacy actions you can take in the community to foster healthier lifestyles for schoolaged children? Explain how you will play an active role in one of the advocacy plans you stated.
- How can you develop a campaign to enhance exclusive breastfeeding for a minimum of six months? Where would you gather information to support your return on investment for this campaign?
- Describe a multifactorial plan you will put in place for management of obesity as an ANP? How will you monitor and measure effectiveness?

## Case Study 1

Billy is age six and his mother brings him into the pediatrician's office because he has a complaint of a sore throat for three days and an associated fever. During the checkin procedure, Billy is noted to weight 90 lb. and have a BMI of 36 kg/m2. As an APN, do you address the weight or ignore it because the visit is for his sore throat and you will only get paid for one complaint during the sick visit?

As a concerned practitioner, you trend his weight chart over the past three years and you see he was always >100% percentile and there are no documented notes about his weight and activity patterns. You are waiting for the rapid streptococcal test results, so you have a discussion with Billy and his mother. What are some critical elements to discuss in this conversation?

Mom does not seem engaged in the conversation and states all four children are overweight and she thinks it is hereditary from their father. How would you manage this conversation and start to evaluate the food patterns, dietary intake, Billy's exercise level (amount of television, video games, book reading), any sports, any opportunities to increase activity level, small changes to start to implement in the family diet, etc.?

When would you reschedule Billy for a follow up weight check?

## Case Study 2

Elizabeth is 39 years old and presents to the office because she has vaginal irritation and itching and is complaining that she is thirsty, stating that she has been drinking more water. Her checkin includes the following:

Height 63 inches (5′ 3″)
Weight 245 pounds
Blood pressure 148/90 mm Hg
Temperature 98.8°F
A finger stick glucose is done and the result is 285.

The APN goes in to complete a full history and assessment and orders a full set of labs, including A1C, complete metabolic panel, lipid panel, complete blood count, and thyroid panel. The history includes her statement that she is in good health, is a little depressed at times as she recognizes she is not as fast at work as she used to be, and does not have the same energy to be with her three children running errands and participating in their activities. Some nights, dinner is a chore and she has resorted to more fast foods than in past years.

On physical examination, heart sounds includes an S3, peripheral edema bilaterally in her lower extremities, and a vaginal yeast infection is noted.

- We each have cared for a patient like this. What are the top five priorities on her problem list?
- What would you have on her treatment plan?
- What are several measures you will put in place to set her up for success for working towards healthier lifestyles?
- Are there any resources you can provide her to set her up for success?
- How would you manage the elevated blood glucose?
- What would be your first choice of medical management for the hypertension?
- In what time frame would you have her rescheduled for a followup appointment?
- If you scheduled an appointment for a onemonth follow up and she did not show up, what steps could you take to build a sense of her personal ownership for health management?
- If she came back for a followup appointment in one month having lost five pounds and her fasting glucose was 225, what would be your response? How would you encourage her to continue her journey for success?

## References

Boddy, L.M., Hackett, A.F., & Stratton, G. (2010). Changes in fitness, body mass index and obesity in 9-10 year olds. *Journal of Human Nutrition & Dietetics, 23*, 254–259, doi:10.1111/j.1365-277X.2009.01025.x

Bucha-Torre, S., Akre, C., & Suris, J. C., (2010). Obesity prevention opinions of school stakeholders: A qualitative study. *Journal of School Health. 80*(5), 233–239.

Cadmus-Bertram, L., Marcus, B., Patterson, R., Parker, B. & Marcy, B. (2016). Randomized trial of a fitbit-based physical activity intervention for women. *American Journal of Preventive Medicine, 49*(3), 414–418.

Carey, N. (2012). Beyond DNA: Epigenetics deciphering the link between nature & nurture. *Natural History*. Retrieved from http://www.naturalhistorymag.com/features/142195/beyond-dna-epigenetics

Centers for Disease Control and Prevention (2010). Retrieved from https://www.cdc.gov/obesity/

CPG: Clinical Practice Guidelines. (2017). Retrieved from www.clinicalpracticeguidelines.gov

Darweish, S. (2012). Obesity in children and teenagers. *Primary Health Care, 22*(7), 28–31.

Eilerman, P., Herzog, C., Luce, B., Chao, S., Walker, S., Zarzabal, L & Carnahan, D. (2014). A comparison of obesity prevalence: military health system and United States populations, 2009–2012. *Military Medicine 179*(79), 462–470.

Eyler, A., Nguyen, L., Kong, J., Yan, Y., & Brownson, R. (2012). Patterns and predictors of enactment of state childhood obesity legislation in the United States: 2006–2009. *American Journal of Public Health, 102*(12), 2294–2302. doi:10.2105/AJPH.2012.300763

Faraz, A. (2010). Clinical recommendations for promoting breastfeeding among Hispanic women. *Journal American Academy Nurse Practitioners, 22*(6), 292–9. doi: 10.1111/j.1745-7599.2010.00510.x

Finkelstein, E., Trogdon, J., Cohen, J. & Dietz, W (2012). Obesity and severe obesity forecasts through 2030. *American Journal Preventative Medicine, 42*(6), 563–570.

Ghouse, M., Barwal, S. & Wattamwar, A. (2016). A review of obesity. *Health Science Journal, 10*(4), 1–5.

Gill, S. (2009). Breastfeeding by Hispanic women. *Journal Obstetrical Gynecologic Neonatal Nursing, 38*(2), 244–52. doi:10.1111/j.1552-6909.2009.01013x

Goode, V., Phillips, E., DeGuzman, P., Hinston, I., Rovnyak, V., Scully, K. & Merwin, E. (2016). A patient safety dilemma: obesity in the surgical patient. *AANA 84*(6), 404–412.

Han, J., Lawlor, D., & Kimm, S. (2010). Childhood obesity. *The Lancet. 375*, 1737–1748. doi:10.1016/S0140-6736(10)60171-7.

He, Y., Pan, A., Yang, Y, Ma, X. (2016). Prevalence of underweight, overweight, and obesity amongst reproductive-age women and adolescent girls in rural China. *American Journal Public Health, 106*(12), 2013–2110.

Kelly, T., Yang, W., Chen, C., Reynolds, K., & He, J. (2008). Population burden of obesity in 2005 and projections to 2030. *International Journal of Obesity, 32*(9), 1431–7. Retrieved from http://dx.doi.org/10.1038/ijo.2008.102

Kornides, M., Kitsantas, P., Yang, Y.T., & Villarruel, A. (2011). Factors associated with obesity in Latino children: A review of the literature. *Hispanic Health Care International, 9*(3), 127–136. doi:10.1891/1540-4153.3.127

Lee, K., Moser, D., Lennie, T., Pelter, M., Nesbitt, T., Southard, J. & Dracup, K. (2017). Obesity Paradox: Comparison of Heart Failure Patients with and Without Comorbid Diabetes. *American Journal of Critical Care, 26*(2), 140–148.

Li, J., & Hooker, N. (2010). Childhood obesity and schools: Evidence from the National survey of children's health. *Journal of School Health, 80*(2), 96–103.

Lovold-Mostad, I., Langaas, M. & Grill, V. (2014). Central obesity is associated with lower intake of whole-grain bread and less frequent breakfast and lunch: Results from the HUNT study, an adult all-population survey. *Applied Physiological Nutrition Metabolism, 39*, 819–828.

Marteau, T. (2011). Judging nudging: Can nudging improve population health? *BMJ (Formally known as British Medical Journal), 342*, 263–265.

Perryman, M., (2011). *Ethical family interventions for childhood obesity.* Center for

Disease Control and Prevention. Retrieved from www.cdc.gov/pcd/issues/2011/sep/11_0038.htm

Phillips, F. (2012). Facing up to childhood obesity. *Practice Nurse, 41*(11), 14–17.

Popkin, B., Adair, L., & Ng, S.W. (2011). Population nutrition transition and the pandemic of obesity in developing countries. *Nutrition Reviews. 70*(1), 3–21. doi:10.1111/j.1753-4887.2011.00456.x

Rooney, B., Mathiason., M., & Schauberger, C., (2011). Predictors of obesity in childhood, adolescence, and adulthood in a birth cohort. *Maternal Child Health Journal, 15,* 1166–1175. doi:10.1007/s10995-010-0689-1

Sanderson, K., Patton, G., McKercher, C., Dwyer, T., & Venn, A. (2011). Overweight and obesity in childhood and risk of mental disorder: A 20-year cohort study. *The Royal Australian and New Zealand College of Psychiatrists, 45,* 384–392. doi:10.3 109/00048674.2011.570309

Schlickau, J., & Wilson, M. (2010). Breastfeeding as health-promoting behavior for Hispanic women: Literature review. *Journal of Advanced Nursing, 52*(2), 200–10. doi:10.1111/j.1552-6909.2009.01013x

Seppala, T., Mantyselka, P., Saxen, U., Kautiainen, H., Jarvenpaa, S., & Korhonen, P., (2014). Weight change and health related quality of life: Population-based longitudinal study of the effects of health-related quality of life on the success of weight management. *Journal of Community Health, 39,* 349–354.

Stewart, L. (2012). Managing and preventing obesity in infants. *Practice Nursing, 23*(4), 200–203. doi:10.1111/j.1365-277X.2008.00938.x

Trotter, G. (2016). *Reducing the Trends and the Stigma of Obesity.* The Kansas Nurse, October 2016, 9–12.

United Nations (UN). (n.d.). The United Nations- Millennium development goals. Retrieved from http://www.un.org/millenniumgoals/bkgd.shtml

U.S. Department of Health and Human Services (USDHHS). 2011. The Surgeon General's Call to Action to Support Breastfeeding. Retrieved from http://www.surgeongeneral.gov.

Wang, Z. (2014). Age and the impact of obesity on mortality. *American Journal of Public Health. 104*(4), e3.

Wang, Y. C., McPherson, K., Marsh, T., Gortmaker, S. L., & Brown, M. (2011). Obesity 2: Health and economic burden of the projected obesity trends in the USA and the UK. *The Lancet, 378*(9793), 815–25.

Water, T. (2011). Critical moments in preschool obesity: The call for nurses and communities to assess and intervene. *Contemporary Nurse, 40*(1), 60–70.

World Health Organization (2012). Face to face with chronic illness. Retrieved from http://www.who.int/features/2005/chronic_diseases/en/index.html

Wright, K. (2011). Influence of body mass index, gender, and Hispanic ethnicity on physical activity in urban children. *Journal for Specialists in Pediatric Nursing 16,* 90–104. doi:10.111/j.1744-6155.2010.00263.x

## CHAPTER 12

# Population Health in Trauma and Mental Health

MELISS V. BATCHEN, DNS, RN, CFN

MARY A. BEMKER, PhD, PhyS, LADC, LPCC, CCFP, CCTP, CNE, RN

## Population Health in Trauma and Mental Health

**P**OPULATION HEALTH is a term that continues to evolve in definition. The concept of population health is a common term used in
Canada, but even at its point of origin, a unified definition of population
health cannot be agreed upon by healthcare organizations and providers
there. Kindig and Stoddart (2003) defined population health as health
outcomes of a group of individuals that should include health outcomes,
patterns of health determinants, and policies and interventions that link
these two concepts. Population health differs from public health in that
population health addresses healthcare and concerns for specific groups
within a public grouping, whereas public health addresses healthcare
and concerns for overall populations.

Fawcett and Ellenbecker (2015) proposed a conceptual model of
nursing as it intersects with population health. It was noted that multiple
definitions of the term population health created confusion, incorporating concepts of epidemiology, public health, and community health, or
relied on elements defined by geography or common characteristics, using entire groups instead of focusing on the actual concept of the health
of a given population for individuals and determinants of health within
that population. The focus of the proposed model was the "attainment
of the highest possible quality of life for aggregates of people by means
of nursing activities" (Fawcett & Ellenbecker, 2015, p. 290). As nursing
incorporates a focus on caring for the whole patient versus a medical

291

model focused on the identification and treatment of disease or disorder processes, nursing's approach to population health should be teamed with the concepts of interdisciplinary caregivers to effectively address the needs of the various populations.

In 2006, Radzyminski proposed the importance of population health as a framework for forensic nursing and its emerging curriculum. She noted that common curricula were based on the general concept of the patient and advanced nursing practice in the traditional setting. A population health framework allowed forensic nurses to develop aggregate assessment skills applicable to patients/clients in like situations, with the goal of maximizing the health of any given population. Forensic nursing has been addressing population health for more than a decade, with specialties such as sexual assault nurse examiners (SANE), forensic nurse death investigators (FNDI), forensic mental health nurse practitioners, correctional facility nurses, and legal nurse consultants (LNC). These nurses' practices focus on specific populations and the inherent issues that may accompany the populations and care addressing their needs. SANEs perform rape examinations and evidence collection working with victims of sexual assault. Some of these nurses specialize in pediatric sexual assault examinations. Considering the horrific nature of the purported crime, the nurses have special training and regular debriefing to allow for discussion of techniques, needs of the populations, and professional collaboration for development of increased public safety knowledge. The FNDI usually works with a medical examiner or coroner's office and may be a primary or coinvestigator (Vessier-Batchen, 2007). These nurses bring critical nursing knowledge to a scene, using assessment skills and critical decision making to clarify aspects of a scene. Forensic mental health nurses may practice in various settings from criminal psychiatric facilities to outpatient clinics. These nurses must work with various mentally ill patients who have committed crimes and with those patients who are unable to function within the confines of the law, but do not warrant incarceration. Correctional nurses work with a particularly unique population in dealing with prisoners. The nurses must consider safety issues while incorporating safe and complete practice for varied offenders. The legal nurse consultant brings legal knowledge combined with nursing knowledge to aid in providing direction for attorneys working with medical malpractice and for nursing professionals who may be facing legal action related to practice.

According to Christopher (2014), a focus on community-based

nursing could effectively address the growing importance of population health management, noting that population health competency has become a critical variable in successful transformation of healthcare for these groups. The Visiting Nurse Service of New York (VNSNY) collaborated with Duke University's School of Nursing and New York University College of Nursing to understand and improve population-care-management knowledge in nursing staff and leaders. Focusing on identification and recognition of emerging trends in patient populations could effectively help nurses to identify and use tools that would help patients to manage chronic and complex health issues. This approach could also help nurses to improve patient outcomes by helping interprofessional teams to communicate positively with patients, with the intent of avoiding unnecessary emergency visits and hospital readmissions.

Population health is also used to reference vulnerable populations. These populations have become a burden for many American communities, ultimately leading to economic instability, improper or inadequate healthcare services, and social ignorance regarding the specific healthcare needs of the populations (U.K. Essays, 2015). Determining the vulnerability and identity of these populations requires knowledge and supportive resources to provide appropriate needed services. Hahn and Cella (2003) examined health outcomes assessments in vulnerable populations to better identify challenges in healthcare for these populations and to provide recommendations for better communication of needs and care for any identified populations. They highlighted the importance of assessing the literacy of any given population to ensure effective understanding and communication of the health issues and care needed at the time of the encounter. Recommendations included specificity and simplification of any resource and information materials, culturally appropriate communication interventions, and use of multimedia approaches such as pictures, graphics, and computers to convey information regarding healthcare and needs of the individual/population accurately. Further, DeGuzman and Kulbok (2012) explored the concept of "built environments," population health, and nursing's impact on the provision of care in given populations. Their development of a framework to identify influential levels of optimal health achievement in populations is primarily focused on the walkability (the accessibility of various activities within walking distances) of the built environment to access work, healthcare, and recreation. The alteration of walkability, by each of the populations and their environments, may affect health outcomes and behaviors. Advanced practice nurses (APNs) may be able to address those limitations and decreased walkability by providing education and direction for these populations.

Guzys, Kenny, Dickson-Swift, and Threlkeld (2015) explored the implications of a population health literacy assessment and populations' abilities to capably communicate and understand symptoms and needs to achieve optimal health. The authors were attempting to develop a working model of population health and an appropriate and complete assessment of any group's ability to convey those critical elements that lend to decreased health or the inability to meet health needs, or to obtain and use health-optimizing aids, such as medications, durable medical devices and equipment, and direct or indirect healthcare. Assessing and measuring literacy in an individual or population is a critical element of accurate assessment of healthcare needs. Care and teaching are important elements of ongoing healthcare optimization, but doing so on an appropriate level for the patient/population is paramount to success.

Many of the problems that directly or indirectly affect victims of trauma and mentally ill patients create functional limitations (Holtslag *et al.* , 2008). The study focused on the emotional, mental, and physical symptoms experienced by victims of trauma because of auto accidents. The authors examined the differences between injuries and disabilities versus fatalities by survivors of the trauma or of survivors who lost loved ones because of the auto accident, not only at the individual level, but also as a whole population of survivors. People who experience trauma or ongoing mental health issues may have difficulty maintaining employment, affording housing and utilities, and appropriately caring for self and/or family. As difficulties increase, functionality may continue to erode.

## Survivor Populations

### Trauma Populations

Trauma victims are referred to as survivors in many situations (Vessier-Batchen & Douglas, 2006; Vessier-Batchen, 2007). These trauma victims may be survivors of the loss of a loved one by homicide, suicide, or accident. Other survivors may have survived a direct trauma, including, but not limited to, survivor's guilt in an accident or event, major injury related to a trauma, rape, robbery and being held or confronted with a weapon, natural disasters, and physical/mental abuse. These types of losses and experiences can lead to traumatic aftereffects requiring medical and mental healthcare, medication, and hospitalization. Throughout the literature regarding trauma survival, post-traumatic stress disorder (PTSD) is a prominent diagnosis associated with these populations. The disorder, while mental and emotional, can lead to many physical health issues. Many sufferers report experiencing complications related to anorexia, self-harming (cutting, dangerous activities, etc.), drug use and dependence, and self-initiated denial of and isolation from other human contacts. Signs and symptoms of persons suffering from the aftereffects of trauma could include the appearance of disorientation and/or withdrawal, ongoing anxiety without a direct or visible link, night terrors, edginess, irritability, poor concentration, and mood swings (Psycheguides.com, n.d.). The person may become physically or verbally confrontational. These symptoms may appear hours, days, weeks, or months after the traumatic event. Active and retired military personnel may experience many of the same health issues of survival relative to their military assignments and deployments (discussed in detail in Chapter 9).

According to Victimsofcrime.org (2008), trauma following any type of victimization is a direct reaction to the aftermath of crime. Victims can suffer a tremendous amount of physical and psychological trauma categorized as primary or secondary injuries. Primary injuries include physical, financial, and emotional injuries, whereas secondary injuries, which may manifest for various reasons including lack of receipt of appropriate support and interventions, may result in PTSD. Physical injuries may include cuts, bruises, and broken bones, but may also include extreme fatigue, insomnia, and appetite changes. Financial harm may include theft of money and jewelry, property damage, or medical insurance that does not cover the cost of all expenses related to the trauma. Additional financial burdens may come when related funeral expenses may result from the trauma. Emotional injury can result in immediate and long-term reactions to victims, their loved ones, and friends. Recognizing the immediate, lingering, and long-term effects of trauma on the survivor could increase the effectiveness of treatment.

Cody and Beck (2014) studied the association of development of PTSD symptoms and physical health effects on survivors of two types of trauma, motor vehicle accidents (MVA) and interpersonal violence (IPV), and medications used to mediate symptoms. They noted an age disparity between the groups, with the IPV group being younger than the MVA group, on average. It was found that the more severe the injuries experienced by survivors in either type of trauma, the greater the incidence of use of pain and psychiatric medications by those survivors.

Medication and drug use and dependence may become another issue for these survivors. Medications, in conjunction with other treatment modalities, may be used to assist a patient through difficult periods as the patient finds or develops effective coping strategies related to the experience. When coping continues to elude the patient, other means of coping with the trauma may become prominent. The medications designed to assist the patient may become the means of coping for the patient. If these medications are closely monitored as required, the prescriber may note the problem and begin decreasing the availability of the drugs. In these cases, patients may turn to illegal or illicit drugs to obtain the same level of relief, euphoria, and numbness. The cycle of addiction could begin.

Post traumatic stress disorder (PTSD) has become a recognized disorder following a witnessed and/or an experienced traumatic event. There is no clear explanation for why some people develop the disorder, whereas others do not. The Mayo Clinic (n.d.) reports that causes of the disorder may be complex and may include inherited mental health risks, life experiences, inherited aspects of the person's personality, and the way in which the brain regulates chemicals and hormones released by the body in response to stressors, because of some trauma. Although there may be some mental health aspects of trauma, the mental health disorders that result from a traumatic experience usually differ from those issues faced by populations with mental illnesses. It is important for family and friends to be aware of and recognize the possible signs and symptoms of complications following trauma, but even more important for healthcare providers to recognize that their patients are not able to sufficiently cope with the experience. Regardless of the time that has passed since the experience, the patient may be unable to process the events psychologically or find an effective coping method to process the events of the experience.

PTSD is identified by parameters that help healthcare providers to isolate the disorder to treat its symptoms effectively. According to the Anxiety & Depression Association of America (ADAA, 2016), symptoms of PTSD may not appear until several months or years after a trauma. The person experiences symptoms for at least one month. Those symptoms may include re-experiencing the trauma through intrusive, distressing recollections of the event; emotional numbness; avoidance of places, people, and activities that serve as reminders; and increased stimulation or excitement leading to difficulty sleeping, concentrating, or sitting still.

When medications are used to help patients deal with the aftermath of trauma, an untoward effect may be drug addiction (Adshead & Ferris, 2007; Langman & Chung, 2013; Mayo Clinic, n.d.). Helping patients to find other means of coping with the trauma may not be effective enough, and medications may be necessary. When medicating the patient becomes necessary, meticulous monitoring is necessary to ensure the pharmacological intervention is effective and the patient is taking medications as prescribed. Medications used may include antidepressants, anti-anxiety medications, and prazosin, a drug used to reduce or suppress nightmares. Each of these medications has beneficial properties to help trauma survivors work through their experiences when used with corresponding treatments. However, each of these medications has the potential to become addictive and misused by these patients. The feelings of temporary relief for some patients using these medications may become overwhelmingly comforting, leading to the misuse and possible addiction. According to Adshead and Ferris (2007), PTSD in trauma survivors is usually a comorbid disorder, accompanying other survivor ailments such as depression, anxiety, panic and phobia disorders, and substance misuse. The authors also noted that personality disorders increased the possibility of PTSD development for some patients experiencing trauma. The study further highlighted the effects of treatment of trauma for patients and function in the home, at work, and in the patient's social circle. In assessing someone for the aftereffects of trauma, ask the question, and listen to the answer. Ask the patient about the trauma, regardless of the time elapsed since the trauma. This is especially important if months or even years have passed, but the patient is still experiencing problems that may otherwise have no explanation or cause. Listen to the answer. Allot time to provide an unencumbered answer by the patient, free of time constraints. Adshead and Ferris (2007) also recommended that the patient be advised that history taking and assessment would occur in two stages, a general psychiatric history and an account of the trauma and any post-trauma experiences and events. The patient may become overwhelmed and unable to relay all of the information completely in one visit. The patient could require a return visit to share the events of the experienced trauma fully.

Langman and Chung (2013) examined the correlation between medication misuse and drug addiction and trauma, specifically forgiveness, spirituality, traumatic guilt, and PTSD. The authors discussed the evidence of a high rate of PTSD and psychological comorbidity coexisting with other types of psychological difficulties. They hypothesized that a type of hypersensitivity may develop in trauma survivors, leaving them more vulnerable to dependency on medications and illicit drugs to suppress memories and triggers that cause reliving of the trauma. The examination of the elements of forgiveness, spirituality, and guilt were also revealed to correlate with a higher or lower probability of developing a drug addiction. The study revealed a possible correlation of forgiveness to health but not to development of an addiction to medications or illicit drugs. The aspect of spirituality was shown to demonstrate a stronger correlation to facing addiction, but not necessarily avoiding drug addiction after a trauma. Not surprisingly, feelings of guilt were most strongly correlating with development of PTSD and a higher risk of developing an addiction to medications following a trauma.

There are still no clear indicators to predict the outcomes for survivors of a trauma, but several signs and symptoms may help healthcare providers identify difficulties and lack of adequate coping mechanisms in survivors of trauma. Healthcare providers knowing about and using tools designed to help identify signs and symptoms of PTSD and ineffective coping skills in trauma survivors may possibly decrease the incidences of drug addiction, development of violent outbursts and long-term health issues, and further trauma for the survivor and loved ones exposed to the aftermath.

### Case Vignette

Cindy experienced a car accident in which her best friend was killed. Cindy was driving to a party with her friend when another driver swerved into their lane, resulting in a head-on collision. Cindy suffered severe injuries and was not able to attend her friend's funeral. She was released from the hospital after two months and continued with rehabilitative care for one more month. She also attended physical therapy during that time. She is now physically able to drive a car again, but is unable to sit behind the steering wheel. She begins to sweat, shake, and reports feeling nauseated. She has reported that she experiences nightmares about sitting in the car next to her friend and trying to wake her up. She has been referred by her primary care provider to an advanced practice registered nurse–psychiatric mental health (APRN-PMH) to address PTSD.

From your previous readings, what symptoms would you identify to indicate the development of PTSD? As a primary care provider, what would you say to the individual once PTSD is suspected? Why, as the primary care provider, would you refer this patient instead of trying to treat the presenting symptoms? How would you recommend the patient communicate with you in order to stay informed about treatments and care by the APRN-PMH?

## Mental Health Populations

In populations with mental illnesses, similar groupings occur within the types and symptoms of mental illnesses and diagnoses of patients, i.e., schizophrenia, bipolar disorders, depression, behavioral and substance abuse disorders, and anxiety. According to MedicineNet.com (2015), mental health is not confined to the absence of mental illness, but is more of an optimal level of thinking, feeling, and relating to others. This is a simple, but inclusive, definition of mental health. Addressing the needs of these populations has proven difficult in the past, as there are no visible or concrete symptoms as in medical illnesses. Symptoms may be subtle, presenting at varying times or in specific situations.

Difficulty in identifying the mental health needs of these population groups is underfunded and frequently overlooked. Recent crime statistics reported by many cities with large homeless populations have cited untreated mental health issues and inconsistent care for those committing crimes or becoming victims of crime (VessierBatchen, 2007). APNs and nurse-managed clinics could sufficiently provide availability of care and outreach for homeless patients and for those homeless victims who also have mental illnesses. For many patients in these populations, services and medications are scant or unavailable. Identifying those patients in need would be necessary. Care, monitoring, and ongoing treatment would be necessary to help these patients maintain pharmacological levels and overall health.

*Case Vignette*

Donald has a history of bipolar disorder and non-compliance with medications and therapy. Donald comes into the clinic complaining of an episode of extreme mania, stating that he stole his sister's credit card and bought several items costing several hundred dollars. Donald is exhibiting a heightened sense of accomplishment and reports that he is unstoppable in achieving his goals.

As the APRN-PMH, what would your initial counsel be to Donald regarding medication maintenance and therapy? How could you encourage him to maintain his medications and attend his therapy sessions regularly? What would you consider avoiding in discussion with Donald at this time to avoid confrontation with him? What would you need to know from Donald to ensure that he could safely be allowed to leave your practice?

## Population Needs

Populations may tend to group together because of the ability to better relate to the situations and/or aftermath of a particular type of trauma or illness, creating unique health needs within that population or group. Identifying specific health needs within each of these groups is critical in providing optimal care and direction of services and resources. MacDonald, Newburn-Cook, Allen, and Reutter (2013) posited that the concept of embracing population health in nursing research would provide opportunities to explore individuals' health outcomes influenced by complex social, political, and economic forces, as well as by knowledge, behaviors, and communities. The authors discussed nursing's central core concern and role to facilitate, support, and assist individual, families, and communities, but also discussed the need for attention to multilevel determinants of health as crucial. The proposed population health framework provides for a broader base for nursing research, melding synergistically with the holistic view of humans encompassed by the nursing profession.

Mandated insurance to support healthcare for Americans has taxed the current healthcare system without providing better reimbursement for healthcare providers or increasing the number of healthcare providers available to deliver care to the masses. Iglehart (2013) explored the roles of APNs and limitations/restrictions that hinder full and logical use of practitioners fully capable of greater authority, responsibilities, and functions. According to an earlier Institute of Medicine (IOM, 2010) report [as cited in Iglehart, 2013], 16 states and the District of Columbia allow APRNs to diagnose, treat, and refer patients and prescribe medications without physician supervision. Nine states require physician oversight for APRNs to prescribe, and 24 states require physician involvement/oversight for APRNs to diagnose and treat patients and prescribe medications. States regularly consider reasonable expansion of scope-of-practice regulation to use the APRN workforce available effectively. The level of APRN practice autonomy is changing regularly. Another limitation that is critical to using APRNs effectively is the restrictions and policies of reimbursement for services used by public and private payers. These policies limit coverage for services provided by APRNs and payment reimbursement rates, may be determined by APRN designations as primary care providers, and may include or exclude APRNs as independent practitioners in or out of the healthcare network.

The American Association of Colleges of Nursing (AACN, 2016), the overseer and accrediting body for baccalaureate, master's, and doctoral nursing education, categorizes nurse practitioners (NPs), certified nurse midwives (CNM), clinical nurse specialists (CNS), and certified registered nurse anesthetists (CRNA) as advanced practice nurses. The question posited by this organization is whether an APRN should be providing primary care and, based on several studies, the answer is overwhelmingly yes. The organization cited many myths and untruths identified by the American Medical Association (AMA) regarding education and clinical knowledge of APRNs that disqualifies these practitioners from practicing independently. Clarity is provided and supported to distinguish NPs from physicians and the effect of using APRNs to enhance and embellish healthcare availability for the masses versus limiting care because of restrictions and misinformation.

## Trauma Populations and Advanced Practice Nursing

### *Impact on the Populations*

Advanced practice nursing requires extensive and advanced knowledge of pathophysiology, pharmacology, and physical assessments, providing an extension of care to populations that may otherwise receive less specialized care needed to address their issues. According to Kartha *et al.* (2014), using APNs allows increased care access with similar outcomes in primary care and surgery. The authors examined the use of physician assistants (PA) and APRNs by the Veterans Health Administration (VHA), noting that both specialists are used for inpatient care. The authors compared backgrounds, training, regulation, reimbursement, and a long-standing preference for PAs versus APRNs by the VHA, noting that APRNs and PAs were widely used throughout the hospital system and provided valuable extensions of care and resources.

### *Physical and Emotional Symptoms*

Trauma survivors may experience physical symptoms as they deal with an incident, event, or loss. There may also be emotional symptoms that emerge, which can be triggered by an environment, sounds, or a memory. Any of these triggers may be caused by a one-time event, i.e., an accident, natural disaster, or violent attack; by repeated triggers, i.e., an ongoing battle with a life-threatening illness or living in a high-crime area; or by situational events, i.e., impending surgery, sudden death of a loved one, or a humiliating or disappointing experience (Helpguide.org, 2016). When a PTSD event occurs, the person may not immediately be identified as a PTSD patient or trauma survivor. Medical identification bracelets and/or pet service companions are becoming increasingly used for trauma survivors, which can help first responders to provide appropriate care for these patients.

According to Mims and Waddell (2016), the goal of animal-assisted therapy is to provide long-term therapy to survivors of trauma, whether to a group or an individual. Kruger and Serpell (2010) and Sussman (1985) [both as cited by Mims & Waddell, 2016] noted improved blood pressures, decreased use of medications, and the psychological benefits of reduced anxiety and stress in human-animal interactions, sufficient to warrant consideration of their use on a regular basis with trauma survivors. Dietz, Davis, and Pennings (2012) examined situations with children who suffered various types of trauma showing significant decreases in trauma symptoms in therapy sessions, including therapy animal versus therapy sessions conducted without therapy animals.

The emotional aftermath of trauma may also lead to self-treatment and selfmedication using prescriptive medications beyond physician instructions and intended use, illicit drugs, and/or alcohol to decrease and dampen thoughts and memories of the trauma. An investigation into this method of treatment was conducted by Ertl, Saile, Neuner, and Catani (2016), in which they referred to the self-treatment as selfmedication hypothesis. The study revealed that cross-sectional and longitudinal studies in this area reported a link between trauma-exposure and substance abuse.

*Methods of Meeting Needs*

Some recommended ways advanced practice nurses could assist victims or survivors of trauma to begin or continue a healing process might include using movement, avoiding isolation, learning to self-regulate the nervous system, and maintaining and taking care of health (Helpguide.org, 2016). Movement may include exercising or physical activities. The APRN should remind the patient to focus on the body's activity or to tune into the rhythm of the activity, and not allow distracting thoughts. Withdrawal from people and activities is common, but creates a negative space to remember or relive the event. There may be fear that explanations will be solicited or that the victim may have to "entertain" the person or people or answer questions about the trauma. Reminding the victim that the activities and discussions are not determined by anyone else may empower the victim to allow support without fear of becoming overwhelmed. Other ways of minimizing isolation could include volunteering, joining a support group, reconnecting with old friends, and participating in social activities.

Learning to self-regulate the nervous system may sound difficult, but could be as simple as participating in yoga or tai chi classes, allowing feelings to be experienced without suppression or hiding, or using calming activities such as listening to music, walking, or spending time with a pet. Making health maintenance and care a priority is crucial to building a strong road to recovery. Developing a sleep and wake routine, avoiding drugs and alcohol, eating a well-balanced diet, and reducing stress will help the victim to maintain health while finding and developing effective coping methods to aid in recovery and resolution.

Continued support and/or availability of support is a critical element of helping trauma survivors achieve levels of resolution, which allow them to move forward in life with increased positive outcomes. Physical and mental healthcare meeting the needs particular to these populations can facilitate a fuller recovery for the survivors and their surrounding support persons (victimsofcrime.org, 2008). These activities can be presented and supported by the APN, providing direction for the victim/survivor, while assisting with processing the loss and feelings associated with the event.

As APRNs expand their areas of practice, using resources to provide appropriate and effective care for trauma survivors should include ongoing and current methods of treatment and care for the survivors. The Office of Violence Against Women (2014) provides courses that educate healthcare providers by helping them improve their ability to address types of violence and the repercussions of that violence. A course is available that teaches about the history of violence and sexual assault in Native American tribes. Courses are also available for professionals that provide information about trauma care programs.

### Case Vignette

Michael was robbed at gunpoint and beaten by the robber. The police brought him to the ER for his injuries. The APRN on duty examined Michael and found that he had a suspected concussion, several lacerations, and a broken rib. Michael is withdrawn and appears fearful when someone approaches him to provide care.

As the APRN, what would you say as you approach Michael to discuss his injuries and care? In order to re-assess Michael, what would be the best way to approach him to conduct a physical examination for him without causing further trauma or fear? Who else would you, as the APRN, call to provide support and consultation for Michael?

## Mental Health Populations and Advanced Practice Nursing

*Impact on the Populations*

Mental health issues are an ongoing discussion in the media and in inpatient and outpatient care environments. Violent and nonviolent crimes, committed by or to persons with mental illnesses, bring the issues concerning care and lack of availability and/or affordability of that care into focus. These events often link the incidences of homelessness, inconsistent care, medication administration, and continuity, and invisibility of the problem to the attention of the public. These populations, either grouped together or grouped by illnesses and like symptoms, continue to struggle with perceptions of their illnesses and access to care. As APNs become more specialized, nurses could logically provide needed care for these varied populations, by populating clinics, providing community care in outreach mobile units, and providing education for the community, as well as the patients in need. The American Psychological Association (APA, 2017) and the Agency for Healthcare Research and Quality (AHRQ, 2017) report that approximately one in four patients seen by a primary care provider experiences symptoms of depression. Of the patients seen, only about one-third of the patients are diagnosed with this disease.

The incidences of violence surrounding populations with mental illnesses are more prevalent than previously noted in earlier decades (Amar & Clements, 2011). APNs who specialize in psychiatric nursing may encounter many of these victims and offenders in traditional care settings, delving into forensic psychiatric nursing (correctional or forensic psychiatric facilities) in a nonforensic environment. The medicolegal implications of advanced practice with patients with mental illness are not regularly considered but should be examined by APNs. The broader consideration of what these practitioners do and the patients they treat could maximize treatment of trauma, identification of potential offender behaviors, and implementation of strategies and interventions for all levels of prevention.

Ribe *et al.* (2015) examined the effects of infection and mortality on populations with severe mental illnesses, namely bipolar affective disorder and schizophrenia. The authors attempted to discover why populations with severe mental illnesses had a higher mortality rate within 30 days after a hospital admission with an infection compared to patients with similar admission diagnosis but with no history or evidence of mental illnesses. This study supports the concept that populations with mental illnesses should be considered as vulnerable, both mentally and physically, because higher mortality following medical illnesses, namely infections, was evident for these populations.

*Mental Health Statistics, Issues, and Practice*

People may experience the highs and lows of life on a regular basis, regardless of locale, socioeconomic status, marital status, sexual orientation, or age. For mental health populations, stresses and challenges affect daily lives for children, adults, and the elderly, with varying effects present for each person or group. The severity, duration, and physiological changes in an individual may be greatly impacted when those difficulties are grounded in mental illness.

According to the American Psychiatric Association (2015), mental illness is a health condition that creates differences in thoughts, emotions, and/or actions, which may, in turn, lead to unhappiness and despair. The multiple disorders, syndromes, and diseases in these populations can cause problems with functioning in settings in which others are involved and may become most noticed in social, family, and work settings.

Although mental illnesses are treatable, many portions of these populations are ashamed to seek out care and assistance until the issues become major factors in their lives. They may not be able to maintain employment, stable family dynamics, or effective communications, especially when attempting to express feelings of anxiety or depression associated with some illnesses. Additionally, approximately 40% of all reported disabilities worldwide are related to mental illness. Depression, bipolar disorder, and obsessive-compulsive disorders are the primary diagnoses of those noted illnesses identified among patients seeking disability support (National Alliance on Mental Illness, 2017).

Most individuals who have a mental illness can function. Although overall the vast majority of the public perceive patients with mental illness as being homeless or deranged, that is typically not the case. It may be difficult to obtain data about patients with mental illnesses because symptoms may be mild and/or intermittent and because these patients may function normally in living environments and circumstances, making it important for primary care providers to screen for mental health issues routinely.

Comorbidity is often noted when other manifestations of illness are identified in addition to the mental health issues the patient/client is presenting. Discovery of mental health issues may be more commonly identified when an individual presents with an identified disease or disorder. A thorough assessment may be the most effective means for determining comorbidity of illness/disease and mental illness. Examples of corresponding events could include lingering flu or cold symptoms and anxiety and depression, repeated headaches or migraines and depression and substance abuse, or a previous trauma, such as an automobile accident and PTSD and substance use disorders (Substance Abuse and Mental Health Services Administration, 2016). Substance use disorders are discussed in detail in Chapter 13.

The prevalence of populations with mental illness in the United States (U.S.) has become more widely recognized. Over 45 million adults have been diagnosed as having some form of mental illness in the past year. At least 11 million of those patients are diagnosed with a serious mental illness (National Institute of Mental Health, n.d.). Nearly 25% of all adult stays in a nonpsychiatric, civilian hospital are related to depressive disorders, schizophrenia, bipolar incidences, or some other mental health or substance use disorder (American Psychological Association, 2017).

The Centers for Disease Control and Prevention (CDC) determined that individuals with severe psychological distress increased between 2007 and 2011 (2.7% to 3.4%, respectively) in the United States. In 2012, there was a slight decrease to 3.0%. However, from 2013 to 2016, no significant findings have been reported regarding adults reporting severe psychological distress within the previous 30 days prior to a hospital admission (Centers for Disease Control and Prevention, 2016a).

With the inclusion of mental health services in the Patient Protection and Affordable Care Act (also referred to as the Affordable Care Act, or ACA), findings indicate that more patients in these mental health populations are seeking treatment for mental health conditions; however, among those seeking treatment for mental health conditions, more patients are turning to primary care providers for these services instead of services provided by specialized practitioners (Lowes, 2016).

The Global Burden of Disease Study (last updated in 2015) is supported by the National Institute of Mental Health (NIMH) and the Global Alliance for Chronic Disease, who collaborated with more than 650 organizations interested in mental health to identify neuropsychiatric disorders and populations with mental illnesses as a disease burden. The ongoing study continues to collect and update data regarding mental illnesses as a grouping and considering mental health and behavioral and neurological disorders, which comprise 10% of the disease burden. Even though this combination of health concerns is prominent for these identified populations, few resources are noted globally to address the issues (National Institutes of Health, n.d.). The most common mental health disorders noted among adults include anxiety, depression, bipolar disorder, schizophrenia, dementia, and developmental disorders (World Health Organization, 2016). As many of these patients present to general practitioners and health clinics, it is important to screen patients carefully and make referrals to the appropriate care providers. Recognition of specific mental health problems is important for proper treatment and although many conditions may look similar, treatment regimens and drug combinations are often required to treat many disorders.

It is imperative, as a provider, that an overall assessment be conducted and to know the populations that are being served. An individual presenting with joint pain may be depressed because of that pain. Another patient may speak about a situation that is causing depression and anxiety. If it can be linked back to a situation, then the individual may have an adjustment reaction rather than depression. With all these variables and nuances, it can be important to screen and refer, considering the need for medication as a possibility and the need for psychotherapy in more severe and complex cases. In some cases, both may be warranted. For specific criteria related to the various types of depression, please consult the *Diagnostic and Statistical Manual of Mental Disorders, Fifth Edition* (DSM-5) (APA, 2013).

Anxiety disorders are evidenced by excessive fear continuing beyond a time that appears to be reasonable. Anxiety is differentiated from fear, as fear is the emotional and physical responses associated with a past event that occurred. Anxiety may generate the same dynamics, but they are connected to the belief that something negative might happen in the future. What specifically that future event might be is the differentiating factor associated with specific anxiety disorders (American Psychiatric Association, 2013; SAMHSA, 2016). Cultural factors should be considered when screening for anxiety disorders. It is also important to address point of origin, because many anxiety disorders developed during childhood and persist into adulthood. Anxiety disorders should be diagnosed only after the physiological etiology of a reaction is eliminated. Screening tools for anxiety include the Generalized Anxiety Disorder 7-Item (GAD-7) and the Primary Care Post-Traumatic Stress Disorder Screen (PC-PTSD) (SAMHSA, 2013).

Patients with bipolar and bipolar-related disorders experience manic, hypomanic, and depressive symptomatology. During the manic stage of this disease, patients may exhibit such symptoms as irritable mood, hyperactivity, pressured speech, flight of ideas, uncontrolled involvement in activities that have a high potential for injury, delusions of grandeur, and a decreased need for sleep (American Psychiatric Association, 2013; World Health Organization, 2016). Even if depressive etiology is not evident, an individual may be bipolar (World Health Organization, 2016). The depressive dynamics evident with bipolar disorder mimic those of someone with depression. The difference is that both the manic and hypomanic stages and the depressive state (with five or more depressive criteria) would be noted within two weeks of occurrence of each stage (American Psychiatric Association, 2013). Diagnosis rather than screening is needed to make an accurate determination of the disease. As previously stated, it is important to assess the situation. A thorough history, including life events, is imperative to accurately screen and diagnose mental health issues. Tools used for screening include the STABLE Resource Tool Kit, and the Mood Disorder Questionnaire (Substance Abuse and Mental Health Services Administration, 2013).

*Treatments and Therapies*

Treatment for mental health conditions tend to be focused on medication or psychotherapy alone. However, combining pharmacotherapy with psychotherapy has proven to be more effective than either treatment used alone. This difference was especially prevalent with a patient presents with major depression, panic disorder, or obsessive-compulsive disorder (OCD) (Cuijpers *et al.*, 2014). The ability to differentiate needed therapies is an important consideration for any practitioner. Many times, patients want medications to remedy deep-seated and/or neurological problems. It is difficult for these issues to be managed with medication alone.

The largest gain in prescription medications for mental health issues continues to be antidepressants and medications to treat anxiety (Grohol, 2013). Antidepressants are the third most prescribed medications by U.S. physicians, following prescriptions for analgesics and antihyperlipidemia agents (Centers for Disease Control and Prevention, 2016b). Because many patients seek these medications from their primary care providers, it is important to screen for depression and treat accordingly. Most patients do not associate antidepressants with addiction and may assume that these medications are perfectly safe. However, the Physician's Desk Reference (2017) stipulates criteria for prescribing and the contraindications and potential side effects that occur. When anti-anxiety medication is discussed, dependency is one concern noted. Regardless of the type of medication considered, it is important to do a thorough history and consider the physical and mental ramifications of the medication on the patient's overall health.

When addressing prescriptions for mental health issues and illnesses, correct diagnosis from an experienced mental health clinician is important. The practitioner should also know and understand the rationale for medications prescribed. In recent decades, medications originally prescribed for one diagnosis have been found to be useful in treating other illnesses, referred to as off-label prescribing, so the practitioner must be aware of the diagnosis for which a medication has been prescribed. The rise in the practice of off-label prescribing, and the rise in patient requests for specific medications from primary care providers, has been linked to advertising by the pharmaceutical companies. Caution must be maintained when prescribing off-label, especially when treating vulnerable populations (Smith, 2012). Additional treatments that have proven useful for patients with mental illnesses include individual and group talk therapy, hypnosis, and eye movement desensitization and reprocessing (EMDR). Cognitive-behavioral therapy is another useful tool in treating some mental illnesses. The goal of this treatment modality is to shift negative thoughts and feelings into a healthier and more positive direction. By doing so, behaviors are more positive, generating greater productive behaviors in patients (Beck & Haigh, 2014).

If people believe themselves to be powerless to become healthier because of chronic disease, there is no motivation to attempt change. These patients may develop a mindset that nothing will work. They may feel that they have tried multiple methods for overcoming the moods and changes without success. Depression is almost inevitable and expected. Practitioners and therapists could help these patients realize their limitations and steps to be taken to achieve a higher level of health (Deeley, 2017).

Shapiro and Forrest (2016) examined EMDR as a means of therapy that allows the patient to obtain issues and resolutions for feelings generated by a traumatic or detrimental life event. Through this modality, negative thoughts can be refocused and reframed, distress can be eliminated, and physiological responses to the event or series of events can be eliminated. During this treatment, the individual is requested to follow movements with the eyes, listen to specific sound patterns, and/or feel tapping in a neutral area of the body. Through this process, the traumatic memories are partnered with bilateral attention activation.

Adams, Koop, Quan, and Norris (2015) explored predictors of admissions, hospital lengths of stay, emergency department wait times, and costs of readmissions and care in older adults with and without diagnoses of mental illnesses in two provinces of Canada. It was discovered that, of those older adults with diagnosed mental illnesses, hospital admissions and lengths of stay were significantly longer than for those older adults with similar medical diagnoses but no diagnoses of mental illnesses. The authors discovered discrepancies in correct and appropriate physician or care referrals, test delays, and lack of home care and community services for older adults with mental illnesses, leading to an increased use of resources, and lengthened recovery for these adults.

In instances of mental illness in children, the signs and symptoms may not become evident until later in a child's development. With incidences of bullying becoming more widely evident and suicide ranked as the third leading cause of death in 10 to 24 year olds, diagnosis and care of children with mental illnesses is of greater concern for psychiatric nurses (Cooper, Clements, & Holt, 2012). The authors discussed the correlation of bullying and suicide in children with and without mental illnesses. The extensive review of current literature revealed a strong relationship between bullying and adolescent suicides with or without diagnoses of mental illnesses. Some literature noted greater propensity for suicidal actions in males more than females, whereas other studies revealed the greater differences noted more in methods versus gender. Although this study focused on bullying in childhood groups, bullying can be a factor in suicidal ideation in populations with mental illnesses, because these populations are considered vulnerable and may be more visible for varied reasons, leaving them susceptible to verbal and physical attacks.

Keyes, Dhingra, and Simoes (2010) examined changes in levels of mental health as predictors of future risk of mental illness. The authors concluded that gains in mental health decreased the odds of incidence of mental illness. They also explained that losses of mental healthcare availability increased the odds of incidences of mental illness. A patient's previous history of mental illness is a good predictor of future mental illness; however, the authors believe that tools for monitoring mental health and illness should be further evaluated to improve diagnosis of, response to, and treatment for mental illness at a population level. The research revealed that moderate mental health is a good predictor of continued mental health and languishing is a stronger predictor of future mental illness.

## Methods of Meeting Needs

As APNs develop specialty practice roles, there is a great opportunity to meet the needs of patients with mental illnesses. These patients may not require hospitalization but may require ongoing monitoring and treatment, medication adjustments, and evaluations to determine increasing treatment needs.

One in four Americans live with and/or experience mental illness. With the paucity of mental health and addiction care providers, APNs specializing in psychiatric mental healthcare are critical to support healthier outcomes and greater care consistency for these populations (Hanrahan, Delaney, & Stuart, 2012). The authors recognized psychiatric nursing as one of the oldest nursing specialties and more than 15,000 APRNs-PMH certified in the field. Although this number seems significant, it is scant when measuring the number of people with diagnosed mental illnesses and lack of available care. The authors examined the APRN-PMH workforce, difficulties faced and continuing for the practitioners, aging out of current practitioners, need for support and leadership recognition within the field, and need for recruitment and retention of practitioners in the specialty. The average age of the APRN-PMH workforce is 51 years, with only 8% of the workforce reportedly below the age of 40 years. Within 10 years, half of these practitioners will be eligible for retirement. These practitioners also lack visibility and note of value and importance in the nursing workforce. Policy documents regarding mental healthcare often omit the psychiatric nurse and NP while addressing psychiatrists, psychologists, and social workers. This practice may exclude or inadequately address critical information and knowledge particular to nurses, such as patient safety issues. A lack of support for APRN-PMH specialists leads to frustration, burnout, and loss of continued commitment to the specialty. Hanrahan *et al.* (2012) outlined strategies to address the crisis of a shortage of these specialty practitioners. They noted that these practitioners would be able to provide the greatly needed care for the underserved population and its health needs and should include expanding the concept of recovery and endorsing peer support to continue recovery, which has long been central to APRN-PMH practice. The authors also highlighted the need for implementing strong recruitment strategies at different levels of nursing practice and on federal, state, and local levels; fostering leadership development throughout the workforce; and enhancing support of these practitioners.

Keyes *et al.* (2010) noted that measures and diagnostic criteria of mental health might be useful as monitoring and clinical screening tools for the practitioner. They noted that, based on their 10-year study, the prevalence of mental illness increases independent of baseline findings, highlighting the implications for development of effective interventions and support for specific mental health populations. Addressing the specific needs of mental health populations may further positive health promotion and protection for these vulnerable groups.

According to Cusack, de Crespigny, and Athanasos (2011), many areas of the country experience extreme weather conditions, but heat is one of the most predominant weather conditions found in most parts of the country. Although the authors focused their study in Australia, this same study criteria is applicable in the United States, i.e., the southern states and southern California experience very little winter weather. Prolonged and extreme heat heightens drug and alcohol conditions and exacerbates mental illnesses. Heat-related illnesses can create overwhelming clinical needs and healthcare management issues. Practitioners must understand and appreciate the complications that can be created by such extreme weather conditions. Understanding how heat affects the body and why people with mental health and substance use conditions are more susceptible to health risks in such situations will help the practitioner to effectively treat such conditions and address the issues. The average person exposed to the heat of a season for a prolonged period may experience heat stress as the body works to regulate temperature. For those populations on psychiatric medications or that use alcohol and/or drugs that can interfere with normal heat regulation of the body, a greater risk of heat-related problems may occur. The practitioner should be aware of the thermoregulatory side effects of many medications and some street drugs to treat a patient who may experience more difficulty in the heat more effectively. Awareness of the effects of older and newer generations of neuroleptic and anticholinergic medications have been associated with heat-related emergencies, such as heat intolerance and stroke, because of their effects on the body's natural thermoregulation. The authors also noted that these patients may not be able to cope with and adapt to changes in temperature because of physical and/or mental impairments. Practitioners should note that increased monitoring of these patients is needed in order to avert heat-related emergencies.

*Case Vignette*

Zeke was brought into the emergency department (ED) by police because of erratic behavior at his workplace. His boss told police that Zeke was "not acting right" and the other employees became frightened. The ED's APRN-PMH on staff was called in to examine Zeke. After the initial examination, you, as the APRN-PMH, discover that Zeke has a previous diagnosis of schizophrenia. He reports that he has had the flu and is not sure that his medication is working.

As the ED APRN-PMH, what would you recommend initially as care for Zeke? What tests would you consider ordering to help Zeke regain stabilization? Who would you contact to ensure Zeke's continuity of care with other care providers? What immediate interprofessional collaborations would you recommend in this situation?

## Overlapping Issues Between the Populations

Although the effects of trauma may be acute or chronic and could require long-term care and medications, symptoms and treatment of mental illnesses usually require lifelong, ongoing care, treatment, medication administration and adjustments, and monitoring. It may be difficult to separate traumatic emotional disturbances and difficulties and actual mental illnesses in overburdened emergency departments and quick clinics because of patient loads and time constraints. Determining one condition from another requires time, true listening, and accurate assessments to help these patients.

Trauma can have a major impact on a person's life. If that person experiences a traumatic event and has a mental illness, the effects of that trauma may be increased and without effective treatments commonly used. The person may be less likely to process and adapt to the address stressors physically, psychologically, socially, and/or emotionally. Martins, Baes, Tofoli, and Juruena (2014) examined the effects of the trauma of emotional child abuse to the adult development of severe and chronic depression. Bernstein *et al.* (2003) and Butchart (2006) [as cited in Martins *et al.*, 2014] examined and discovered a significant correlation between traumatic events that occur during childhood and adolescence referred to as early-life-stress (ELS) and unfavorable long-term health outcomes in adulthood. For persons with a mental illness experiencing trauma, the practitioner must consider that these individuals may or may not have the resiliency to effectively use or benefit from common treatments and may need combinations of treatments, including additional medications, to recover from a traumatic event.

The potential for not addressing feelings and emotions following a traumatic experience may be a foundation for the development of a mental illness. Examples of mental disorders related to trauma include social engagement disorders, PTSD, and reactive attachment disorders. Reaction to stressors and traumatic events are varied and dependent on multiple factors. Whether the individual first experienced the trauma or the mental health issues, the practitioner must consider that if a patient or client is experiencing delayed, prolonged, or intermittent responses to a traumatic event, it is important to provide support and assistance to address the issues. Support and assistance may come in the form of a support group, trauma support professional, psychiatric mental health NP, psychotherapist, counselor, or psychiatrist. Medications can support an individual for a time; however, it is important that treatment be augmented with additional support. The potential for the development of a substance addiction could be perpetuated (Smith, 2012). Although various medications are utilized for the treatment of mental illness and trauma, the practitioner should be aware that an individual previously diagnosed with a specific mental health condition might require special considerations before medication is prescribed for an extended time. With some diseases, such as bipolar disorder and schizophrenia, clinicians with clinical expertise and advanced education specific to mental health diseases offer a professional diagnosis and treatment protocol for safety and effective treatment outcomes. Many patients routinely seek ongoing care with a primary care provider. Although treatment and monitoring with these professionals is appropriate in many instances, care of patients with mental illness, mild or severe, may not be as thorough. The importance of effectively using referrals and consultations to specialists when indicated can enhance the care of patients by all professionals involved.

## Financial Impact of Trauma and Mental Illness

The burdens of overcoming the effects of trauma or the ongoing needs of mental healthcare are increased by the financial strain that may accompany care (Grossmeier, Terry, Anderson, & Wright, 2012). For those victims/survivors who can continue to work, employer insurance may or may not cover the cost of ongoing care. For those victims/survivors who hold only part-time work or are unable to work at all, the cost of care may be prohibitive, leading to unchecked symptoms and inadequate to no care.

According to Insel (2015), the World Economic Forum reported that global, mental health costs were estimated at $2.5 trillion in 2010 with a projected cost of $6 trillion by 2030. This cost is one of the largest among diseases in the world. According to the National Alliance on Mental Health (2017), approximately 44 million American adults, or nearly 19% of the population, experience some form of mental illness in any given year. About 10 million adults have a mental illness that interferes or limits major life activities (National Alliance on Mental Illness, 2017; National Institute of Mental Health, n.d.). Twenty-five percent of American adults experienced anxiety or depression during the last year, some of which were related to PTSD. Among adolescents, approximately 21% experience a severe mental disorder at some point during their lives (National Alliance on Mental Illness, 2017). Although many of these individuals reside in homeless shelters or are incarcerated, many more individuals suffer life difficulties and obstacles due to mental health dynamics. Only 41% of populations with a mental health condition received services in the past year. Among those patients and clients who use mental health services, most are identified as Caucasians. African Americans and Hispanic Americans used mental health services at approximately half the rate of Caucasians, whereas Asian Americans used mental health services at approximately one-third of the rate of Caucasians. Fifty percent of chronic mental illnesses begin by age 14 and 75% of chronic illnesses are evidenced by age 24. In spite of what is currently known about mental illness and the need for treatment, it could be decades between initial presentation of the first symptoms and initial treatment (National Alliance on Mental Illness, 2017). The cost of mental illness and treatment was approximately $193 billion in lost earnings. These financial burdens were ultimately placed on society, employers, families, and individuals. Portions of these financial considerations comprise Social Security Disability benefits (SSI and

SSDI) that are paid to individuals disabled due to mental disorders. In 2012, it was reported that approximately 5.3 million people 65 years of age or younger received SSI and SSDI benefits due to their mental health status. This constitutes approximately 70% of individuals who receive these benefits on a yearly basis (Insel, 2015).

Of patients seen and treated by a primary care provider, approximately one in four patients experience symptoms of depression (Agency for Healthcare Research and Quality, 2017; American Psychological Association, 2017). Only about one-third of these patients/clients are diagnosed with this disease (American Psychological Association, 2017). In addition, those patients with a serious mental illness have an increased risk of developing other chronic conditions. In the United States, young adults 18 years of age or older and with treatable, but undiagnosed, mental health issues, die 25 years earlier than persons of the same age group without any mental health issues when a medical condition or situation occurs. Additionally, adolescents with mental health issues struggle in school environments. If placed in a special education environment while in school, students with mental health issues are found to have the highest dropout rate (37%) of any disabled population in school (National Alliance on Mental Illness, 2017).

## Summary

Evidence supports the effectiveness and quality care attributed to the skill and knowledge of APRNs (Manion & Odiaga, 2014). High levels of patient satisfaction have also been reported by patients working with APRNs. The critical need for liberalization of the full scope of practice laws in all states would help practitioners to achieve the goal of legal autonomy and to increase the availability and affordability of healthcare services for more populations. Practitioner led health clinics have proven to be successful and cost-effective, providing high-quality care in areas less served and to populations that do not access traditional healthcare settings for multiple reasons. Such clinics have demonstrated success in meeting the health needs of patients in various populations who might have avoided seeking help, even if the need was recognized. These clinics also aid the community in addressing unrecognized health needs, augmenting services that might otherwise be provided through emergency departments and urgent care clinics.

The economic impact of healthcare has changed in past years. Although patients seem to have more access to healthcare cost coverage, some physicians and other primary care providers are leaving practices, unhappy with government regulations. This crisis creates longer patient wait times for evaluation and receipt of care. Emergency departments are overwhelmed and hospitals face financial crises. Practicing APRNs currently outnumber family practice practitioners and should be recognized as an integral element of the complex solution to affordable healthcare (Manion & Odiaga, 2014).

## Tool Kit and Resources

The tools and resources available to practitioners in aiding patients in recovery from trauma or maintenance of stability in mental illnesses are many. For survivors of trauma, there may be physical injuries to overcome, requiring medical interventions, short- or long-term care, multiple surgeries and/or physical therapy, and possible rehabilitation. These consequences following a trauma can lead to prolonged need for medical interventions, possible medication dependency to treat physical pain, and alcohol and/or drug overuse and abuse. Another aspect of trauma is the psychological and emotional injuries that may occur. Being told to move on or get over it does not help the survivor resolve these more complex issues. Knowing where to get the needed help is as critical as realizing that help is needed. For survivors of trauma, PTSD is a real and frequent consequence of trauma, but not all survivors develop this disorder. Finding appropriate coping methods and outside help to deal with symptoms and events can be as daunting as the disorder. Some forms of psychotherapy may help some survivors, whereas psychotherapy and medication may be needed for more extreme cases (Mayo Clinic, n.d.). Informal groups may be another alternative for many survivors, using support groups as a means to express grief, anger, confusion, or sadness more readily and safely. For APNs working with these populations, knowing the physical implications of the trauma and possible psychological and emotional implications will be critical in providing support and treatment.

Jacobs, Jones, Gabella, Spring, and Brownson (2012) reviewed tools available to encourage and enhance the implementation of an evidence-based approach of caring in public health. These tools could be adapted to address care of the health needs of target populations specifically. The Council for Training in Evidence-Based Behavioral Practice was formed using experts in medicine, nursing, public health, social work, psychology, and library sciences to produce training using a transdisciplinary model of evidence-based practice facilitating communication and collaboration. A critical component of development of useful tools is training of the professionals who would be responsible for using the tools for evaluation and formulating and providing recommendations for these populations. Key elements of the training were identified as engaging the community in assessment and decision making, using data and information systems systematically, making decisions on the best available peer-reviewed evidence, applying program planning frameworks based in health behavioral theory, conducting sound evaluation, and disseminating what is learned. Collecting data relevant to evaluation and care of the target population provides the foundation for development/identification of the appropriate evaluation tools, ultimately providing a more complete picture of the population health needs. Once the appropriate data are identified, the practitioners should select the best available evidence by using tools that synthesize, interpret, and evaluate the literature. With this information, practitioners can develop evidence-based guidelines for evaluation and treatment recommendations for the targeted population. An operational framework, and evaluation and dissemination of the program structure, function, and process, can be implemented.

Incorporating scientific evidence available to practitioners can help these professionals meet the demands for a systematic approach to public and population health problems that should yield measurable outcomes.

Substance Abuse and Mental Health Services Administration - Health Resources and Services Administration (SAMHSA-HRSA, 2017) noted that even with a high prevalence of mental health and substance abuse problems, too many Americans are untreated - in part because of undiagnosed conditions, disorders, or diseases. Earlier identification of mental health and substance abuse disorders translates into earlier and, possibly, better care and intervention. Screening is imperative for all patients, including children and the elderly. The organization's website provides information and access to many assessment tools for mental health practitioners. It should be noted that many of these tools can be used to evaluate trauma and mental health patients, and some tools or portions of those tools require specific licensure for use in evaluation, i.e., The Healthy Living Questionnaire. The information is organized into resources, screening forms, depression, drug and alcohol abuse, bipolar disorder, suicide risk, anxiety disorders, and trauma. Although the last section is specific to trauma, several other tools may also be valuable to evaluating the effects of trauma on patients.

With the high incidence of depression among the general population, patients seeing their primary care provider may present with symptoms associated with depression. Those who are depressed may speak about sadness, hopelessness, and/or an irritable mood (primarily heard from adolescents). Interests and pleasures previously obtained from activities may be absent. It would be important during the interview to ascertain the types of activities and the changes in engagement and enjoyment. Changes in weight and sleeping habits may also be a key indicator; however, it is important to rule out a physical reason for any changes. In the DSM-5 (APA, 2013), fatigue, feelings of excessive worthlessness or inappropriate guilt, difficulty with concentration and decision-making, and recurring thoughts of death are associated with depressive mood. In addition, joint pain, back pain, and other similar manifestations may be associated with depression. Common screening tools for depression include the *Hospital Anxiety and Depression Scale, Geriatric Depression Scale,* and the *Edinburgh Postnatal Depression Scale* (Aetna, 2017).

When addressing population health, and working with patients with mental health and trauma issues, hypnotherapy has become a useful tool to help patients unlock subconscious and unconscious thoughts to address memories and/or traumatic events that may be catalysts for depression and disturbances. This same treatment modality has been used to assist with behavioral changes such as smoking cessation and overeating because of the patient's heightened state of suggestion (Deeley, 2017).

The Emotional Freedom Technique (EFT), which may also be known as Thought Field Therapy (E. Rooney, personal communication, February 28, 2017), is defined and described as a noninvasive, clinical procedure for the relief of psychological and physical distress that patients may experience after a trauma or traumatic event or during active events in a mental illness (Rancour, 2016). The procedure is considered a branch of comprehensive energy psychology that has evolved since the 1970s and can be used in addressing health needs in either of these populations, producing a >90% effective rate in reducing anxiety, depression, and many types of pain. Benor, Rossiter-Thornton, and Toussaint (2017); Feinstein (2010); Gaesser and Karan (2017); and Patterson (2016) conducted studies using the technique for multiple populations, including nursing students, and found statistical significance regarding the efficacy of the technique in reducing anxiety and pain levels and depression. The technique uses noninvasive tapping demonstrated by the trained nurse and self-performed by the patient on key acupuncture sites. There has been a 98% efficacy rate reported with the use of this therapy documented in more than 60 studies in peer-reviewed journals. The therapy is based on the premise that the cause of all emotional and physical disease stems from a disruption in the body's energy system; therefore, the memory of an event is not the trigger for a patient's pain; instead the memory becomes a disruption in the body's energy flow, causing the symptoms. The EFT utilizes tapping on specific anatomical landmarks to "reset" the body's energy. The nurse begins by asking the patient to recall the event causing the symptomatology, and rate that pain, just as the patient would do with any pain scale. The nurse guides the patient through the tapping sequence and asks the patient to recall the memory and rate the pain again. The EFT can be used as many times as needed to aid the patient in achieving a lower level of distress and is consistently gaining acceptance as a holistic, self-administered method of achieving control and calm in the turbulent aftermath of a traumatic event or mental health episode. One of the greatest benefits to this technique is the ability of the patient to use it between sessions to minimize episodes of depression and anxiety until the next therapy session.

*Discussion Questions*
- When a person is admitted to an ER following a traumatic event, what other treatments should be considered and may be necessary in addition to physical injuries following initial evaluation?
- When an individual presents with a possible mental health issue, what other factors must be considered as part of the diagnostic process?
- What types of preventative efforts could be initiated in a community clinical setting that would promote positive health and well-being?
- In high-risk crime areas, how can the APRN help vulnerable populations in the community maintain safety and health?

*Assignments*
- Identify a specific mental health or traumatic event that an APRN may encounter in practice. Evaluate and determine three websites that could be used for patient and family education. Provide rationales for your choices.
- Develop a personal tool kit that includes resources that an APRN would utilize in practice. Include resource ID and summary of content.
- An APRN is presented with a patient who has experienced a trau-

matic event or mental health episode. Describe the specific dynamics of the event or episode. Identify three individuals with whom you would collaborate and provide rationales for the decided collaborations.

## Case Study 1
## By Camille McNicholas, PhD, APRN

*Trauma*

Barbara P. is a 28-year-old, school health nurse practitioner. Barbara has been working in pediatrics for seven years, and she became a school nurse because there were less demanding pediatric health concerns in a school setting. She felt she could do much good focusing on prevention and aiding the students to develop a healthy lifestyle. Barbara has been working in an elementary school for the last three years, and she is very content there.

In the spring, Barbara lets students go outside during their health class. She hears shooting midway through the class and sees a young man run around the corner of the school, knock down a teacher, and enter the school. He is armed with at least two guns that Barbara sees. The students start to cry and run toward the school. Barbara gathers the students and takes them to the house next to the school. The house belongs to the principal and her husband. Stephon James, the principal's husband, is retired, and he takes them to the basement. They continue to hear shooting. She asks Mr. James to call 9-1-1, and she tells the students to stay with Mr. James.

Concerned for the safety of the students and staff at the school, Barbara returns upstairs to assess what she can from the James' house. She notes that Ms. Janice Marshall, the crossing guard, is running toward the school. Halfway there, she stops and grabs her chest. Barbara does not see that Ms. Marshall has been shot, but the crossing guard drops to the ground and is moaning. Janice is within 20 feet of the school and 100 feet from Barbara.

Barbara immediately runs to the crossing guard to assess the situation. She knows that Janice has high blood pressure. Barbara has spoken with Janice previously regarding her health, and she knows Janice recently changed her blood pressure medication. She also knows that the students like Janice, and she feels they will be doubly traumatized if something happens to her. Janice indicates that, "My chest and side of my face are aching. I am also really sick to my stomach."

Barbara lifts Janice from under the shoulders to a standing position. They move away from the school with Janice leaning on Barbara. Barbara calls 9-1-1 and states they have a potential heart attack victim outside of the school. EMS is concerned about coming in with an ambulance because the school is "hot" with shooting. The police have the building surrounded, but shooting is still heard from the building.

Barbara takes Janice's pulse. It is regular, so she gives Janice three children's aspirin that she had in her pocket.

- What would you do next if you were in Barbara's situation? Are the children a priority at this time?
- Should Barbara attempt to move Janice further from the school so that an ambulance can reach her?
- Should Barbara make herself available for the potential trauma victims in the school? Should she proceed to the hospital once the situation is contained to help there?

### Case Study 2

*Trauma*

Donna C. was raped during a party she attended at a friend's house. She admitted to having two alcoholic drinks but didn't remember many details about party events after the second drink. She remembered putting her second drink down to go to the bathroom. When she returned, her drink didn't seem to be moved and didn't taste any different. Donna reported that she began to feel sick and dizzy after finishing the second drink, sat down on the sofa in the room, and woke up a few hours later in the guest bedroom with her clothes disheveled. No one at the party admitted seeing Donna being moved or moving her to the bedroom or any change in her behavior.

Donna shared these details with a friend, who urged her to go to the emergency room (ER). Once in the ER, the physician recommended that Donna allow a rape kit to be collected, that the police should be contacted, and a police report filed. Donna agreed. The hospital uses Sexual Assault Nurse Examiners (SANE) for rape examinations and evidence collection. The SANE on call arrived within 15 minutes of notification. She introduced herself to Donna, explaining her role, expertise, and the reason she was called to conduct the examination. The nurse asked if Donna had showered or otherwise washed herself since the suspected assault. Donna said that she had not bathed because she didn't realize what happened to her. The nurse explained that a sterile sheet would be placed on the floor behind a dressing screen and Donna should stand in the center of the sheet to undress completely, dropping the clothes onto the sheet and stepping off the sheet. Donna should put on the hospital gown and come to the examination table.

The SANE began the examination, explaining each step of the examination before and as she conducted the steps. Donna became emotional when the nurse prepared to collect pubic hair comb samples. The nurse paused in the process and explained what she was doing and why she was collecting the sample with a comb and paper. The nurse explained that she was doing this so that any stray hairs from an alleged attacker would also be collected. Her hair would be eliminated, and any additional hairs could be assessed for DNA and possible identification.

The rape examination revealed that Donna had a sexual experience, as semen was present, and that sex was likely unprotected. Internal trauma was also noted in the vaginal wall, but this could not be substantiated as forced sexual intercourse. The SANE recommended that Donna agree to further testing for venereal diseases and possible HIV infection. The nurse practitioner requested Donna consider steps to inhibit pregnancy, such as taking the Plan "B" pill (morning after pill), if she desired.

The SANE practitioner provided Donna with contact information for the Rape Relief/Crisis Center. Here she will receive counseling and support. The SANE further indicated that Donna might begin to experience varied emotions and feelings that could lead her to believe this event was somehow her fault. The SANE assured Donna that these feelings were common, but untrue. The SANE also recommended that Donna seek out counseling as soon as possible if these feelings begin to occur.

Donna is confused as to why you as a practitioner are doing this examination. As an APN, what would you communicate to Donna regarding your credentials and the procedures you are utilizing to examine her for potential sexual assault?

- If you were the SANE, what would you do if Donna chose to take the morning after pill?
- How would you counsel her with regard to expectations regarding this morning after pill?
- In providing support for Donna, what information from this chapter would you utilize in counseling her as to future expectations and processing of this experience?

## Case Study 3

*Mental Health*

John H. is a homeless man with a history of bipolar disorder. He has been arrested for violent outbursts against pedestrians walking near his tent. He has also been hospitalized for three previously attempted suicides—two attempts by hanging and one attempt by throwing himself in front of a passing tractor trailer. Each incident resulted in brief hospitalizations and reordering of medications. There is a local outpatient clinic for mental health patients, but John states that the people "look at him funny" and that he feels like a "charity case" going there for medicines and treatment.

John presented to the nurse at the community health center stating that he is very excited about his birthday. At the center, the staff sang happy birthday and presented a cake to everyone who had a birthday that month. John became more and more animated during this presentation. As others wished him a happy day, his speech became pressured and he asked to speak to the nurse alone.

He stated that he started to feel manic and that this happens often when he gets "too many good things at once." The program at the community health center has been wonderful for him, and he did not expect anyone to be so nice to him about his birthday. He stated that he is becoming concerned because, even though he is taking his medications, he is starting to feel as if he is becoming manic. He stated "this is not a good thing." If you were the APN at this site, what would be the top three priorities you would choose to do when assessing John? What is your rationale for this?

- What community supports would you utilize to assist in addressing this mental health issue? How would you determine what resources are needed and how John would access them?
- With what you know, is John a threat to himself or others? What assessment would you do to ascertain if John is safe to leave the center and seek support later?

## References

Adams, L. Y., Koop, P., Quan, H., & Norris, C. (2015). A population-based comparison of the use of acute healthcare services by older adults with and without mental illness diagnoses. *Journal of Psychiatric and Mental Health Nursing, 22,* 39–46. doi:10.1111/jpm.12169

Adshead, G., & Ferris, S. (2007). Treatment of victims of trauma. *BJ Psych Advances, 13*(5), 358–368. doi:10.1192/apt.bp.105.000844

Aetna. (2017). Primary care physicians on front line of depression screening. Retrieved from https://news.aetna.com/2016/12/primary-care-doctors-on-the-front-lines-of-depression-screening/

Agency for Healthcare Research and Quality. (2017). Clinical guidelines and recommendations. Retrieved from http://ahrq.gov

Amar, A. F., & Clements, P. T. (2011). Psychiatric forensic connections: 6 degrees of separation [Guest editorial]. *Journal of the American Psychiatric Nurses Association, 17*(2), 110–111.

American Association of Colleges of Nursing. (2016). Expanded roles for advanced practice nurses. Retrieved from http://www.aacn.nche.edu/media-relations/fact-sheets-apn-roles

American Psychiatric Association. (2015). What is mental illness? Retrieved from: https://www.psychiatry.org/patients-families/what-is-mental-illness

American Psychological Association. (2017). Data on behavioral health in the United States. Retrieved from http://www.apa.org/helpcenter/data-behavioral-health.aspx

American Psychological Association. (2013). *Diagnostic and statistical manual of mental disorders* (5th ed.; DSM-5). Washington, D.C.: Author.

Anxiety & Depression Association of America (2016). Symptoms of PTSD. Retrieved from https://www.adaa.org/understanding-anxiety/posttrraumatic-stress-disorder-ptsd

Beck, A. T., & Haigh, E. A. (2014). Advances in cognitive theory and therapy: The generic cognitive model. *Annual Review of Clinical Psychology, 10*, 1–24. doi: 10.1146/annurev-clinpsy-032813-153734

Benor, D., Rossiter-Thornton, J., & Toussaint, L. (2017). A randomized, controlled trial of wholistic hybrid derived from eye movement desensitization and reprocessing and emotional freedom technique (WHEE) for self-treatment of pain, depression, and anxiety in chronic pain patients. *Journal of Evidence-Based Complementary & Alternative Medicine, 22*(2), 268–277. doi: 10.1177/2156587216659400

Centers for Disease Control. (2016a). Early release of selected estimates based on data from the National Health Interview Survey, January–March, 2016. Retrieved from: https://www.cdc.gov/nchs/data/nhis/earlyrelease/earlyrelease201609_13.pdf

Centers for Disease Control (2016b). Therapeutic drug use. Retrieved from: https://www.cdc.gov/nchs/fastats/drug-use-therapeutic.htm

Christopher, M. A. (2014). The role of nursing and population health in achieving the triple aim: How nurses are helping to drive patient-centered, community-based care. *Home Healthcare Nurse, 32*(8), 505–506.

Cody, M. W., & Beck, J. G. (2014). Physical injury, PTSD symptoms, and medication use: Examination in two trauma types. *Journal of Traumatic Stress, 27*, 74–81. doi:10.1002/jts

Cooper, G. D., Clements, P. T., & Holt, K. E. (2012). Examining childhood bullying and suicide: Implications for school nurses. *The Journal of School Nursing, 28*(4), 275–283. doi: 10.1177/1059840512438617

Cuijpers, M., Sijbrandij, M., Koole, S. L., Andersson, G., Beekman, A. T., & Reynolds, C. F. (2014). Adding psychotherapy to antidepressant medication in depression and anxiety disorders: A meta-analysis. *World Psychiatry, 13*(1), 56–67. doi: 10/1002/wps.20089

Cusack, L., de Crespigny, C., & Athanasos, P. (2011). Heatwaves and their impact on people with alcohol, drug, and mental health conditions: A discussion paper on clinical practice considerations. *Journal of Advanced Nursing, 67*(4), 915–922. doi:10.1111/j.1365-2648.2010.05551.x

Deeley, Q. (2017). Hypnosis as therapy for functional neurologic disorders. *Handbook of Clinical Neurology, 139*, 585–595. doi: 10.1016/B978-0-12-801772-2.00047-3

DeGuzman, P. B., & Kulbok, P. A. (1012). Changing health outcomes of vulnerable populations through nursing's influence on neighborhood built environment: A framework for nursing research. *Journal of Nursing Scholarship, 44*(4), 341–348.

Dietz, T. J., Davis, D., & Pennings, J. (2012). Evaluating animal-assisted therapy in group treatment for child sexual abuse. *Journal of Child Sexual Abuse, 21*(6), 665–683.

Ertl, V., Saile, R., Neuner, F., & Catani, C. (2016). Drinking to ease the burden: A cross-sectional study on trauma, alcohol abuse, and psychopathology in a post-conflict context. *BMC Psychiatry, 33*(2011), 1975–1980.

Fawcett, J. & Ellenbecker, C. H. (2015). A proposed conceptual model of nursing and population health. *Nursing Outlook, 63*(3), 288–298. Retrieved from http://dx.doi.org/10.1016/j.outlook.2015.01.009

Feinstein, D. (2010). Rapid treatment of PTSD: Why psychological exposure with acupoint tapping may be effective. *Psychotherapy Theory, Research, Practice, Training, 47*(3), 285–402. doi: 10.1037/a0021171

Gaesser, A. H., & Karan, O. C. (2017). A randomized controlled comparison of emotional freedom technique and cognitive-behavioral therapy to reduce adolescent anxiety: A pilot study. *The Journal of Alternative and Complementary Medicine, 23*(2), 102–108. doi:10.1089/acm.2015.0316

Grohol, J. (2013). Top 25 psychiatric medication prescriptions for 2013. Retrieved from http://psychcentral.com/lib/top-25-psychiatric-medication-prescriptions-for-2013/

Grossmeier, J., Terry, P. E., Anderson, D. R., & Wright, S. (2012). Financial impact of population health management programs: Reevaluating the literature. *Population Health Management, 15*(3), 129–134.

Guzys, D., Kenny, A., Dickson-Swift, V., & Threlkeld, G. (2015). A critical review of population health literacy assessment. *BMC Public Health, 15*, 215.doi:10.1186/s12889-015-1551-6

Hahn, E. A., & Cella, D. (2003). Health outcomes assessment in vulnerable populations: Measurement challenges and recommendations. *Archives of Physical Medicine and Rehabilitation, 84*(Suppl. 2), 35–42.

Hanrahan, N. P., Delaney, K. R., & Stuart, G. W. (2012). Blueprint for development of the advanced practice psychiatric nurse workforce. *Nursing Outlook, 60*, 91–106. doi:10.1016/j.outlook.2011.04.007

Helpguide.org. (2016). *Emotional and psychological trauma.* Retrieved from http://www.helpguide.org/articles/ptsd-trauma/emotional-and-psychological-trauma.htm

Holtslag, H. R., van Beeck, E. F., Lichtvled, R. A., Leenen, L. P. H., Lindeman, E., & van der Werken, C. (2008). Individual and population burdens of major trauma in the Netherlands. *Bulletin of the World Health Organization, 86*(2), 111–117.

Iglehart, J. K. (2013). Expanding the role of advanced nurse practitioners-risks and rewards. *The New England Journal of Medicine, 368*, 1935–1941. doi: 10.1056/NEJMhpr1301084

Insel, T. (2015, May 15). Mental health awareness month: By the numbers [Web log post]. Retrieved from https://www.nimh.nih.gov/about/directors/thomas-insel/blog/2015/mental-health-awareness-month-by-the-numbers.shtml

Jacobs, J. A., Jones, E., Gabella, B. A., Spring, B., & Brownson, R. C. (2012). Tools for implementing an evidence-based approach in public health practice. *Centers for Disease Control and Prevention, Previous Chronic Disease, 9*. doi:http://dx.doi.org/10.5888/pcd9.110324

Kartha, A., Restuccia, J. D., Burgess, Jr., J. F., Benzer, J., Glasgow, J., Hackenberry, J., Kaboli, P. J. (2014). Nurse practitioner and physician assistant scope of practice in 118 acute care hospitals. *Journal of Hospital Medicine, 9*(10), 615–620. doi: 10.1002/jhm.2231

Keyes, C. L. M., Dhingra, S. S., & Simoes, E. J. (2010). Change in level of positive mental health as a predictor of future risk of mental illness. *American Journal of Public Health, 100*(12), 2366–2371. doi:10.2105/AJPH.2010.192245

Kindig, D., & Stoddart, G. (2003). What is population health? *American Journal of Public Health, 93*(3), 380–383.

Langman, L., & Chung, M. C. (2012). The relationship between forgiveness, spirituality, traumatic guilt and posttraumatic stress disorder (PTSD) among people with addiction. *Psychiatric Quarterly, 84*, 11–26. doi:10.1192/apt.bp.105.000844

Lowes, R. (2016). Is mental health treatment shifting to primary care doctors? Retrieved from http://www.medscape.com/viewarticle/862907

MacDonald, S. E., Newburn-Cook, C. V., Allen, M., & Reutter, L. (2013). Embracing the population health framework in nursing research. *Nursing Inquiry, 20*(1), 30–41. doi: 10.1111/nin.12017

Manion, A. B., & Odiaga, J. A. (2014). Health care economics and the advanced practice registered nurse. *Journal of Pediatric Health Care, 28*(5), 466–469. http://dx.doi.org/10.1016/j.pedhc.2014.04.009

Martins, C. M. S., Baes, C. V. W., Tofoli, S. M. d. C., & Juruena, M. F. (2014). Emotional abuse in childhood is a differential factor for the development of depression in adults. *The Journal of Nervous and Mental Disease, 202*(11), 774–782. doi: 10.1097/NMD.0000000000000202

Mayo Clinic. (n.d.). *Post-traumatic stress disorder (PTSD)*. Retrieved from http://www.mayclinic.org/diseases-conditions/post-traumatic-stress-disorder

Medicinenet.com (2015). *Mental health and mental illness facts*. Retrieved from http://www.medicinenet.com/mental_health_psychology/article.htm

Mims, D., & Waddell, R. (2016). Animal assisted therapy and trauma survivors. *Journal of Evidence-Informed Social Work, 13*(5), 452–457.

National Alliance on Mental Illness. (2017). Mental health by the numbers. Retrieved from http://www.nami.org/Learn-More/Mental-Health-By-the-Numbers

National Institutes of Health. (n.d.) Grand challenges in global mental health. Retrieved from https://www.nimh.nih.gov/about/organization/gmh/grandchallenges/index.shtml

National Institute of Mental Health (2017). Mental health information. Retrieved from http://nimh.nih.gov

National Institute of Mental Health. (n.d.). Serious mental illness (SMI) among adults. Retrieved from http://www.nimh.gov/health/prevalence/serious-mental-health-smi-among-us-adults.shtml

Office of Violence Against Women. (2014). The importance of understanding trauma-informed care and self-care for victim service providers. Retrieved from http://www.justice.gov/ovw/blog

Patterson, S. L. (2016). The effect of emotional freedom technique on stress and anxiety in nursing students: A pilot study. *Nurse Education Today, 40*, 104–110. http://dx.doi.org/10.1016/j.nedt.2016.02.003

PDR Network. (2017). *Physician's desk reference* (71st ed.). Montvale, NJ: Author

PsychGuides.com (n.d.). Trauma symptoms, causes, and effects. Retrieved from http://www.psychguides.com/guides/trauma-symptoms-causes-and-effects

Radzyminski, S. (2006). Population health as a framework for forensic nursing curriculum. *Journal of Forensic Nursing, 2*(1), 33–41.

Rancour, P. (2016). The emotional freedom technique: Finally, a unifying theory for the practice of holistic nursing, or too good to be true? *Journal of Holistic Nursing*, 1–7. doi: 10.1177/089801016648456

Ribe, A. R., Vestergaard, M., Katon, W., Charles, M., Benros, M. E. Vanderlip, E., ... Laursen, T. M. (2015). Thirty-day mortality after infection among persons with severe mental illness: A population-based cohort study in Denmark. *American Journal of Psychiatry, 172*(8), 776–783. doi:10.1176/appi.ajp.2015.14901100

Shapiro, F., & Forrest, M. S. (2016). *EMDR: The breakthrough "eye movement" therapy for overcoming anxiety, stress, and trauma.* New York: Basic Books.

Smith, B. L. (2012). Inappropriate prescribing. *Monitor in Psychology, 43*(6), 36. Retrieved from http://www.apa.org/monitor/2012/06/prescribing.aspx

Substance Abuse and Mental Health Services Administration (SAMSHA). (2016). Common comorbidities. Retrieved from https://www.samhsa.gov/medication-assisted-treatment/treatment/common-comorbidities

Substance Abuse and Mental Health Services Administration (SAMSHA). (2013). Screening tools. Retrieved from http://www.integration.samhsa.gov/clinical-practice/screening-tools

Substance Abuse and Mental Health Services Administration—Health Resources and Services Administration. (2017). SAMHSA—HRSA screening tools. Retrieved from http://www.integration.samhsa.gov/clinical-practice/screening-tools#TRAUMA

U. K. Essays. (2015). Vulnerable population health. Retrieved from http://ukessays.com/essays/health/vulnerable-population-health.php

Vessier-Batchen, M., & Douglas, D. (2006). Coping and complicated grief in survivors of homicide and suicide decedents. *Journal of Forensic Nursing, 2*(1), 25–32.

Vessier-Batchen, M. (2007). *Life after death: A comparison of coping and symptoms of complicated grief in survivors of homicide and suicide decedents* (Doctoral dissertation). Retrieved from ProQuest Digital Dissertation. (UMI 3269582)

Victimsofcrime.org (2008). The trauma of victimization. Retrieved from http://www.victimsofcrime.org/help-for-crime-victims

World Health Organization. (2016). Mental disorders. Retrieved from http://www.who.int/mediacentre/factsheets/fs396/en/

## CHAPTER 13

# Substance Use Disorders

MARY A. BEMKER, PhD, PsyS, LADC, LPCC, CCFP, CCTP, CNE, RN
MARY BIDDLE, DNP, RN, CNE, CCFP

## Substance Abuse and Addiction

SUBSTANCE ABUSE and addiction are well evidenced in our society. It is difficult to watch a news report, read a news magazine or view movies without being faced with the issue of substance use disorders. Substance use disorders is the term that encompasses what was known previously as substance dependence and substance abuse (American Psychological Association, 2013). This disease impacts more than the individual abusing a chemical substance.

Therefore, this chapter will address the various types of chemical substances that are abused, explore the impact on family and address potential interventions. Focus will be directed toward advanced practice nurses, nurses who are generalists, those working in the emergency department (ED) or other specialty unit, those in the community, and those who work in psychiatric or mental health facilities.

## Substance Use Disorders

The *Diagnostic and Statistical Manual of Mental Disorders, Fifth Edition* (DSM-5), stipulates that substance use disorders arise with the recurring use of a chemical substance(s) (alcohol and other drugs) that increases in amount and/or frequency (American Psychological Association, 2013). When tolerance begins to occur, more substance must be used to obtain the same effect. Although it might be assumed this is an easy "yardstick" to use as a means to screen for chemical dependency, many who abuse or are addicted to chemical substances mask this fact. When they have the ability to keep this fact away from the majority of individuals with whom their lives touch, they are considered "functional" alcoholics or functional addicts" (Bienvieu, 2017).

These individuals may be able to meet the majority of their responsibilities, for a given period of time. Health problems, absences from work or school, legal consequences, or some other major life issue eventually become part of the individual's life, and the person has to deal with consequences from such.

*Case Vignette*

Percy is a 53-year-old, white male who has worked for the same company as an accountant for 30 years. He has been married to his college sweetheart for 29 years, and together they raised four children. Percy comes into the office of his primary care provider (PCP), and he shares during his annual examination that his wife needs a new hobby other than complaining about him. He makes jokes about his use of alcohol, and states he only has "a few" to help him relax at night. "Doesn't a man that works as hard as I do deserve this?" Percy asks. Percy's PCP notes that he has an elevated blood pressure, and his spleen is notably enlarged since his last checkup. Tests for liver function are normal, but his liver enzymes are elevated. His palms are red, and he has developed rosacea.

Percy hedges and does not answer directly when asked what type of alcohol he drinks and how many drinks he consumes in the evening? He is evasive when asked how many nights a week he drinks. His PCP is in a quandary as to what needs to happen next, as she is aware alcoholics and addicts may sometimes "disappear" if they disclose too much information about their use too quickly. If you were the PCP, what would you do?

Signs of a functional alcoholic (or other drugs of abuse) might include the following:

- Joke about use of a chemical substance
- Use a chemical substance to relax and deal with stress
- Deny using chemical substances, is evasive or downplays use
- Does not want to take part in social events where alcohol or their drug of choice is not a part of the activity
- Hides chemical substances or become enraged when confronted over use

- Often drinks or abuses another chemical substance by using more often or in larger amounts than they are intended (Bienvieu, 2017; Hancock, 1970)

Based on the 2013–2014 surveillance data for the United States (U.S.), an estimated 4 visits per 1,000 to the Emergency Department were linked to adverse effects of drug use (Shehab, et al, 2016). Many of these issues were not related to mood altering chemical substances. However, abuse of legal substance and illicit use of chemical substances are common among the general public, and therefore is represented among the patient and client population seen by PCPs. Yet only 1 in 6 patients report that they have discussed their drinking with their PCP (Centers for Disease Control and Prevention, 2014). It is important that the healthcare provider start the conversation about drinking or abusing other chemical substances without being accusatory. The conversation needs to contain facts as it applies to the individual, and information needs to be presented in a manner that the patient can understand.

If it is determined that the individual has abused or may be addicted to chemical substances, options as to how the situation is addressed need to be provided. For example, does the individual want to stop using all together, moderate the use patterns, or not change anything (Bienvieu, 2017; Centers for Disease Control and Prevention, 2014). The option to quit or continue to use chemical substances in the pattern currently exhibited is up to the individual. Any attempt to push one's beliefs off on the person can have the opposite of the desired effect on their chemical use.

Those with an addiction will use any excuse to use. Some examples are as follows:

- "It's raining outside, I'll use."
- "It's sunny outside, I'll use."
- "I'm happy, I'll use."
- "I'm sad, I'll use."
- "Others are trying to control me, I'll show them and use more!"

The bottom line is that an individual with a substance use disorder will use regardless of the logic or illogical thinking demonstrated. One has to hit bottom before change can happen, and what a "bottom" may be for one person can totally be different for another.

*Case Vignette*

Clara is a 36-year-old female who has problems with prescription pain medication and alcohol. Clara works five days a week and has little social life. Clara comes home from work, fixes a drink or two, and relaxes. Sometimes Clara cannot remember how many drinks she had or how many pills she took for the pain in her knee.

Clara's father is the district attorney in a small town. Clara has been in rehab multiple times, due to consequences of her drinking. A cousin of hers was paralyzed in a car accident, and Clara was driving. Clara's BAL (blood alcohol level) was twice the legal limit. Clara also hit and killed two of her pets while under the influence, and she has been divorced three times. All of her ex-husbands state Clara is a lovely person when sober, and she is mean and hateful when drunk. (The police were called for domestic disturbances with more than one relationship Clara was in. Sometimes she was the attacker; other times she was attacked.)

Clara moved to a moderate-sized city about five years ago. She resides in an apartment approximately six blocks from where she works. Clara is proud of the fact that she has not gotten behind the wheel of a car intoxicated in five years. (Clara does not own a car.) She indicates she no longer has a problem with alcohol or pain medications, because the pain medications are prescription and she uses alcohol to get rid of all the pain. Clara is lonely, and she reports this causes her to be depressed.

Does Clara continue to have a problem with chemical substances?

If you were dealing with Clara in a professional role, what else would you want to know? Would you attempt to address Clara's problems yourself, or would you refer her somewhere else? If you chose to refer her, where would that be?

**Genetic Implications**

There is evidence that some are predisposed to chemical dependency and addiction. Addictions are moderately to highly inherent. Genetics can account for approximately 50% of the risk for chemical dependence. For example, inheritable potential for hallucinogens is approximately 39%, whereas cocaine has a 72% potential for genetic predisposition (Bevilacqua & Goldman, 2009; National Council on Alcoholism and Drug Dependence, 2016a). In addition, there are multiple examples of genetic compositions that support the development of substance use disorders. For example, most addicted to alcohol or cocaine present the A1 allele of the DRD2 (dopamine receptor gene) (National Institute on Drug Abuse, 2016; University of Utah, 2017a).

Although there have been tests available at major university medical centers regarding the genetic susceptibility of an individual to addiction for a number of years, there are currently tests to provide this information that can be obtained without a prescription. In any case, reliability and validity of the tests need to be considered before the findings can be assessed and utilized. In addition, one must consider how the findings are utilized? Will the findings satisfy mere curiosity, or will the findings support prevention efforts in the cases in which the increased probability of developing an addiction is noted (Saunders & Ashcroft, 2012)?

If the genetic testing indicates little evidence to support a strong genetic predisposition to addiction, will some use these findings as an indication that they have no risk for developing a substance use disorder? This is a real concern, because alcohol and other drug addiction is an equal opportunity disease. With any general make up, there will be some disposition simply because of our histories. No gender, neighborhood, or socioeconomic class is exempt from this potential. Although the rapidity of developing a substance use disorder may vary between persons and substance of choice, if one uses long enough, has a regular pattern of abuse, and uses to make feelings disappear, the individual is prone to develop an addiction (American Psychological Association, 2013).

The question then becomes, is chemical dependency a disease?

As early as 1953, the American Medical Association House of Delegates Proceedings urged insurance companies to treat alcoholism as a disease (American Medical Association, 1953). The disease designation has since been applied to all forms of substance use disorders and is accepted by many professional healthcare boards (American Society of Addiction Medicine, 2011; National Center on Addiction and Substance Abuse, 2016).

For this disease to be evidenced, the following have to be noted:

1. Impaired condition impacting one or more physical systems
2. Unique signs and symptoms
3. Physical harm (American Medical Association, 2016)

It is important to note that subjective reflection within the healthcare profession and society can result from a diagnosis (American Medical Association, 2016). The PCP must be aware of his or her own feelings and biases related to substance use disorders. Otherwise, it can be easy to enable or reject the individual who shares this information. Our own beliefs can get in the way of proper healthcare delivery.

As an example, Jana is a 58-year-old female of Spanish and Caucasian descent. She has been in recovery from alcoholism for 25 years. Jana had an emergency Appendectomy, and her surgeon prescribed narcotics for pain postoperatively. When Jana's spouse questions this, the surgeon states, "You don't really think she still has a problem with alcohol, do you? Look how long it's been since she's been drunk. This won't hurt her." Jana's spouse contacts you immediately. What do you say and do about this?

## Brain Chemistry

A major dynamic noted with substance use disorders is a change in brain chemistry and neurological patterns of transmission that can exist after an individual is no longer under the influence of a chemical substance. Upon use, the brain attempts to counterbalance the physiological impact of the foreign substance that is having an influence on neurotransmission.

The chemical reward system associated with alcohol and other drug use is a key factor in the acute reinforcement of chemical use and abuse, and it is connected to the negative impact of chronic drug abuse as it relates to the reward function. Systems of neurotransmission and neuromodulators (e.g., gamma-aminobutyric acid [GABA]) are also linked to the reinforcement of acute impact of drug use (Cruz, Bajo, Schweitzer, & Roberto, 2008). The physiological and behavioral impact of these changes may be the foundation for repeated drug relapses and extreme drug cravings when a drug related stimuli serves as a trigger. The DSM 5 (American Psychological Association, 2013) indicates categories to consider if a substance use disorder is suspected and if it is linked to impaired control, social impairment, risky use, and pharmacological criteria.

## Impaired Control

With impaired control, tolerance is noted. The individual takes the substance in larger amounts than indicated or takes the substance for a longer period of time than was prescribed or initially intended. The individual is often found obsessing about the substance, and his or her life revolves around the substance—getting the substance, using it, or recovering from using it. The individual may express a continual desire to cut down or regulate their use; however, efforts to do so appear to be unsuccessful. In extreme cases, an individual's daily life may revolve around the substance (American Psychological Association, 2013; Wardell, Quilty, & Hendershot, 2016).

**Social Impairment**

When considering social impairment, it is important to note if the individual may fail to accomplish major life obligations due to chemical use. The individual continues to use chemical substances even though social or interpersonal problems are caused or exacerbated due to their use of chemical substances. Social, occupational, or recreational activities may be diminished so that substance abuse can occur. The individual may withdraw from significant others and activities that they previously enjoyed (American Psychological Association, 2013; Suissa, 2015).

**Risky Use**

With risky use, recurrent use of chemical substances is noted in situations that have the potential to be physically harmful. The individual will continue to misuse substances even when he or she realizes that key areas such as psychological or physical problems are created or escalated due to their use. It is important to note that the individual is aware that their use disorder is causing major problems in their life and they choose to use anyway (American Psychological Association, 2013; Chiauzzi, Dasmahapatra, & Black, 2013).

**Pharmacological Criteria**

When considering pharmacodynamics, tolerance is a key variable. Tolerance occurs when a significantly increased amount of the chemical substance is needed to achieve the desired effect. It is important to note that tolerance is very individualized and can vary based on the substance and individual. Healthcare providers need to be aware that tolerance can be difficult to determine using history alone; therefore, laboratory tests can be valuable when making this determination.

When histories are taken, it is also key to seek clarity as to what the patient or client is stating. For example, an individual who does not consume alcohol on a regular basis may indicate feeling dramatic effects after drinking 2 beers; however, someone with high tolerance may argue they feel no effects when consuming 13 beers. Also, it is important to note that ambiguous terms such as few, some, or every once in while need clarity, because they can mean different things to different individuals. It cannot be hypothesized that our reality is the same as our clients' or patients' (American Psychological Association, 2013).

Withdrawal is noted when blood or tissue concentrations of a substance decrease in an individual who systematically maintains heavy and prolonged use of a chemical substance. To minimize withdrawal symptoms, many individuals consume a lower level than typical to minimize the withdrawal symptoms (hence, the term "hair of the dog"). Withdrawal symptoms vary greatly based on the individual and the type of substance being used.

More rapid absorption into the blood stream occurs with intravenous injection, inhalation, or intranasal absorption. These forms of use result in a more intense and rapid intoxication (Poison Control, 2013; University of Utah, 2017b). Longer acting substances tend to have a prolonged withdrawal period; therefore, it is important to consider the half-life of the chemical substance in order to make a determination about this. Typically, the longer the acute withdrawal period, the less intense the symptoms tend to be (American Psychological Association, 2013; Nielson, Hansen, & Gotzsche, 2012).

Note that if multiple substances are utilized, each will have their own etiology and will need to be considered separately as well as sequentially (American Psychological Association, 2013). For example, it is well known that when combining alcohol and benzodiazepines, the combination of these chemical substances leads to longer impact and enhances the effects of each chemical substance on the central nervous system (Weathermon & Crabb, 1999).

*Case Vignette*

Alice Kang is a 43-year-old Asian female. She was referred to you from a driving under the influence (DUI) program that she is court mandated to attend. Alice has congestive heart failure, and the swelling in ankles and legs are evidenced with visual assessment. Alice claims she was duped when she received this DUI (her second in one year and her tenth in her lifetime).

She stated that she was returning from purchasing groceries and was pulled over by a police officer. Alice stated she had a few drinks the night before and stopped drinking about 10:30 P.M. She indicates she did not drink that morning. Her arrest report indicates that she was transported to the county jail at 11:42 A.M. and that she had a blood alcohol content (BAC) of 0.12%. (In most states, a BAC greater than 0.08% is considered under the influence.)

Upon physical assessment, Alice's BP is 172/93. Her pulse is 80, and her temperature is 98.4. She has a puffy face and broken blood vessels around and across her nose. Her liver is enlarged upon palpitation. What information is important to you from this scenario? What else would you like to know before speaking with Alice about her drinking?

## Alcohol Impact and Related Disorders

Alcohol use is common in the United States. Alcohol prevalence, according to the National Survey on Drug Use and Health (NSDUH), was noted in the majority of Americans 18 years of age and older. Among the population surveyed, 70.1% indicated they had drank an alcoholic beverage within the last year, whereas 7% stated they drank heavily in the prior month to being surveyed (National Council on Alcoholism and Drug Dependence, 2016 b; National Institute on Alcohol Use and Alcoholism, 2017).

Alcohol use disorder was indicated on the 2015 NSDUH survey among 26.9% of those 18 years of age and older (approximately 6% of this age group). Of this population, it is noted that 9.8 million were male and 5.3 million were female (National Institute on Alcohol Abuse and Alcoholism, 2017). Prevalence of this disease is noted most heavily among Native Americans and Alaskan Natives (American Psychological Association, 2013).

Among those 12 to 17 years of age, it was estimated that 623,000 had an alcohol use disorder. Among those surveyed, it is believed that 298,000 were male and 325,000 were female (National Institute on Alcohol Abuse and Alcoholism, 2017). Among this age range, Hispanics, Native Americans, and Alaskan Natives have higher incidence of alcohol use disorders (American Psychological Association, 2013; Substance Abuse and Mental Health Services Administration, 2016).

In most cultures, alcohol is typically the most utilized abused substance. It contributes greatly to morbidity and mortality, with an estimated 5.9% of all global deaths resulting from alcohol abuse (National

Institute on Alcohol Abuse and Alcoholism, 2017). The World Health Organization (WHO) and other health focused organizations indicated that consumption of alcohol was linked to more than 200 injury-related conditions and diseases, including cirrhosis of the liver, cancers, and alcohol related injuries (Alcohol Related Liver Disease, 2016; World Health Organization, 2014).

Issues related to excessive alcohol use in the United States cost nearly $249 billion in 2010 as based on incidence and price. The U.S. Government paid approximately 40.0% of this cost (Centers for Disease Control and Prevention, 2016; Sacks, Gonzales, Bouchery, Tomedi, & Brewer, 2015). This economic burden stemmed predominantly from binge drinking (four or more drinks for a woman and five or more drinks for a man per function or sitting). Nearly 88,0000 people die from alcohol-related deaths in the United States annually (National Institute on Alcohol Abuse and Alcoholism, 2017).

Two diagnostic tests that provide a direct measure related to blood alcohol levels (BACs) are gamma-glutamyltransferase (GTT) and carbohydrate-deficient transferrin (CDT) (American Psychological Association, 2013). Interpretation of tests that assess BACs typically indicate the following as measures and interpretations:

- blood ethanol concentration of > 30 mg/dL is a good indicator that an alcoholic beverage has been consumed
- blood ethanol concentration of > 80 mg/dL is the legal limit in most states
- blood ethanol level ≥ 400 mg/dL is potentially lethal (Mayo Clinic, 2017b).

These examples of alcohol blood concentration diagnostic tests can assist with measurement of BACs. Blood alcohol levels are important for diagnostic purposes.

Alcohol use disorder is related to the risk of accidents, violence, and suicide. It is believed that alcohol use disorders are correlated to increased intensive care admissions. When alcohol is used by individuals with antisocial personality disorders, criminal acts such as homicides are elevated. There is an increased incidence of depressive symptoms that can lead to suicide attempts (American Psychological Association, 2013). Delirium Tremens, linked to withdrawal from alcohol in individuals with a high alcohol intake lasting a month or more, is typified by rapid confusion, irregular heart rate, sweating, auditory and/or visual hallucinations, high body temperature and/or seizures. Benzodiazepines and admission to a psychiatric or intensive care unit is warranted when DTs begins or as a preventative measure with medical withdrawal (Schuckit, 214; Weintraub, 2017).

*Case Vignette*

Josh Mansfield is a 23-year-old who just began a new job. Josh is liked by most, as he is "the life of the party" when he and his work friends go out. He entertains the office staff with his stories of his escapades in college, and he indicates he has turned over a new leaf now that he is out of school and employed.

Josh is very proud that he is not an alcoholic. He notes that he does not drink except on Friday and Saturday nights. He states he does not drink alone, and he always leaves his car at home so he won't get locked up for driving while intoxicated.

Upon further investigation, it is determined that Josh drinks between 10 and 15 beers when he is out. He estimates that he generally gets to the bar around 11:00 P.M. and closes the place down at 4:00 A.M. If he drinks mixed drinks, he estimates that he has about 10 to 12 mixed drinks over the same time period. He is quick to indicate that he does not mix hard liquor with beer, and he states he never drinks wine.

As Josh speaks about his drinking, he notes that there are times when he does not remember what happens when he is out. On Monday, when others allude to what he might have done over the weekend, he laughs and makes general remarks because he does not remember. He also states he cannot predict how many drinks he will have once he starts drinking.

Is Josh an alcoholic? What evidence do you have to support your belief? If you were his PCP, would you be concerned about Josh's actions? Do you believe Josh bringing this information up indicates he has a concern about his drinking? Is he a binge drinker? How can you find out? What would you state to Josh about this? What support would you recommend he utilize to address this issue?

## Caffeine Disorders

Caffeine intoxication occurs when an excess of 250 mg of caffeine is consumed in a short period of time. Restlessness, gastrointestinal disturbances, insomnia, tachycardia, and diuresis are some of the symptoms noted when caffeine intoxication occurs. Especially large amounts of caffeine can be consumed with energy drinks, weight loss aids, and specialty coffees and teas. Caffeine is often added to vitamins, medications, and food products as a supplement to provide a synergistic response. Like the diagnosis of alcohol induced disorders, it is important to not rely solely on historical summation of caffeine use. Caffeine blood levels can provide a more accurate evidenced-based measurement for diagnosis and treatment (American Psychological Association, 2013).

There is a variety of symptoms noted with caffeine withdrawal. These symptoms can be as extreme as flulike symptoms or evidenced as mild fatigue and headache. Withdrawal symptoms usually occur between 12 and 24 hours and peak after 1 to 2 days of last use. Withdrawal symptoms can be eliminated with ingestion of caffeine. Heavy use of caffeine is often seen concurrent with other chemical abuse disorders. Caffeine use is contraindicated with some medical disorders, medical procedures, and pregnancy (American Psychological Association, 2013; Rogers, Heatherley, Mullings, & Smith, 2013).

The U.S. Food and Drug Administration (FDA) has issued a safety advisory related to caffeine powder. Large quantities are readily available through the internet and are often sought for those wanting to lose weight, for those who have a desire to stay awake for long periods or to assist with alertness. One teaspoon of caffeine power is equivalent to approximately 25 cups of regular coffee. It is important to consider caffeine use when diagnosing other disorders such as anxiety and sleep disturbances (National Institutes of Health, 2015). Caffeine overdose can lead to an erratic and fast heart rate, vomiting, diarrhea, disorientation, seizures, and death (American Psychological Association, 2013; National Institutes of Health, 2015).

*Case Vignette*

You work in the emergency department of a hospital. Over the past six weeks, you have noted an influx of high school students complaining of rapid heart rate, feeling irritable, and not wanting to sit still. Most indicate that they need to drink a beer or two to go to sleep at night and complain of persistent headaches. After reviewing several charts, you note that the majority of patients attend the same high school.

What specific diagnostic information would you need to determine if these instances are caffeine addiction? If you determined that caffeine was being abused, what would be your next step in dealing with the problem? Would you speak to the school nurse about this issue? Would that be breaking confidentiality?

## Tobacco

Tobacco use disorders are linked to cigarettes, cigars, vaporized nicotine (eCigarettes), nicotine medications, and smokeless tobacco. These disorders are exemplified by daily tobacco use or use of nicotine medications on a daily basis. Tolerance occurs when symptoms from nicotine consumption are no longer evidenced (for example, nausea and dizziness), and feelings of being "a little down" and tired occur where not employed (American Psychological Association, 2013; U.S. Department of Health and Human Services, 2017). Many with tobacco use disorders smoke or otherwise use tobacco or nicotine to avoid or relieve withdrawal symptoms.

When a major life event is predicted to limit the individual's ability to smoke at will, the smoker may limit social activities. Instead of attending a party at a friend's house who does not smoke, the individual will stay at home or spend much of the time away from the party smoking. Individuals will continue to use tobacco even when the potential for harm is present (e.g., smoking in bed or while oxygen is in use). Individuals who have a nicotine or tobacco use disorder will report smoking or using tobacco products upon waking, waking at night to use tobacco, or increased daily tobacco consumption. Cancers and cardiac, skin, and pulmonary disorders are commonly seen among tobacco users (American Psychological Association, 2013; Caldeira, Garnier-Dyhstra, Vincent, Picksworth, & Arria, 2012).

The prevalence of nicotine use is noted more among Native Americans and Alaskan Natives than among any other ethnic population (American Psychological Association, 2013). In spite of this being noted, tobacco use is significant enough among the general population that all patients and clients need to be screened for tobacco use.

Nicotine can be consumed in multiple forms. Using a water pipe, commonly known as a hookah, is increasing throughout the world. Adolescents and young adults are the primary users in the United States of this mode of nicotine consumption. Many of the same chemicals noted in cigarettes are also seen in hookah smoke. Nicotine, hydrocarbons, carbon monoxide, and aldehydes are just a few of the chemicals noted (Eissenberg, 2013). Withdrawal symptoms and relapse concerns are also similar to cigarette smokers.

Ecigarettes, electronic nicotine devices, or vapor cigarettes have also recently come into common use among the general population. Little is known about the consumption of nicotine from this modality;

however, there have been noted incidents of burns associated with e-cigarettes exploding while in possession of an individual. These devices are not controlled by the U.S. FDA as a smoking cessation tool; therefore, it cannot be assumed they can be used for this benefit. E-cigarettes contain carcinogens (nitrosamines and formaldehyde). They also emit toxins that create a potential for health concerns related to secondhand smoke (American Psychological Association, 2013; Bell & Keane, 2012; Oncology Nursing Society, 2015).

Over 90% of those who use nicotine or tobacco products are smokers. It is commonly known that tobacco use can lead to problems with the cardiovascular system (e.g., increased blood pressure and heart rate, increased incidence of coronary artery disease and myocardial infarction), cancer (e.g., lung cancer, cancer of the mouth, throat cancer) and respiratory problems (e.g., sinus and ear infections, sore throats, dry hacking cough). However, many are not aware that smoking increases the risk of diabetes, impotence, fertility problems, low birth weight and preterm delivery (American Psychological Association, 2013; Cleveland Clinic, 2014; Khader, Al-Akour, AlZubi, & Lataifeh, 2011).

Secondhand smoke presents health risks for individuals who come in contact with someone while they are smoking. These risks vary depending on the amount of exposure involved. It has been noted that exposure to secondhand smoke increases the risk of cancer and cardiac difficulties developing. Sinus infections, ear infections, and sore throats have been evidenced those exposed to secondhand smoke. Children raised in households in which smoking occurs are more likely to smoke and have respiratory complications such as asthma or increased respiratory infections. Secondhand smoke has been linked to psychological distress in some children and adolescents, and every day respective memory issues have been connected to being exposed to passive smoke. Ability to spend time with a parent can be altered if the parent is a smoker (in some cases where parents are not living at the same residence). Exposure to secondhand smoke has decreased in response to smoke-free legislation (American Psychological Association, 2013; Cleveland Clinic, 2014; Fisher & Kraemer, 2015; Hawkins & Berkman, 2014; Hefferman & O'Neal, 2013; Jarvis & Feyerabend, 2015; in re Julie Anne, 2002; Leung, Leung, & Schooling, 2015; Padron, Galan, & Rodriguez-Artalejo, 2014)

Cultural variables differ as to acceptance of tobacco use. This variance provides different messages to individuals based on ethnic dynamics. Other factors, such as geographic locale and family beliefs and practices, also can have an influence. Considering ethnic backgrounds, including questions related to family and friends, smoking practices, ability to smoke in others' homes, etc., can prove useful in understanding this dynamic in patient's and client's lives.

The vast majority of individuals attempt to quit the use of tobacco products at least once in their lifetime; however over half relapse within one week of quitting. Those with an external locus of control, substance users and those with hyperactive disorders are more prone to tobacco use. Use and progression of tobacco consumption is influenced and increased by genetic predisposition. All of these factors need to be considered when addressing tobacco use and cessation (American Psychological Association, 2013; Kocak *et al.*, 2015).

Withdrawal symptoms occur when tobacco is not used on a regular basis or if chain-smoking is a common practice. Some continue to use tobacco even though physical symptoms or diseases from tobacco use emerge (e.g., chronic obstructive pulmonary disease) (American Psychological Association, 2013; Leyro, & Zvolensky, 2013; Limsanon, & Kalayasiri, 2015).

Withdrawal symptoms can mimic those of many other substances. Removing nicotine from the system can create a myriad of responses. Mood changes, difficulty thinking and acting in what is a "typical manner," and weight gain are a few of the changes associated with nicotine withdrawal. Tobacco withdrawal symptoms often begin within the first two to three hours of the individual being nicotine free. The withdrawal period typically does not exceed three weeks; however, the craving or memory of smoking may extend well beyond this, especially if triggers are presented to a former user (e.g., smell of burning tobacco). Therefore, it is prudent that prior to admitting a patient to a smoke-free facility or treatment center that the issue of smoking is broached and alternative options are considered if the patient is a smoker (American Psychological Association, 2013).

### Case Vignette

Nathan Whitecloud comes to your smoking cessation workshop at the community health center. Being 18 and getting ready to go away to college, Nathan decides he wants to stop smoking. After the workshop, Nathan confides in you that he fears quitting smoking, and he is concerned about what will happen to him if he doesn't.

Nathan shares that he used to be on the track team at his high school, but he becomes short of breath when he exerts himself for any period of time. He states his grandfathers on both side of his family died of lung cancer, and he wants to stop before he deals with the stresses of moving away and attending college. When asked about the reason he might want to continue smoking, Nathan explains the last three times he attempted to quit smoking, he became anxious or lethargic, "ate everything in sight", didn't know what to do with his hands and was irritable. He said he had problems focusing as well. The longest absence from smoking was reported to be 12 days.

Is there any additional information you would like receive from Nathan? What plan would you put together to support Nathan if he decides to quit smoking? Do you need to consider any supports for him at the university where he will attend this coming year?

## Cannabis

Cannabis use disorders include bio-psycho-social dynamics related to substances associated with the cannabis plant or chemically similar compounds. Cannabis and synthetic equivalents are prescribed for medical purposes. For example, cannabis has been prescribed for glaucoma, muscular dystrophy, human immunodeficiency virus (HIV), anorexia and to relieve the symptoms of side effects linked to chemotherapy (Bonn-Miller, Oser, Bucossi, & Trafton, 2014; Deutsch Rosse, Connor, Murphy, & Fox, 2008; Parmer, Forrest, & Freeman, 2016; Lutge, Gray, & Siegfried, 2013).

Medical marijuana is available in many states, and the legal use of marijuana for recreational purposes is growing. Typically, marijuana or its synthetic alternative (e.g., Marinol, Cesamet) is dispensed through approved government site for such use (Lamarine, 2012). Many continue to purchase the drug illegally for recreational use (National Institute of Health, 2017).

Potency of cannabis (delta-9-thc) is available in various concentrations that range from 1% to 20% (American Psychological Association, 2013; Lamarine, 2012). Cannabis is most often smoked but can be ingested orally by mixing it into food. Outside of the United States, a combination of cannabidiol and tetrahydrocannabinol (THC) is available in a spray and is distributed under the brand name Sativex (Lamarine, 2012). When THC is vaporized or smoked, the impact occurs at a greater rate than when it is ingested (National Cancer Institute, 2017).

Withdrawal symptoms can occur when cannabis use is stopped. These symptoms can mimic an anxiety disorder. Anxiety, restlessness, hair pulling, anhedonia and irritability are often associated with cannabis withdrawal (American Psychological Association, 2013; Katz, Lobel, Tetelbaum, & Raskin, 2014; Substance Abuse and Mental Health Services Administration, 2010).

In the United States Native Americans and Alaskan Natives are two of the most prominent racial ethnic subgroups noted for using cannabis. In addition, African Americans are noted in the top three subgroups for adults and Latino Americans are noted in the top three subgroups for adolescents for cannabis use. (American Psychological Association, 2013). A higher incidence among males than females has historically been noted with the use of cannabis; however, differences among genders are less common among adolescents. With adolescence, energy levels, eating patterns, and mood are the most observed changes when cannabis is used. Alcohol, cannabis and tobacco are typically noted as the first substances utilized by adolescents (the reason these are identified as "gateway" drugs). Use among adolescents and adults can range anywhere from occasional to daily use, often with peers. Risk factors associated with cannabis use include academic failure, unstable family atmosphere, family history of substance use disorders, and availability of the substance (American Psychological Association, 2013; Substance Abuse and Mental Health Services Administration, 2016).

Screening for cannabis includes biological tests for cannabinoid metabolites. One of the most well-known side effects of cannabis use is amotivational syndrome. This reduction in goal-related activity is linked to school failure and employment problems. Social relations, accidents related to potentially dangerous situations, and onset of other mental disorders have been noted as well (American Psychological Association, 2013; Volkow *et al.*, 2016).

Acute psychotic episodes have been linked to cannabis use with some individuals. When accessing for disorders such as depression and delusion disorders, it is wise to rule out cannabis use. Some over-the-counter substances are taken by individuals to mask the impact of cannabis use. This needs to be considered when using urine tests for diagnosing cannabis usage (American Psychological Association, 2013).

Symptoms associated with cannabis withdrawal may begin 24 to 72 hours after last use. These symptoms often peak within one week and can last up to 45 days or more (American Psychological Association, 2013; Substance Abuse and Mental Health Services Administration, 2010). Withdrawal symptoms are often seen with greater severity among adults than adolescents; however, the quality of the drug, amount smoked or ingested, and frequency of use impacts the severity of symptoms experienced with cannabis withdrawal. It is important to remember that cannabis withdrawal symptoms can be similar to other substances (e.g., alcohol), some mental disorders, or a medical condition. Screening needs to be specific so that correct diagnosis can be determined (American Psychological Association, 2013).

*Case Vignette*

Melanie Artez is a 15-year-old female who has been in treatment for cannabis use. When she appears in your office, she is angry, anxious, and appears to have difficulty concentrating. Melanie was released from inpatient treatment for cannabis use disorder three days ago. She was a patient on the substance treatment unit for 10 days. (Her father, who came with Melanie, stated that is the maximum time her insurance provider would pay for inpatient treatment on his plan). Since being home, Melanie and her father both indicate she is exercising more and that tends to relieve stress. She indicates she has difficulty eating, even things she generally likes. Melanie attributes this to her not being hungry.

A referral was made from her school for Melanie to be assessed for ADHD, and it was implied that she might have been self-medicating with this drug. When asked how long she had smoked marijuana and how much she typically smoked at one time, Melanie was evasive. Her father continues to try and prompt her to share more specific information with you.

As a provider, what is the next thing you would want to do in addressing Melanie's marijuana use as this scenario evolves? What information would you want to obtain from the treatment facility regarding her diagnostic information?

If you were to test for chemical substances, what tests would you utilize with Melanie? What precautions would you take to make certain you had an accurate sample? Are there any other questions you would like to ask Melanie? What developmental considerations, if any, would you include in your assessment and treatment considerations? What additional information might you want to obtain from her school?

## Hallucinogens

Phencyclidine (PCP) and ketamine were originally marketed as preanesthetic agents; however, they were removed from the pharmaceutical market when hallucinogenic side effects were noted. These chemical substances produce a dissociative quality in low doses. In high doses, stupor, coma or death can occur. Typically smoked or ingested orally, these drugs can also be snorted or injected (American Psychological Association, 2013; Dunn & Bruno, 2010; Greenberg, Segal, & Jacobs, 2016.).

Total elimination from the body can take 8 days or longer. Hallucinogenic effects can last weeks and can trigger a persistent psychotic episode similar to schizophrenia. Withdrawal symptoms are diverse and therefore cannot be noted. This chemical substance is used by approximately 2.5% of the population with less than 0.5% of this number being used among those 12 to 17 years of age (American Psychological Association, 2013).

Little is known with regard to risk and ethnically related diagnostic issues. The majority of users appear to be male. This is evidenced through the fact that approximately 75% of all that present to the ED with a phencyclidine issue are male. Phencyclidine can be identified in the urine up to 8 days post ingestion (American Psychological Association, 2013; Maxwell, 2014).

Memory, speech, and cognitive impairments have been noted several months post chronic phencyclidine use. Hyperthermia or hypothermia, seizures, and catalepsy are a few of the cardiovascular and neurological results of phencyclidine intoxication.

Intracranial hemorrhage, respiratory problems, and cardiac arrest can also result from phencyclidine use. Many times this drug has been added to other substances such as cannabis and can make diagnosis difficult. This use disorder needs to be eliminated prior to diagnosing schizophrenia, major conduct disorder, or major personality disorder (American Psychological Association, 2013; Parrott, 2013).

Other hallucinogens include mescaline, Ecstasy (MDMA), psilocybin, Lysergic Acid Diethylamide (LSD), and morning glory seeds. These chemicals are typically taken orally; however, some can be smoked, snorted, or injected. The effects of these hallucinogens vary and can depend upon the quality and amount consumed. LSD and MDMA, for example, can influence the individual several hours to several days after use. Others are more short acting. Tolerance to hallucinogens develops with chronic use, and individuals who use these drugs may have long-term autonomic and psychologic effects (American Psychological Association, 2013; Weaver, Hopper & Gunderson, 2015).

Many new drugs continue to appear on the market as novel psychoactive substances (NPS), and their inherent hallucinogenic effects mirror those of illicit drugs that provide the same physiological responses. Once the amalgamation becomes known and regulated, a new correlative substance appears on the scene (Zawilska & Andrzejczak, 2015). These products are sold under the guise of being bath salts, air fresheners, or some other equally placid substance (e.g., Locker Room).

The prevalence of hallucinogens is one of the least common among substance use disorders. However, there has been a growing interest and use of NPS in the United States. White males are the typical users of these chemical substances. They tend to reside in lower socioeconomic areas within urban communities (Palamar, Martins, Su, & Ompad, 2015). Use of hallucinogens is noted to be nearly equal among Native American, Alaskan Native, Hispanic, and Caucasian adolescents and adults (American Psychological Association, 2013). The effects of hallucinogens need to be differentiated from other substances such as amphetamines as part of the diagnostic process. Schizophrenia and other potential disorders—such as panic disorders, bipolar disorders, depressive disorders, metabolic disorders, seizure disorders, and alcohol or other sedative withdrawal—need to be differentiated from the initial impact of using an hallucinogen during the diagnostic process. Collateral reports from family and friends, clinical history, physical examination, and toxicology are all part of the diagnostic process. (American Psychological Association, 2013).

One significant difference with hallucinogens is that the perceptual disorders can be re-experienced when the individual is sober. Perceptual disturbances; geometric hallucinations; intensified colors; disturbances of peripheral vision; persistent palinopsia (positive after images); and perceptions of moving objects, halos, and shadows are some of the visual disturbances associated with hallucinogenic use. Other medical conditions—such as other drug effects, brain injury or lesions, seizure, migraine aura, and preexisting psychosis—need to be ruled out as part of the diagnostic process (American Psychological Association, 2013; Fraunfelder, Fraunfelder, & Chambers, 2014).

*Case Vignette*

Ronald Jefferson is a 66-year-old male who moved to the United States from Jamaica at the age of six. He served in the Vietnam War, and he continues to speak about the lack of respect he was shown when he returned from Vietnam. He was referred to your practice because he was having trouble attending a DUI group. (Group participation is a state requirement due to Ronald getting a third DUI within five years.)

Ronald states that he is fine until he sits across from a particular picture in the group room. He states that the picture reminds him of the terrain in Vietnam, and the picture begins to move when he looks at it. He says he sees things moving, like the water and the trees. At times he states he sees someone coming toward him with a gun from out of the picture. At that point he states he begins yelling, gets down on the ground looking for his rifle that is not there. Because of the disruption that this causes, he has been asked to get a physical assessment before he can return to the group.

Ronald denies using any hallucinogens in the last 30 years. He states that he used LSD regularly when he returned from Vietnam. He also indicated that he used MDMA when he attended heavy metal concerts in the past. Ronald indicates that currently, the only thing he does for "entertainment" is drink beer.

As a provider, what diagnostic criteria would you seek to provide some insights into the dynamics being described? What additional information, if any, would you seek from Ronald? What potential concerns would you have with regard to Ronald's health and well-being? What considerations would be included in your treatment plan?

## Inhalant Use Disorders

Inhalant use disorders are one of the most prevalent types of substance use disorders in the United States (American Psychological Association, 2013; Bowen, Howard, & Garland, 2016; Nguyen, O'Brien, & Schapp, 2016). Inhalant abuse occurs when a hydrocarbon-based, inhalant substance is sniffed to the point where significant impairment or distress occurs. Hydrocarbons are toxic gases emitted from some glues, paint, fuel (gasoline and lighter fluid), and other similar substances. Most compounds that are inhaled are a combination of several substances that create psychoactive effects. Therefore, it may be difficult to determine the exact substance responsible for this disorder (American Psychiatric Association, 2013; National Institute on Drug Abuse, 2012; Nguyen, O'Brien, & Schapp, 2016).

Diagnostic features of inhalant use disorder include motor impairment, negative impact on learning ability, memory and operant behaviors, missing school or work, inability to perform responsibilities associated with school or work, and continued use of inhalants even though it causes social or interpersonal problems (American Psychological Association, 2013; Konghom *et al.*, 2010; Nguyen, O'Brien, & Schapp, 2016; van Amsterdam, Nabben, & van den Brink, 2015).

Standard drug screens do not pick up inhalant abuse. Therefore, the practitioner needs to look to specific behavior and causal consequences for a diagnosis. These may include possession (especially large amounts), lingering odors from substances inhaled, glue-sniffers rash around the mouth and nose, association with other inhalant users, and paraphernalia. Suicide attempts have also been reported among inhalant users. About 4% of American adolescents demonstrate a pattern of inhalant abuse; among those, prevalence is highest among Native Americans and lowest among African Americans. Among adults, 0.1% or less are considered inhalant users. There is no significant difference in adolescent abuse patterns by gender. Almost no adult females are known to abuse inhalants (American Psychiatric Association, 2013).

Consequences from inhalant use disorders may result in "sudden sniffing death" resulting from cardiac arrhythmia (American Psychiatric Association, 2013; Kimura-Kataoka, Fujihara, Yasuda, & Takeshita, 2015). In addition, distorted perception and other neurological issues; gastrointestinal, cardiovascular and pulmonary problems; increased risk of communicable diseases, such as tuberculosis and sexually transmitted diseases (STDs); mood disorders, and anxiety and suicide are noted (American Psychological Association, 2013; Garland & Howard, 2011).

Mortality can occur from respiratory depression and asphyxiation, gastric-induced pulmonary aspiration, cardiac abnormalities, and risk related injuries. Inhalant abuse can occur in combination with other substance use disorders (American Psychological Association, 2013; Garland & Howard, 2011). The symptoms may be indistinguishable or overlapping; therefore, it is important to investigate use of other substances prior to making a diagnosis. Physical manifestations could include renal, gastrointestinal, blood, cognitive, spinal, and neurological disorders. If an individual presents themselves for care and exhibits symptoms as described, it is important to rule out inhalant abuse (American Psychological Association, 2013).

*Case Vignette*

Madison Sinclair is a 5-year-old female who was brought in by her parents to be seen in your facility. According to parental reports, Madison's older neighbor (12-years-old) thought it would be funny to see Madison huff gasoline. The neighbor reported Madison huffed paint three times in his presence. (The last time was two days ago.) Upon interview, Madison stated that she really liked to play with the neighbor, and she liked it when his Mommy watched her for her parents. She stated he was fun, and he did not treat her like a kid. She indicated she did not know how many times she "smelled that rag," and she reported waking up dirty after one incident. She reported that things moved funny, the ground was flatter and people did not look "right" after she smelled "that rag". She could not determine how long she was exposed to the gasoline rag or how long the influences from such lasted.

From her description of huffing experiences, it appears that she has a distorted reality that created much confusion and left the parents with little understanding as to what actually happened.

As a healthcare provider, what steps would you take to address the situation as presented? What would be the appropriate diagnostic steps at this point in the intervention? In addition to the inhalant abuse, what other concerns might you have and how would you address them?

## Opioid Use Disorders

Opioids are a class of chemical substances that are related and interact with opiate receptors in the central and peripheral nervous system (e.g., nociceptive pathways) and that produce morphine-like effects. There is also evidence of opioid influence on the neuroendocrine and gastroenteric systems (Hemmings & Egan , 2013; Sacerdote, Limiroli, & Gaspani, 2013). Most often prescribed for pain relief, opioids are also used for other maladies such as cough suppression (Erdogan, Aktas, Celebioglu. Krakaya, & Kalyoncu, 2016).

Opiate use disorders occur when opiate substances continue to be consumed illegally or in amounts that exceed recommended dosages. Opioids are obtained through legal sources when they are prescribed to address a specific medical condition. They can also be obtained from illegal sources. This can occur when symptoms are falsified or exaggerated with healthcare providers, simultaneous prescriptions are obtained from multiple providers (in states that do not monitor such activity), or when the individual seeks out unscrupulous healthcare providers that will support their substance use disorder. Individuals may steal prescription pads and use fraudulent or shared identities to obtain prescriptions. Individuals with an opioid use disorder have been known to steal from individuals who legitimately need the medication. Healthcare professionals who have an opioid use disorder have been known to illegally obtain medications from their place of employment. There is also an increased incidence of theft and violence in an effort to obtain opioids, with increased surveillance and monitoring of narcotic distribution (Illinois Criminal Justice Information Authority, 2016; NBC News, 2017; The Economist, 2015).

Since 2000, the rate of overdose deaths associated with opioid use disorders has increased by 200%. In 2014, nearly 29,000 deaths in the United States were linked to overdoses of opioids. Heroin was responsible for approximately 37% of these deaths, and other opioids (including prescription pain killers) were linked to the remainder (Substance Abuse and Mental Health Services Administration, 2015b).

To address these complex dynamics linked to opioid use disorders, state sponsored prescription monitoring programs have been put into place in 47 states and one U.S. territory. Most monitor Schedule II medications. Some also include Schedules III, IV, and V. These programs gather information related to dispensing of controlled substances by state. Information collected include prescriber, dispensing pharmacy, medication dosage, and quantity. Information can be obtained by prescribers, pharmacists, law enforcement, and state medical boards. (Green & Pfenning, 2015; National Association of State Controlled Substances Authorities, 2017; Substance Abuse and Mental Health Services Administration, 2015a; U.S. Department of Justice, 2016).

A history of criminal activity, such as embezzlement, burglary, and forgery, are associated with opiate abuse. Some evidence indicates that criminal mindset and substance abusers are very similar in their thinking processes. Others however note that criminal activity may be linked to their abuse and addiction (Sadoff, Drogin, & Gurmu 2015).

Problems with social and occupational endeavors are often noted with opioid use disorders across occupations and professions. Prevalence of opioid abuse is estimated at between 26 and 36 million abusers worldwide, with an estimated 2.5 million abusers of heroin and prescription medications in the United States. Statistically males' rates of use are significantly higher than those for females; however, female adolescents have a greater potential for developing opioid use disorders (American Psychological Association, 2013; Volkow, 2014).

Among healthcare providers, opioid use disorders can result in termination from a current position, legal implications and possible incarceration, and problems with licensing boards. Having a history of opioid abuse can limit the ability to be hired in positions where actual and potential access to opioids exists. While many state boards have programs to support the impaired health professional and offer monitoring of those that qualify once their licenses reinstated, licenses are often limited to prevent access to narcotics. This limitation is dependent upon personal and professional behavior, criminal conviction and state laws (California Board of Registered Nurses, n.d.; LARA, n.d.; KY Board of Pharmacy, n.d.; New York State Department of Health, n.d.).

Opioid use disorders are noted equally across most races and ethnic populations (American Psychological Association, 2013). Individuals who abuse opioids typically have a very high tolerance, and abrupt discontinuation of opioid use leads to withdrawal. Triggers to opioid abuse often last well past detoxification (American Psychological Association, 2013; Volkow & McLellan, 2016).

Withdrawal symptoms can occur when opioid use is curtailed or administration of an opioid antagonist is present. (An antagonist such as naloxone reduces the dependence and analgesic tolerance to opioids.) Presenting withdrawal symptoms may include complaints of aches and pains especially in the back and legs, restlessness, irritability, nausea, gastrointestinal disturbances, hyperhidrosis, pupillary dilation, insomnia, and fever. As with other use disorders, symptoms must not be attributable to any other chemical substance or medical malady. Speed and severity of opioid withdrawal will depend on the specific substance utilized. Withdrawal from short-acting opioids could begin in 6 to 12 hours after last use, whereas withdrawal from long-acting opioids may not present for 1–2 days after last use. Less acute withdrawal symptoms such as insomnia may last for weeks to months. A variety of withdrawal treatments have been noted in the literature, including buprenorphine, methadone, clonidine, and naloxone (American Psychological Association, 2013; Shippenberg, Chefer, & Thompson, 2009; Steele & Cunningham, 2016; WebMD, 2016).

Routine urine tests can screen for opioid drug use, as much as 12 to 36 hours after administration. Increased incidence of decreased gastrointestinal motility, HIV, hepatitis, and decreased liver function are seen in opioid use. Assessment findings, such as injection tracks with possible infection and pinpoint pupils, are commonly seen with opioid use disorders. Tetanus and other infections can also be associated with opioid use. Depending on the route of choice, the opioid user could exhibit irritation of the nasal mucosa and/or perforation of the nasal septum. Some users inject directly into the subcutaneous area of the skin, which results in scarring and infection. Increased risk for suicide, accidents, and violence are also associated with opioid use and should be kept in mind while assessing this population. (Suicide may be linked to intoxication or withdrawal with opioid use disorders.) Children born to mothers with a history of opioid use should be evaluated prior to and after delivery for exposure and physiological dependence (American Psychological Association, 2013).

Opioids are less likely to generate symptoms that are often confused with mental disturbances compared with other drug classifications. However, opioid use disorders can mimic alcohol intoxication and hypnotic and anxiolytic intoxication. This needs to be considered during the diagnostic phase (American Psychological Association, 2013).

*Case Vignette*

Jamal Gilkon is a 38-year-old male. He is married with three children, and he currently works as an auto mechanic. While working to restore a classic car, a chain broke and the car's engine fell. The engine hit Mr. Gilkon in the back, breaking three of his vertebra.

Mr. Gilkon had surgery to correct this problem three years ago, and he reported that he continues to experience pain in his lower back, making it difficult to work and sleep. As his PCP, you prescribed an NSAID and administered an epidural steroid. In addition, you prescribed aquatic and physical therapies to address the muscle tightness in his back. Mr. Gilkon was last seen two months ago for a routine examination, where he requested opioids to deal with the pain. He indicated that he drank several mixed drinks every evening to get to sleep and that this practice was making him groggy in the morning.

You note that Mr. Gilkom has lost 20 pounds since his last visit. This is explained by the patient as the outcome of a recent bout of flu. Mr. Gilkon states he had not worked since his last appointment, and his wife adds that when he sucks on a lollipop, that seems to help the nausea. (Main complaint at time of office visit is nausea and vomiting.) He is sweating, and his wife reports that he has "shakes" in the evening when he comes home from work (when he is able to work) and right before he goes to bed. He complains his ankles and feet are swollen, and he has pitted edema upon examination. At times, he appears distracted or is unfocused. There are no signs of needle marks upon skin inspection.

As his PCP, what additional information would you seek as you diagnose the symptoms evidenced by this patient? Are there any clarifying questions you might ask Mr. Gilcon or his wife during this visit? What diagnostic tests would be appropriate?

How would you determine if these symptoms are related to opioid abuse?

## Sedative Use Disorders

Sedatives and hypnotics are generally divided into benzodiazepine and nonbenzodiazepine receptor agonists; these medications are prescribed when a patient presents with anxiety disorders or insomnia (Kaufmann, Spira, Depp, & Mojtabi, 2016). This category also includes hypnotic and anxiolytic substances, which may be obtained illegally or by prescription (American Psychological Association, 2013).

These chemical substances are brain depressants and can have rapid onset. Longer-acting substances may be used for intoxication. Misuse of these substances often occurs in conjunction with use of other substances. This practice is most noted when there is a desire to change the overall impact of the other substance. For example, a sedative can be used to boost the effects of an opioid. Another use employed could be the combination of sedatives and stimulants to decrease the effects of the later. This combined use of medications can cause an untoward outcome referred to as a "yo-yo effect." Depending on the current presentation of the patient/client, this may make it more difficult to diagnosis (American Psychological Association, 2013).

As is the case with many of these categories, absence from school or work, neglect of family responsibilities, decreased socialization, lack of participation and withdrawal of previously enjoyed activities, and operation of a motor vehicle under the influence are often seen with sedative abuse disorder (American Psychological Association, 2013; Barnhart, Makela, & Latocha, 2004; Hansen, Boudreau, Ebel, Grossman, & Sullivan, 2015; Padala, Padala, Monga, Ramirez, & Sullivan, 2012).

This class of chemical substances may be prescribed for legitimate medical conditions; however, because of increased tolerance, dependence may result. Therefore, it is imperative that the practitioner evaluate if drugs previously prescribed were used appropriately or were obtained and/or used under fraudulent conditions.

The prevalence in this category of chemical substances is seen predominately with Caucasians, African Americans, and Hispanics; however, it is most noted among Alaskan Natives and Native Americans in the adult population (American Psychological Association, 2013).

Psychological determinants often increase the abuse of these chemicals. As tolerance ensues, it is easy for an individual to increase the dosage or frequency of administration based upon the original symptoms that were presented. Antisocial behavior and personality disorders have an increased incidence of sedative use. Cognitive impairment, depression, neurological hyperactivity, gastrointestinal disturbances, and neuromuscular impairment similar to alcohol abuse disorder symptoms are often seen during withdrawal from these chemical substances. Withdrawal symptoms diminish when a sedative-hypnotic agent is taken (American Psychological Association, 2013; Lader, 2002). Withdrawal symptoms include anxiety, insomnia, postural hypotension, nausea, vomiting, tremor, incoordination, restlessness, blurred vision, sweating, hyperpyrexia, anorexia, seizures, and delirium.

Significant areas of daily functioning may be disturbed when sedative use disorders are noted. Social, family, and work duties are often ignored, and issues with lack of motivation and concern might be evidenced as well. Detoxification best occurs under medical supervision. Severe withdrawal is more likely to occur with long-term use and high medication levels (American Psychological Association, 2013; Lader, 2002).

*Case Vignette*

Monica Moralez, a 53-year-old female, is a Vice President of Human Resources. Due to the stress generated from this position, Ms. Moralez is taking prescription sleeping medications prescribed by her previous PCP. She is seeing you for the first time with a refill request for her sleeping medication. Her BP is 110/60, her temperature is 98.4, and her pulse is 60. Her skin is pink and warm to the touch. On physical examination, Ms. Moralez flinches where her stomach and large intestines are palpated. The patient explains that she was in a major car accident a few weeks ago that could be the cause of the GI discomfort. (Note: No bruising or discoloration were noted in these areas upon examination.) She also complains about being easily distracted and having difficulty following conversations at times. Ms. Moralez indicates this has been an ongoing issue, but has worsened within the last few weeks.

When you look at the previous provider's name, it is one that is known within the medical community for freely writing prescriptions. Although the provider has been under investigation by their professional board, no charges have been brought forth.

As the current PCP, what are the next steps that need to be taken with treating Ms. Moralez? What will need to be determined in order to ascertain if her symptoms are linked to sedative use or to some other dynamic? As her new provider, will you continue to prescribe prescription sedatives to this patient? What will you tell Ms. Moralez is the reason behind your decision related to writing a prescription refill for her sleeping medication?

## Stimulants

Stimulants are usually taken orally or intravenously; sometimes, however they are crushed and snorted. This class of medication is typically prescribed for conditions such as attention-deficit hyperactivity disorder (ADHD) (Laver-Bradbury, 2013), narcolepsy (Scammell, 2015), and obesity (Smith & Campbell, 2011). Although many take these medications as intended, some abuse the prescriptions provided. Others may obtain these substances illegally. Stimulant use disorders can develop in as little as one week depending on the amount and frequency used. Stimulant use can result in a feeling of well-being and unrealistic confidence. Use of stimulants can create social isolation, aggression, and sexual dysfunction. Presenting symptoms of stimulant usage may include rambling speech, headache, and tinnitus. Paranoid ideation, auditory and tactile hallucinations, and aggressive behavior may accompany these symptoms.

Depression, thoughts of suicide, and difficulty concentrating are common symptoms of withdrawal from the medication (American Psychological Association, 2013; Davidson, 2016; Spiller, Hays & Aleguas, 2013).

Use rates are similar among males and females in adults and are higher in female adolescents compared with male adolescents. Usage rates in adults are highest in Native Americans and Alaskan Americans. For adolescents, usage rates are higher for whites and African Americans (American Psychological Association, 2013).

Some report stimulant use to control or decrease weight or to improve overall abilities in school, work, or athletics (Jeffers & Benotsch, 2016; White & Noeun, 2016). Use patterns may be episodic (binge use) or noted daily. Individuals diagnosed with antisocial personality disorder, bipolar disorder, or schizophrenia may have increased susceptibility to stimulant use disorders. Unstable home life, psychiatric conditions, and environmental association increases the probability of stimulant use disorders. Prenatal cocaine exposure and childhood exposure to community violence increase the probability of cocaine use among teenagers (American Psychological Association, 2013; Kobulsky, Minnes, Min, & Singer, 2016; Singer, Min, Lang, & Minnes, 2016).

Medical conditions associated with stimulant use disorder include respiratory and nasal disorders (American Psychological Association, 2013), skin disorders related to tracking (American Psychological Association, 2013), HIV infection (American Psychological Association, 2013; Wright *et al.*, 2007), STDs (American Psychological Association, 2013; Stahlman, Javanbakht, Stirland, Guerry, & Gorbach, 2013), hepatitis (American Psychological Association, 2013; Nyamanthi *et al.*, 2012), weight loss (American Psychological Association, 2013; Jeffers, Benotsch, & Koester, 2013), altered nutrition (American Psychological Association, 2013), tuberculosis (American Psychological Association, 2013), cardiovascular complications (American Psychological Association, 2013; Kratochvil, 2012), and neurological and seizure disorders (American Psychological Association, 2013). Stimulant use can also be related to the "yoyo effect" when used in combination with sedatives to reduce the stimulant effects.

Withdrawal from these substances may be evidenced by excessive sleeping, an enhanced appetite, generalized dissatisfaction with life, and depressive symptomatology. Comorbidity often occurs, and other determinants for symptoms presented need to be eliminated before stimulant use disorders are diagnosed (American Psychological Association, 2013; Lee *et al.*, 2013).

*Case Vignette*

Lee Park is a 28-year-old female who recently transferred to your city. She is petite, and upon initial observation appears anxious. Ms. Park shared that she has problems with her weight and that is the reason she is coming to see you today. Ms. Park indicates that she is large for a woman of Asian descent, and she fears it will impact her standing with her current employer (who is originally from China). She states she has abused laxatives in the past to the point where she had to be hospitalized. Ms. Park is in tears as she states this, and she clenches her fist while juggling her legs rapidly. She states she needs something to help keep her weight down, or she is afraid she will go back to using laxatives.

From the information above, what do you expect to find on examination?

How will you determine the difference between laxative abuse, an eating disorder, substance use disorder, and/or another issue? What will you need to rule out to make a diagnosis that would include stimulant abuse? What would you need to include to diagnose this patient with stimulant abuse disorder?

## Eating Disorders

Food addictions and eating disorders are based on psychological needs and physiological changes generated by consumption of certain foods. Fat and sugar are often identified as the culprits linked to eating disorders, such as bulimia and gross overeating (Appelhans *et al.*, 2012). Research supports that low level–attentional biases are related to obstacles associated with healthy eating (American Psychological Association, 2013; Gearhardt, Treat, Hollingsworth, & Corbin, 2012).

Signs and symptoms vary depending upon the type of eating disorder noted. Lack of body fat, obsessive thinking, and ritualized eating are often noted with those diagnosed with anorexia. The list of "acceptable" foods are often limited, and the individual will believe they are grossly overweight when the scale and visual assessment indicate otherwise. There is an unrealistic fear of gaining weight, and thin is the ultimate goal that is never achieved. Self-esteem is linked to body image, and there is generally a denial as to the severity of current weight (National Institutes of Health, 2014).

Medical complications derived from anorexia may include osteopenia or osteoporosis; brittle and dry hair, skin, and nails; chronic constipation; loss of muscle mass and weakness; mild anemia; infertility; slowing of major organs reflective in blood pressure, pulse, and respirations; and multi-organ failure (National Institutes of Health, 2014).

Binging and purging are key factors linked to bulimia nervosa. Individuals with this disease typically eat copious amounts of foods and then vomit or use excessive amounts of laxatives or diuretics to eliminate the food from their bodies (National Institutes of Health, 2014). If the individual purges through vomiting, he or she typically eats foods that are high in sugar and fat but are easy to regurgitate (e.g., ice cream). It is important that the practitioner to be cognizant of signs of vomiting, such as an inflamed throat, worn tooth enamel, persistent hoarseness, and acid reflux, as a possible indication of purging (National Institutes of Health, 2014; Sansone & Sansone, 2012).

Those with bulimia nervosa typically have a normal body weight, or they may even be slightly overweight. They typically have a negative body image and are consumed with the need for weight loss. They too are dissatisfied with the way that they look. Shame and disgust often accompany purging; however, it has been noted for some to purge multiple times a day. In addition to the previously named symptoms, those with bulimia may also have intestinal distress, severe dehydration, and an electrolyte imbalance (National Institutes of Health, 2014).

Those that choose to eat substances with high processed sugars and additional fats may experience difficulty due to being obese. Even if their metabolism allows for such food ingestion, food tends to be the center of their existence, and it is often noted how they comfort themselves. Food consumption is typically linked to stress, mood, and amount and type of food chosen. It is important to evaluate the types of food eaten and the impact that food has on patients and clients. This information can be used for educating the patient or client and in monitoring their physical and psychological conditions (Blasio, Steardo, Sabino, & Cottone, 2013; Clark & Saules, 2013; Singh, 2014).

### Case Vignette

Lydia Domanique is a 23-year-old female that is in the entertainment industry. Ms. Domanique is 5′ 8″ tall, and she weighs 110 pounds. Upon seeing the weight on the scale, she immediately steps down and starts pacing the room. When you ask what she is doing, she states she needs to get in her 10,000 steps on her wrist instrument. You ask how many steps she has so far that day, and she states 27,323.

Ms. Domanique indicates that she can only eat certain foods. Foods that she eats most are cheese and crackers, celery, and radishes. She states she sometimes eats peanut butter and crackers. She reports eating a half-gallon of ice cream in one sitting at times. She indicates that she immediately throws up the ice cream because it "unsettles my stomach."

Ms. Domanique is not able to tell you how often she eats ice cream other than to say this generally happens when she is stressed. She states that she likes to get her steps in, so she generally eats while she is walking. Her favorite place to walk is around the parameter of her basement. She gauges how much to eat based on how long it takes her to walk around the basement one time.

Upon examination, you note that her ribs, clavicle, and hips are pronounced. Her skin is brittle, and there is little rebound. Her BP is 90/50, pulse 56, and respirations 16. She continues to discuss how much she weighs and how this distresses her since she is in the public eye.

As her provider, what would you suspect is the issue with Ms. Domanique?

What would you need to do to determine a proper diagnosis? What would need to be ruled out prior to making such a diagnosis?

## Steroid Abuse

Anabolic steroids are another substance that does not fit within any of the previous classifications of chemical substances. Anabolic steroids are synthetic derivatives that mimic testosterone in the body. They are typically taken to increase muscle mass and/or enhance physical/athletic abilities.

Use of steroids are often noted in the following terms:

- *Cycling*—Different combinations of steroids are used over a 6- to 12-week period to attempt to reach peak performance (National Institutes of Health, 2006).
- *Stacking*—Two or more different type of steroids are taken at the same time (National Institutes of Health, 2006).
- *Pyramiding*—Varying dosages of one or more steroids are used to increase overall effectiveness while minimizing side effects (National Institutes of Health, 2006).

Administration can be via an oral or IM route. Side effects may include mood swings, GI disturbances, acne, aggressive comments and threatening behaviors, impotence, voice pitch changes, cardiac complications, liver disease, feminization (among adolescent males), and testicular atrophy (Brooks, Ahmad & Easton, 2016).

### Case Vignette

John Brown has been boxing for several years. This 20-year-old male is looking to enter the Welterweight division, and he has been bulking up on protein shakes. He has increased workout routines that are directed toward building muscle. In addition, Mr. Brown reports that he is getting less sleep and is under more pressure from his manager to succeed in this venture.

You note that Mr. Brown has severe acne on his face and neck. When asked about this, he states it is a reaction to some vitamin that his manager adds to his protein shake. He said he can live with it, if it means he can move up a weight category in boxing. With that classification, his manager has assured him of more sponsors and possibly television commercials.

Mr. Brown becomes agitated during your time with him. He makes many disparaging remarks toward others, and at one point he hits himself so hard that he leaves a bruise on his thigh. He says that you are asking stupid questions, so you must be a stupid person.

What would you do at this point in your encounter with Mr. Brown?

What strategies would you use to make a diagnosis and offer treatment? Are there any other responsibilities that you might have with the information presented?

## Addiction to Activities

Addictions have been linked to activities as well as chemical substances. The results of addictive behavior have led to negative consequences, such as academic, social, and occupational impairment. Regardless of the process, all addictions include tolerance, withdrawal symptoms, and absence of withdrawal symptoms when the activity is initiated. This is the same as is noted with substance use disorders (American Psychological Association, 2013; Sharma, 2016). Examples of addiction to activities have been linked to sexual encounters, excessive shopping, computer games and technological communication practices (e.g., texting, emailing, social media).

In recent times, individuals have come out and stated they have a sex addiction and are seeking treatment. Some are addicted to shopping, and they shop to relieve stress or feel an exhilaration that cannot be met in any other manner. Others have a cyber addiction (e.g., video gaming, sexting, etc.) or communicate predominantly through their phones and computers (even when others are physically present with them).

When addressing a possible addiction to an activity, it is important to address individual and pathological problems noted that can lead to poor impulse control. Discussing the process, including the "high" obtained from planning and participating in the events, can support diagnosis and can be the start of a conversation leading to treatment and recovery (Suissa, 2015). Some research addresses the psychosocial conditions (e.g., low self-esteem, week social ties, hyperindividualism) (Wiederhold, 2016) and potential personality disorders (e.g., vulnerable narcissism and social networking addiction) that can be seen with these kinds of addictions (Casale, Fioravanti, & Rugal, 2016). If noted, these can be an indication for further exploration.

*Case Vignette*

Stan Lee Grout is a commercial pilot. He is the senior aviator on transatlantic flights. This is a highly stressful endeavor for him and, because of drug testing and the need to be alert, he cannot take prescription medications to allay his symptoms.

Mr. Grout comes to see you because of irritated genitalia. He states that he knows his wife has a healthy sexual appetite, so she probably cheats on him while he is gone. (No concrete proof of this accusation was forthcoming.) He therefore can see no reason why he "can't have a little fun."

After testing Mr. Grout for STDs, further questioning offers additional insights into his practice. Mr. Grout indicates he will orgasm at least 12 times every day he is away from home and not flying. This experience may be with one person or multiple partners and can include masturbation. He states he is pressed to continue with the sexual act even if he can no longer orgasm that day; his penis is rubbed raw, and pressing activities are often neglected.

Considering what you know about addiction, do you believe Mr. Grout has an addiction? What considerations must be addressed in addition to the sexual behavior? What would you recommend for Mr. Grout in response to the sexual behavior he admits makes him feel out of control and shamed?

## Gambling

Gambling also falls into this category of addictive activities. An individual who is addicted to gambling is often preoccupied with chasing the losses and making the "big win" that will rectify it all. Betting something in hopes of obtaining something more is the foundation of gambling. An individual with a gambling addiction may gamble when troubled, be unsuccessful in reducing money and time spent gambling, and assume others will provide funds necessary to replace what was lost gambling (e.g., pay utility bills, rent, provide food) (American Psychiatric Association, 2013; Mayo Clinic, 2017a).

According to Gamblers Anonymous (2017), there are three stages to gambling addiction. The winning stage occurs when an individual might win a substantial amount of money and feel a euphoria that is invalid. (At this point, the gambler may assume that the money he is now betting belongs to the casino, racetrack, etc., but it is not; it is HIS or HER money! They won it from the establishment, and it now belongs to them.) The gambler will increase betting and the amount of each bet.

During the losing phase, the gambler will continue to bet in hopes of recovering losses. Money may be borrowed, and credit cards may be taken out to cover losses (many times the bills go to a post office box where others associated with the gambler are unaware). Withdrawal from social activity and significant others are noted during this time; in fact, the gambler typically gambles alone during this downturn. He or she may become nostalgic about the "good times" when winning occurred, and may believe that they will develop a strategy to be on top again (Gamblers Anonymous, 2017; Murch & Clark, 2016).

Finally, the desperation phase of this model evolves. Here the gambler is hopeless and may feel suicidal. Substance use disorders may develop, family and other significant relationships may disband, legal consequences of actions can develop, and time is often spent gambling or contriving means to obtain money to continue gambling. The gambler uses events and others as a means to justify their behavior, while responsibilities and financial demands are often ignored (Gamblers Anonymous, 2017; Murch & Clark, 2016).

Signs and symptoms of compulsive gambling might include the following:

- Preoccupation with gambling
- Unsuccessful control over gambling activities
- Feeling irritable, restless, anxious, etc., if trying to control gambling behavior
- Use gambling to escape problems
- Lying to family members over gambling activities or outcomes (losses and wins) of gambling
- Putting significant relationships (work, family. friends, school) in jeopardy because of gambling
- Take part in criminal activity (embezzlement, fraud, theft) to secure funds for gambling
- Seeks out enabling relationships from others who will "bail them out" of problems or events linked to gambling  (Mayo Clinic, 2017a; New York Council on Problem Gambling, n.d.)

Risk factors associated with a gambling disorder include:

- Bipolar disorder, obsessive compulsive disorder, and ADHD

- Substance use disorders, personality disorders, depression, or anxiety
- Gender (more males that female tend to gamble)
- Association with compulsive gamblers
- Taking drugs that are dopamine agonists
- Being highly competitive, impulsive, or easily distracted or bored (Mayo Clinic, 2017a)

*Case Vignette*

Janice Williams, a 67-year-old widow, comes to see you for some advice. She states she is lonely and gets depressed now that her husband of 30 years has died. (He has been dead for four years.) She states that her daughters are concerned that she "goes to the boat" and has a good time once a month when her "check comes in." She states her favorite game is slots, and she goes alone so as not to be distracted.

Mrs. Williams talks about how her daughters are just greedy, and they want everything she has when she dies. She does not understand why they might get mad if she has to ask them to help out with bills every once in a while. Mrs. Williams is evasive as to how often she must ask for financial assistance and how much is needed. She does say that "going to the boat" is the only thing that has made her happy since she retired and her husband died. "Without that, life is not worth living," she tells you.

What additional information do you need to determine health concerns in Mrs. Williams life? In what specific areas will you address questions?

If a referral is needed, to what specialists or organizations would you refer Mrs. Williams? Based on what is shared here, would you be concerned for Mrs. Williams safety? Please consider rationale for your answer.

## A Family Disease

Thus far in this chapter, the focus has been placed on the individual with the addiction or use disorder. However, addictive behaviors and use disorders (chemical or otherwise) impact the entire family. Things have to change to support the impaired family member, and part of the reason for this is so that the impaired member feeling as if they have some control.

This type of environment promotes unhealthy behavior on the part of all of the family members, and this type of pressure can have multiple consequences.

Therefore, it is important when treating an individual suspected of having an addiction or a substance use disorder, that the possible health consequences of the remaining family members are not overlooked or discounted.

As an addiction or use disorder evolves in one individual, family roles tend to cement, with each individual playing a part to support that addiction. Even when angry and aggravated, the family and others may enable the behavior that is negatively impacting the family.

The spouse or partner of the individual with the addiction is often the chief enabler. This role can be just as addicting as the chemical or activity of choice happens to be for an alcoholic or gambler. The individual in this role attempts to compensate for what is occurring within the family and their lack of control to alter the outcomes. The person assuming this role is often identified as being codependent, and he or she assumes the demands for all in the family. This will often be exhibited through calling and making excuses for the abuser at work or school, taking on additional jobs to have enough funds to make ends meet, attending all of the children's school functions alone, and making excuses in other ways for the individual with the use disorder (Wegsheider-Cruse, 1976; Wegsheider-Cruse, 1989).

Children in a family where a use disorder is evidenced often assume roles to distract from the "family problem". These children may be living with this individual, or may have been separated from him or her because of an event, such as divorce or incarceration. The parent, sibling or other significant family member may be continuing the behavior that is addictive or abusive. They may be "white knuckling" it, and having a difficult time dealing with their frustrations, anxieties and other emotions that were previously masked with a chemical or activity. The children may not understand the dynamics that are in play, and they could actually believe the irrational and shaming statements made toward them or others for whom they care. Fear created by the instability within the home environment and possible violence that could erupt in families where this type of dynamic is taking place, can actually cause post-traumatic stress disorder (PTSD) among members of the family (Hsieh *et al.*, 2016).

Children in such family environments may avoid the drama within their home by seeking shelter elsewhere. They do not, however, reciprocate by bringing friends to their home. In other instances, children are afraid to leave because of what might happen to a sibling or a parent if they are not there to protect them (Black, 2002; Wegsheider-Cruse, 1976; Wegsheider-Cruse, 1989).

As it can easily be seen, a good deal of physical as well as mental health issues can evolve from family relationships where addiction and use disorders are evidenced. Physical exhaustion, attention seeking behavior, putting others first, and other such unhealthy choices, can lead to stress and stress-related illnesses. Whether a client or a patient, it is important to ask questions that can support an understanding of what is going on in the individual's life when assessing and evaluating factors that impact health.

Statements such as the following are common:

"The dealer that supplied my Dad with drugs told me he was going to molest me or my three-year-old brother as payment for the drugs. It was my choice."

"My mother said she would not leave the house and gamble if I wasn't so clumsy, fat, and ugly."

"My father said he beat me because he loved me."

"The people at school were scared to say anything about me coming to school in dirty clothes, hurt, or without food. My mother was an important person in that town, and they were scared they would lose their jobs if they reported her drinking."

"Neighbors brought over their leftovers after they ate dinner so we would have something to eat. Mom worked the second shift and Dad was passed out by dinnertime. We were to young to cook."

Regardless of how they address the issues within their family, roles, survival roles are exhibited as a means to control an out-of-control family environment. The individual with the addictive behavior becomes the central focus of the family. Others take on specific roles or combinations of roles in order to ensure safety, credibility, and security for all involved. Sharon Wegsheider-Cruse (1989) and Claudia Black (2002) identified specific family roles and the dynamics within such. These roles are noted in childhood, and unless the individual seeks some form of positive intervention, these roles will follow them into adulthood.

The first role noted is that of the "perfect child." He or she is the one often held up for others in the family to emulate. This is the child identified as the one who will bring honor and respect to the family. In that role, he or she is the designated family hero and is the responsible one in the family. He or she often helps the other parent care for others in the family. This individual is a leader and may excel in academics, sports, and/or community action (Black, 2002).

However, the feelings that generate this behavior can be that of low self-worth. Often putting others' needs ahead of their own, this person tries to demonstrate worth through actions. Fearing rejection, he or she continues to seek new quests in which to shine. It is no secret that these individuals have difficulty letting others see the "real person" behind this persona, and thus they have difficulty establishing and keeping close relationships (Black, 2017; West Virginia University, 2017).

The next role to address is associated with the child who determines his or her job is to promote their own chaos and drama in hopes of minimizing the impact of that which is already occurring in their home. Often seen as the problem child, this individual is scapegoated for all of the trouble that is associated with their family. Although independent like the perfect child, this child acts out his or her feelings by taking risks, embracing change, and seeking pleasure. He or she does not like to follow rules and is often an underachiever. He or she tends to exhibit greater honesty, and does not care who is upset by what he or she says. This child does not attempt to hide the fact that there are issues within the family. He or she often has trouble with boundaries and can be defiant. It is little wonder that this child exhibits many problem behaviors throughout childhood that often continue through the remainder of his or her life. Early pregnancy, addiction, legal issues (e.g., stealing, truancy), and dropping out of school are a few ways these behaviors are manifested (Black, 2017; West Virginia University, 2017).

The next role among children of an abusive family is the child who does not want to create any problems. In fact, if this child went unnoticed, he or she would be happy. This child asks for little and is very good at observing what is going on around him or her. He or she is a good listener and works to "keep the peace." Being indecisive, he or she has difficulty understanding options. Therefore, when others lead, he or she does not question and simply follows. This child often withdraws and does not initiate conversations, relationships, or activities (Black, 2017; West Virginia University, 2017).

The final child's role is that of the one to distract by being an attention seeker. This child has a great sense of humor and often uses this talent to get others to forget their troubles. Others are drawn to them and the solid social skills they exhibit. This child can defuse stressful situations and calm those who are angry.

The downside of this role is that the individual gets his or her worth from others' attention. The individual masks his or her low self-worth through being superficial and charming. Often times, this child denies their own feelings and tells others what is believed they want to hear. This individual will often deny knowing what he or she truly feels if put into a situation where they need to express their feelings or thoughts. Often immature, this child does not like to make decisions and will avoid them at all costs. (Black, 2002; Black, 2017; West Virginia University, 2017).

The impact of growing up in a home with a use disorder does not go away with adulthood or moving from the home. According to Woititz (1983), there are some specific characteristics noted with adult children of alcoholics (ACOA). (These same characteristics can be identified in those who grew up in similar environments.) These individuals do not know what healthy happens to be. They will often lie, even if there are no consequences for telling the truth. Experiencing difficulty with close relationships, having fun, or forgiving themselves for not being perfect are often seen among ACOAs. They may procrastinate or exhibit other behaviors that prevent completion of an activity or enterprise. Noted difficulty with change, especially if they feel they have no control over it, is often evidenced. It is difficult for ACOAs to consider options other than the one they have chosen. They tend to have all or nothing thinking. That is the reason they are reported to be hypervigilant or extremely irresponsible when addressing life issues and events.

Ackerman (2002) found that, in addition to these dynamics, adult females tend to feel responsible for everything and everyone around them. They are often drawn to relationships with individuals who are addicted, and there is a high probability they too might become addicted.

Ackerman (1994) noted that adult males often kept feelings and emotions to themselves and had a fear of anyone really getting to know them. Significant relationships could occur, but these men did not share feelings and connection with anyone. Fearful of criticism, these ACOAs often deny any unpleasant events; however, they are often angry.

For more detailed criteria and information, consult the *Diagnostic and Statistical Manual of Mental Disorders, Fifth Edition* (DSM5) (American Psychological Association, 2013).

## Tool Kit and Resources

*Government Agencies*
*American Indian Health*: https://americanindianhealth.nlm.nih.gov/alcoholism.html

*Health Topics—Alcohol and Other Drugs*
*American Academy of Family Physicians*: http://www.aafp.org/patient-care/public-health/alcohol.html

- This is a dedicated page dedicated to information related to alcohol use disorders. An Alcohol Practice Manual is included on this page for reference. Additional journal articles. Policies and recommendations are included.

*American Indian Health*: americanindianhealth.nlm.nih.gov

- Information related to health needs of the American Indian, including those associated with substance use disorders and gender differences can be found here.

*Centers for Disease Control and Prevention (CDC)*: https://www.cdc.gov

- The nation's health protection agency that provides trends, issues and interventions in health related areas in the US and worldwide.

*Drug Enforcement Agency (DEA)*: https://www.dea.gov/index.shtml

- Information linked to drug patterns, legal issues, enforcement and community needs are noted at this site.

*National Institute on Alcohol Abuse and Alcoholism (NIAAA)*: https://www.niaaa.nih.gov

- Information linked to alcohol abuse, research and trends can be found at this site.

*National Institute on Drug Abuse (NIDA)*: https://www.drugabuse.gov

- Research and information related to substance use disorders, patterns and interventions appropriate for the healthcare professional and those that are in their care.

*National Institutes of Health (NIH)*: https://www.nih.gov

- General information source related to research and evidence based care related to a wide array of health concerns.

*NIDAMED*: https://www.drugabuse.gov/nidamed-medical-health-professionals

- A science based resources to help healthcare professionals manage the health needs of patients at risk for substance use disorders

*SBIRT*: http://www.masbirt.org/sites/www.masbirt.org/files/documents/toolkit.pdf

- A step by step guide for screening and intervening for Unhealthy Alcohol and Other Drugs Use (Clinician's Tool Kit included)

*Substance Abuse and Mental Health Services (SAMHSA)*: https://www.samhsa.gov

- General information on a federal level regarding articles, statistics and information on alcohol and other drugs.

*Substance Abuse and Mental Health Services (SAMHSA)*: https://www.samhsa.gov/workplace/toolkit

- A drug-free workplace tool kit is included at this site. Information on programs, campaigns, grants and treatment options are included.

*U.S. Department of Veterans Affairs:* https://www.mentalhealth.va.gov/substanceabuse.asp

- This link addresses mental health and substance abuse issues specific to veterans.

*U.S. Food and Drug Administration (FDA):* https://www.fda.gov

- Information regarding food packaging and safety, drug approval and potential issues linked to prescription medications.


*Professional Organizations and Resources*

*American Association for the Treatment of Opioid Dependence (AATOD)*: http://www.aatod.org

- Information specific to opioid use disorders can be obtained at this site.

*American Psychological Association.* (2013) Diagnostic and Statistical Manual of Mental Disorders, Fifth Edition (DSM-5): https://www.psychiatry.org/psychiatrists/practice/dsm

- A manual with specific criteria related to substance use disorders and other mental health disease.

*mhGAP Intervention Guide—WHO*: http://apps.who.int/iris/bitstream/10665/250239/1/9789241549790-eng.pdf

- The apps.who.int mhGAP Intervention Guide Mental Health Gap Action Programmed Version 2.0 for mental, neurological and substance use disorders in non-specialized health settings can be found here.

*International Nurses Society on Addictions (IntNSA)*: http://www.intnsa.org

- This nursing organization focuses information related to treating those with addictions.

*National Association of Children of Alcoholics (NACOA)*: http://nacoa.org

- An organization with a focus toward the adult needs of children who grew up in homes with an alcoholic or someone with similar attributes. Support with reading materials, meetings, and other support measures can be found here.

*National Council on Alcoholism and Drug Dependence (NCADD)*: https://www.ncadd.org

- Local assistance, immediate assistance and means to get help for alcohol and other drug use is available at this site.

*Prevent Rx Abuse: A CADCA Tool Kit*: http://www.preventrxabuse.org/other-resources/helpful-websites/#.WR9YfhiZNBw

- Multiple resource links are offered at this site. Links include those related to medicine abuse prevention, specific substance abuse prevention and intervention sources, recovery and support, drug take back programs, and legislation.

*Rural Health Information Hub*: https://www.ruralhealthinfo.org/community-health/substance-abuse

- Prevention and intervention substance abuse tool kit for rural communities.

*Support Groups*

*Alcoholics Anonymous* (AA): http://www.aa.org

To find local AA: http://www.aa.org/pages/en_US/find-local-aa

*Al-Anon Family Groups* (Al-Anon and Alateen—family support): http://al-anon.org

To find local meetings: http://al-anon.org/find-a-meeting

*Gamblers Anonymous* (GA): http://www.gamblersanonymous.org/ga/

To find local GA: http://www.gamblersanonymous.org/ga/locations

*GAM-Anon* (family support): https://www.gam-anon.org

To find local meetings: http://www.gam-anon.org/meeting-directory/us-meeting-directory

*Narcotics Anonymous* (NA): https://www.na.org

To find local NA: http://www.naws.org/meetingsearch/

*Nar-Anon Family Meetings*: http://www.nar-anon.org

To find a local meeting: http://www.nar-anon.org/find-a-meeting/

*Related Resources*

*NA Resources for Professionals*: https://www.na.org/?ID=Resourcesfor
    Professionals-content&ID=ResourcesforProfessionals-content

*National Institute for Mental Health*: nimh.nih.gov/index.shtml

*U.S. Department of Veterans Affairs* (Mental Health): mentalhealth.
    va.gov/providers/sud/selfhelp/handouts.asp

*PTSD Military and Veterans*: [ptsd.va.gov] [ninh.nih.gov/healthy/
    topics/post-traumatic-stress-disorder-PTSD/index.shtml] [military.
    com/benefits/veterans-health-care/ptsd]

*Traumatic Brain Injury*: cdc.gov/traumaticbraininjury/get_the_facts.
    html

*Disability Rating Scale*: neuroskills.com/resources/disability-rating-
    scale.php

*VA screening*: benefits.va.gov/PREDISCHARGE/DOCS/disexm58.pdf

*Discussion Questions*
- What are three considerations with prescribing opioids?
- Name three drug classifications and explain the positive and negative
  outcoems that could come from prescribing such medication for an
  adult, a geriatric patient, and an adolescent patient.
- What is the difference between use, misuse, abuse, and addiction.
  Offer an example of each.

## Case Study 1

Juanita Garcia is a 15-year-old female. She tells you that she loves
music and wants to go on a national television show that discovers talent when she graduates. Juanita tells you she loves to twirl and watch
her hands as she dances to music. You note this could be a possible sign
of MDMA use.

- Do you know enough from this conversation to offer this diagnosis?
- Please provide a rationale.

## Case Study 2

James Dayne is a noted jockey. He comes to you complaining of a
sore throat that is persistent. James does not have a temperature, nor are
his white cells elevated. However, when you inspect his throat, you note
an unusual amount of enamel erosion on his teeth. Is this important?

## Case Study 3

Tabatha Wilson is the middle child in a prominent family in the community where you work. Her parents ask you to speak to her as she appears to be very angry. Tabitha is defiant when she comes in to speak with you. She boasts about cutting class, having multiple sexual partners and shoplifting. She speaks of her juvenile arrests as a badge of honor. What might be going on with Tabitha?

What are the next steps in the healthcare process with this patient?

*Definitions*

*Use*—Recreational use with no consequences

*Misuse*—Use with the potential for negative consequences

*Abuse*—Negative consequences occur and use anyway

*Addiction*—Physiological mutation that results in the person feeling "normal" only when using.

## Case Study 1

Ken Mosley-Chang is a 34-year-old who has practiced as an RN for five years. He works in the recovery room and the OR for a rural community hospital. Ken hurt his back three years ago lifting a patient, and he complains of chronic pain. At home, Ken smokes marijuana and drinks a "few" (i.e., 10 to 15) beers when not on call. Ken has sought prescriptions from most of the advanced practice nurses and physicians at his hospital. They are no longer willing to provide him with narcotics for his pain.

Ken seeks out major cases in the OR. He takes calls in the evening when he works both the OR and the Recovery Room. Ken often complains that the narcotics count is wrong when he comes on shift, and the supervisor and other nurses have noted that he tends to not show others when he disposes of unused narcotics. Patients have continued to complain of pain even after Ken has administered narcotics to them. The nurses note this happens more with him than anyone else working in the OR or the recovery room.

A nurse caught Ken with a tourniquet on his arm. Ken stated he was getting ready to draw his blood because he was having a chronic cold. A vial of Fentanyl was next to Ken. He told the nurse it was left out from the previous shift by "that traveling nurse." The nurse also notices

Ken scratching his nose a lot and complaining about it itching; this is one side effect of Fentanyl. In addition, he was noted previously that night stumbling around. He blamed it on his "cold."

- What does the nurse who sees Ken with the Fentanyl near him do next?

- What are the primary concerns of this nurse who finds Ken in the compromising situation?

- What would a nurse manager of the OR need to address?

- What signs and symptoms would need to be paramount, and what assessments would need to be completed?

- What are Ken's rights?

- If he chooses to leave, what can the hospital do legally to address this?

- If Ken is found under the influence, what would be the appropriate next steps?

- As a colleague, what would be your concerns?

- Does there need to a staff meeting to address the OR/Recovery Room situation and feelings nurses may have about this?

- Are there safety protocols that need to be evaluated or put into place? If so, what would they be? (Contributed by Camille McNicholas, PhD, APRN, CRNA)

## Case Study 2

Lydia Brinks is a 29-year-old practicing chiropractor. She is coming to you for tension headaches and states that she knows she is a perfectionist. She has been top in her class from preschool through the latest courses she is taking in culinary arts. Dr. Brinks works six days a week and puts in a minimum of 10 hours each day in her practice. She is married to Mark Brinks, a 37-year-old architect, who decided to quit his job and stay at home with the children once they were born. Together they have three children, ages 3, 4, and 6.

Dr. Brinks takes her role as a parent seriously. She bathes and reads to her children every night. She is taking cooking courses to be able to better serve them quality food. She is writing a children's book on being kind, because she noticed not many parents in her children's classes address such things. She has her children in basketball and soccer and is even the team mother for one of her children's teams.

Dr. Brinks comes to you and explains she is exhausted all of the time. She sees her husband as a slug but defends him if anyone else speaks poorly of him. Dr. Brinks states that 99.5 was considered failing to her, and she has always given it her all. She states that she does not want a lot of medicine, because she said they make her feel out of control when she takes them. She states feeling out of control generates more stress for her.

- Considering what Dr. Brinks shares with you, what considerations would you make in addressing her health concerns?
- What would you need to rule out before addressing any substance use or addiction dynamics impacting Dr. Brink's past or current life?
- What considerations need to be made when planning to discuss any issues related to family with Dr. Brinks?

**Case Study 3**

Rayjay Carson is a 17-year-old high school freshman. Rayjay has been missing school a lot, and his mother complains she smells marijuana on his clothing. Rayjay lacks motivation but is intelligent according to school reports. Recently, Rayjay has been hanging around a known drug dealer that was arrested several times outside of school property.

Rayjay complains his mother "henpecks" him, and he does not see why he needs to graduate from high school. He tells you he will be a man (18) in six months and then he can do whatever he wants. He becomes angry whenever marijuana use is introduced in the conversation, and he brings up the point that it is "legal in most places now anyway, so it is cool if I smoke."

- What would you say to Rayjay about smoking marijuana?
- What other information would you want to obtain from Rayjay?
- What would the next steps be after additional data was obtained?

**References**

Ackerman, R. (2002). *Perfect daughters*. Deerfield Beach, FL: Health Communications Inc.

Ackerman, R. (1994). *Silent sons: A book for and about men.* New York, NY: Fireside Publishing.

The American Liver Foundation. (2016). *Alcohol related liver disease.* Retrieved from http://www.liverfoundation.org/abouttheliver/info/alcohol/

American Medical Association. (1953). *House of Delegates.* Clinical session.v.1953., Subcommittee on alcoholism. p.39. Retrieved from http://ama.nmtvault.com/jsp/viewer.jsp?doc_id=ama_arch%2FHOD00001%2F00000053&query1=&recoffset=0&collection_filter=All&collection_name=1ee24daa-2768-4bff-b792-e4859988fe94&sort_col=Publication%20Date&cnt=0&CurSearchNum=3&recOffset=0

American Medical Association. (2016). *Condition, disease, disorder.* AMA Style Insider. Retrieved from http://amastyleinsider.com/2011/11/21/condition-disease-disorder/

American Psychological Association. (2013). *Diagnostic and statistical manual of mental disorders* (5th ed.). Arlington, VA: American Psychological Publishing.

American Society of Addiction Medicine. (2011). *Definition of addiction.* Retrieved from https://www.asam.org/quality-practice/definition-of-addiction

Appelhans, B., Whited, M., Schneider, K., Ma, Y., Oleski, J., Merriam, P., Waring, M., Olendski, B., & Pagoto, S. (2012). Depression severity, diet quality, and physical activity in women with obesity and depression. *Journal of the Academy of Nutrition & Dietetics, 112*(5), 693–698.

Barnhart, W., Makela, E. & Latocha, M. (2004). SSRI- induced apathy syndrome: A clinical review. *Journal of Psychiatric Practice, 10*(3), 196–199.

Bell, K., & Keane, H. (2012). Nicotine control: E-cigarettes, smoking and addiction. *International Journal of Drug Policy. 22* (3) 242–247.

Bevilacqua, L. and Goldman, D. (2009). Genes and addiction. *Clinical Pharmacology and Therapeutics. 85* (4), 359–361.

Bienvieu, M. (2017). Are you a high functioning alcoholic? Retrieved from http://www.webmd.com/mental-health/addiction/features/high-functioning- alcoholic.

Black, C. (2017). Family roles. Retrieved from http://www.guidingheartswithhope.org/uploads/8/5/8/7/8587840/familyrolesinaddiction.pdf

Black, C. (2002). It will never happen to me: Growing up with addiction as youngsters, adolescents, adults. Minneapolis, MN: Hazelden Publishing.

Blasio, A., Steardo, L., Sabino, V., & Cottone P. (2013). Opioid system in the medial prefrontal cortex mediates binge-like eating. *Addiction Biology 19*, 652–662. 10.

Bonn-Miller, M., Oser, M., Bucossi, M, & Trafton, J. (2014). Cannabis use and HIV antiretroviral therapy adherence and HIV-related symptoms. *Journal of Behavioral Medicine, 37*(1), 1–10.

Bowen, S., Howard, M., & Garland, E. (2016). *Inhalant use disorder in the United States.* Retrieved from https://utah.pure.elsevier.com/en/publications/inhalant-use-disorders-in-the-united-states

Brooks, J., Ahmad, I., & Easton, G. (2016). Anabolic steroid use. *BMJ: British Medical Journal* (online). 355. Retrieved from http://www.bmj.com/content/355/bmj.i5023

Caldeira, K.M., Garnier-Dyhstra, L.M., Vincent, K.B., Picksworth, W.B., & Arria,

A.M. (2012). Cigarette smoking among college students: longitudinal trajectories and health outcomes. *Nicotine & Tobacco Research, 14*(7), 777–785.

California Board of Registered Nurses. (n.d.). What is the intervention program. Retrieved from http://www.rn.ca.gov/intervention/whatisint.shtml

Casale, S., Fioravanti, G., & Rugai, L. (2016). Grandiose and vulnerable narcissists: Who is at higher risk for social networking addiction? *Cyberpsychology, Behavior, and Social Networking. 19*(8), 510–515.

Centers for Disease Control and Prevention. (2014). Alcohol screening and counselling. Retrieved from https://www.cdc.gov/vitalsigns/alcohol-screening-counseling/index.html

Center for Disease Control and Prevention. (2016). Excessive drinking is draining is draining the U.S. economy. Retrieved from https://www.cdc.gov/features/costsof-drinking/

Chiauzzi, E., Dasmahapatra, P., & Black, R. (2013). Risk behaviors and drug use: A latent class analysis of heavy episodic drinking in first-year college students. *Psychology of Addictive Behaviors, 27*(4), 974–985.

Clark S. M., Saules K. K. (2013). Validation of the Yale Food Addiction Scale among a weight-loss surgery population. *Eating Behavior, 14*, 216–219.

Cleveland Clinic. (2014). Smoking: the No. 1 cause of preventable diesease and death. Retrieved from https://my.clevelandclinic.org/health/articles/smoking-and-your-health

Cruz, M., Bajo, M., Schweitzer, P, & Roberto, M. (2008). Shared mechanisms of alcohol and other drugs. *Alcohol Research & Health, 31*(2), 137–147.

Davidson, C. (2016). Developing treatment for stimulant abuse: A brief overview. *East Asian Archives of Psychiatry, 26*(2), 52–59.

Deutsch, S.I., Rosse, R.B., Connor, J.M., Murphy, M.E., & Fox, F.J. (2008). Current status of cannabis treatment of multiple sclerosis with an illustrative case presentation of a patient with MS, complex voice tics, paroxysmal dystonia, and marijuana dependence treated with dronabinol. *Neuropsychiatric Medicine, 13*(5) 393–403.

Dunn, M., & Bruno, R. (2010) Transition to and from injecting drug use among regular ecstasy users. *Addictive Behaviors, 35*(10), 909–912.

Eissenberg, T. (2013), Tobacco smoking using a waterpipe hookah: What you need to know. *AANA Journal. 81*(4), 308–313.

Erdogan, T., Aktas, O.O., Çelebioglu, E., Karakaya, G., & Kalyoncu, A.F. (2016). Codeine for treatment of cough variant asthma. *European Respiratory Journal. 48*; PA3369.

Fisher, F. & Kramer, A. (2015). Meta-analysis of the association between second-hand smoke exposure and ischaemic heart disease, COPD and stroke. *BMC Public Health 15*: 1–18.

Fraunfelder, F.T., Fraunfelder, F.W., & Chambers, W.A. (2014). Drug-Induced Ocular Side Effects. (7th ed.). New York, NY: Elsevier Sanders. Gamblers Anonymous (GA). (2017). Retrieved from http://www.treatment4addiction.com/recovery/12-step-programs/gamblers-anonymous-ga/

Garland, E., & Howard, M. (2011). Adverse consequences of acute inhalant intoxication. Experimental & Clinical Psychopharmacology. 19(2), 134–144.

Gearhardt, A., Treat, T., Hollingsworth, A., & Corbin, W. (2012). The relationship between eating-related individual differences and visual attention to foods high in added fat and sugar. *Eating Behaviors, 13*(4), 371–374.

Green, S., & Pfenning, S. (2015). Optimizing the use of state prescription drug monitoring programs for public safety. *Journal of Nursing Regulation, 6*(3), 4–10.

Greenberg, B. D., Segal, D. S., & Jacobs, B. L. (2016). 9. Hallucinogens: phencyclidine. *Preclinical Psychopharmacology, 343.*

Hancock, D. (1970). *I can't be an alcoholic because.* Center City, MN: Hazelton Publishing.

Hansen, R., Boudreau, D., Ebel, B., Grossman, D., & Sullivan, S. (2015). Sedative hypnotic medication use and the risk of motor vehicle crash. *American Journal of Public Health, 105*(8), e64–e69.

Hawkins, S. S., & Berkman, L. (2014). Identifying infants at high-risk for second-hand smoke exposure. 40(3): 441–445.

Heffernan, T. M., & O'Neill, T. (2013). Exposure to second-hand smoke damages everyday respective memory. *Addiction, 108*(2):420–426.

Hemmings, H. C., & Egan, T. D. (2013). *Pharmacology and physiology for anesthesia: Foundations and clinical application.* New York, NY: Elsevier Health Sciences. p. 253.

Hsieh, Y., Chiung-Tao Shen, A., Wei, H., Feng, J., Huang, S., & Hwa, H. (2016). Association between child maltreatment, PTSD, and internet addiction among Taiwansese students. *Computers in Human Behavior, 56*, 209–214.

Illinois Criminal Justice Information Authority. (2016). A state and national overview of the opioid and heroin crisis. Retrieved from http://www.icjia.state.il.us/articles/ an-overview-of-national-and-illinois-opioid-and-heroin-crisis

In re Julie Anne,121 Ohio Misc2d, 2002- Ohio - 4489

Jarvis, M. J., & Feyerabend, C. (2015). Recent trends in children's exposure to second-hand smoke in England: cotinine evidence from the Health Survey of England, *Addictions 110*(9), 1484–1492.

Jeffers, A., & Benotsch, E. (2016). Non-medical use of ADHD stimulants for appetite suppression and weight loss. In M. Hall, S. Grogan, & B. Grough (eds.) *Chemically Modified Bodies*, UK: Palgrave Macmillan, 149–172.

Jeffers, A., Benotsch, E., & Koester, S. (2013). Misuse of prescription stimulants for weight loss, psychosocial variables, and eating disordered behaviors, 65. 8–13.

Katz, G., Lobel, T., Tetelbaum, A., & Raskin, S. (2014). Cannabis withdrawal-A new diagnostic category in DSM-5. *Israel Journal of Psychiatry and Related Sciences 51* (4), 270–275.

Kaufmann, C., Spira, A., Depp, C., & Mojtabai, R. (2016). Continued versus new prescriptions for sedative-hypnotic medications: United States, 2005–2012. *American Journal of Public Health. 106*(11), 2019–2025.

Kentucky Board of Pharmacy. (n.d.) KY professionals recovery network. Retrieved from http://pharmacy.ky.gov/professionals/Pages/KY-Professionals-Recovery-Network.aspx

Khader, Y., Al-Akour, N., AlZubi, I., & Lataifeh, I. (2011). The association between second hand smoke and low birth weight and preterm delivery. *Maternal & Child Health, 15*(4), 453–459.

Kimura-Kataoka, K., Fujihara, J., Yasuda, T., & Takeshita, H. (2015). Fatal butane inhalation from gas cartridges: a case report and literature review. *Romanian Journal of Legal Medicine.* (23), 115–120.

Kobulsky, J., Minnes, S., Min, M., & Singer, M. (2016). Violence exposure and early substance use in high- risk adolescents. *Journal of Social Work Practice in Addictions, 16* (1-2) 46–71.

Kocak, N,D., Eren, A., Boga, S., Akturk, U.A., Ozturk, U.A., Arinc, S., & Sengul, A. (2015). Relapse rate and factors related to relapse on a 1- year follow-up of subjects participating in a smoking cessation program. *Respiratory Care, 60*(12), 1796–1803.

Konghom, S., Verachai, M., Srisurapanont, M., Suwanmajo, S., Ranuwattananon, A., Kimsongneun, N., & Uttawichai, K. (2010). Treatment for inhalant dependence and abuse. Retrieved from https://www.ncbi.nlm.nih.gov/pubmed/21154379

Kratochvil, C. (2012). ADHD pharmacotherapy: rates of stimulant use and cardiovascular risk. *American Journal of Psychiatry, 169*(2), 112–114.

Lader, M. (2002). Managing dependence and withdrawal with newer hypnotic medications in the treatment of insomnia. *Primary Care Companion to the Journal of Clinical Psychiatry. 1*(4), 33–37.

Lamarine, R. (2012). Marijuana: Modern medical chimaera. *Journal of Drug Education, 42*(1), 1–11.

LARA. (n.d.) Frequently asked questions. Michigan Department of Licensing and Regulatory Affairs. Retrieved from http://www.michigan.gov/lara/0,4601,7-154-72600_72603_27648-43222--,00.html

Laver-Bradbury, C. (2013). ADHD in children: An overview of treatment. *Nurse Prescribing. 11*(12), 597–601.

Leung, C.Y., Leung, G.M., & Schooling, C.M. (2015). Early second-hand smoke exposure and child and adolescent mental health: evidence from Hon Kong's Children of 1997' birth cohort. 110(11):1811–1824.

Lee, N., Pennay, A., Hester, R., McKetin, R., Nielseon, S., & Ferris, J. (2013). A pilot randomized controlled trial of modafinil during acute methamphetamine withdrawal: Feasibility, tolerability and clinical outcomes, *Drug & Alcohol Review, 32*(1), 89–95.

Leyro, T. M., & Zvolensky, M. J. (2013). The interaction of nicotine withdrawal and panic disorder on the prediction of panic-relevant responding to a biological challenge. *Psychology of Addictive Behaviors, 27*(1), 90–101.

Limsanon, T., & Kalayasiri, R. (2015). Preliminary effects of progressive muscle relaxation on cigarette craving and withdrawal symptoms in experienced smokers and acute cigarette abstinence: a randomized clinical trial. *Behavioral Therapy, 46*(2), 1660176.

Lutge, E.E., Gray, A., & Sigefried, N. (2013). The medical use of cannabis for reducing morbidity and mortality in patients with HIV/AIDS. Cochrane Database of Systematic Reviews. Issue4. Art. No. CD005175. DOI:10.1002/14651858.CD005175.pub3.

Maxwell, J.C. (2014). Psychoactive substance: Some new, some old; A scan of the situation in the U.S. Drug & Alcohol Dependence, 134: 71–77.

Mayo Clinic (2017a). Compulsive gambling. Retrieved from http://www.mayoclinic. org/diseases-conditions/compulsive-gambling/symptoms-causes/dxc-20258394

Mayo Clinic. (2017b). Test ID:ACL/ Retrieved from http://www.mayomedicallaboratories.com/test-catalog/Clinical+and+Interpretive/8264

Murch, W. S., & Clark, L. (2016). Games in the Brain Neural Substrates of Gambling Addiction. *The Neuroscientist, 22*(5), 534–545.

National Association of State Controlled Substances Authorities. (2017). Prescription drug monitoring programs. Retrieved from http://www.nascsa.org/rxMonitoring. htm

National Cancer Institute. (2017). Cannabis and Cannabinoids (PDQ)- Health Professional Version. Retrieved from https://www.cancer.gov/about-cancer/treatment/ cam/hp/cannabis-pdq#link/_37_toc

National Center on Addiction and Substance Abuse. (2016). Addiction as a disease. Retrieved from http://www.centeronaddiction.org/addiction/disease-model-addiction

National Council on Alcoholism and Drug Dependence. (2016a). Family history and genetics. Retrieved from https://www.ncadd.org/about-addiction/family-history-and-genetics

National Council on Alcoholism and Drug Dependence. (2016b). Alcohol facts and statistics. Retrieved from https://www.niaaa.nih.gov/alcohol-health/overview-alcohol-consumption/alcohol-facts-and-statistics

National Institute on Alcohol Abuse and Alcoholism. (2017). Alcohol facts and statistics. Retrieved from https://www.niaaa.nih.gov/alcohol-health/overview-alcohol-consumption/alcohol-facts-and-statistics

National Institute on Drug Abuse. (2012). Drug facts: Inhalants. Retrieved from https:// www.drugabuse.gov/publications/drugfacts/inhalants

National Institute on Drug Abuse. (2016, February 1). Genetics and Epigenetics of Addiction. Retrieved from https://www.drugabuse.gov/publications/drugfacts/genetics-epigenetics-addiction

National Institutes of Health. (2006). Anabolic steroid use. Retrieved from https:// www.drugabuse.gov/publications/research-reports/anabolic-steroid-abuse/how-are-anabolic-steroids-abused

National Institutes of Health. (2015). Caffeine powder. Retrieved from https://www. drugabuse.gov/drugs-abuse/other-drugs

National Institute of Health. (2017). What is marijuana? Retrieved from https://www. drugabuse.gov/publications/drugfacts/marijuana

National Institutes of Health. (2014). Eating disorders: About more than food. Retrieved from https://www.nimh.nih.gov/health/publications/eating-disorders/index.shtml

NBC News. (2017). Opioid theft, missing prescriptions prompts investigation of VA hospitals staff. Retrieved from http://www.nbcnews.com/storyline/va-hospital-scandal/opioid-theft-missing-prescriptions-prompts-investigation-va-hospitals-staff-n723291

Neilsen, M., Hansen, E., & Gotzsche, P. (2012). What is the difference between dependence and withdrawal reactions? A comparison of benzodiazepines and serotonin re-uptake inhibitors. *Addiction 107*(5), 900–908.

New York Council on Problem Gambling, (n.d.) About gambling disorder. Retrieved from http://nyproblemgambling.org/resources/gambling-disorder/

New York State Department of Health. (n.d.). Understanding New York's medical conduct program- physician discipline. Retrieved from https://www.health.ny.gov/publications/1445/

Nguyen, J., O'Brien, C., & Schapp, S. (2016). Adolescent inhalant use prevention, assessment, and treatment: A literature synthesis. *International Journal of Drug Policy. 31*, 15–24.

Nyamathi, A., Hudson, A., Greengold, B., Leake, B., Nyamathi, A., Hudson, A., Greengold, B. & Leake, B. (2012). Characteristics of homeless youth who use cocaine and methamphetamine. *American Journal of Addictions, 21*(3), 243–249,

Oncology Nursing Society. (2015). The potential adverse health consequences of exposure to electronic cigarettes and electronic nicotine delivery systems. *Oncology Nursing Forum. 42*(5). 445–446.

Padron, A., Galan, I., & Rodriguez-Artalejo, F. (2014). Research paper. Secondhand smoke exposure and psychological distress in adolescents. *A population-based study. 23*(4): 302–307.

Padala, P, Padala, K, Monga, V, Ramirrez, D, & Sullivan, D. (2012). Reversal of SSRI-associated apathy syndrome by discontinuation of therapy. *Annals of Pharmacotherapy. 46*(3), e8–e8.

Palamar, J.J., Martins, S., Su, M.K., & Ompad, D.C. (2015). Self-reported use of novel psychoactive substances in a US nationally representative survey: Prevalence, correlates, and a call for new survey methods to prevent under reporting. *Drug & Alcohol Dependence. 156*,112–119.

Parmer, JR, Forrest, B.D., & Freeman, R.A. (2016). Medical marijuana patient counseling points for healthcare professionals based on trends in the medical uses, efficacy, and adverse effects of cannabis based pharmaceutical drugs. Research in Social & Administrative Pharmacy 12(4), 638–654.

Parrott, A. (2013). Human psychobiology of MDMA or "Ecstasy": An overview of 25 years of empirical research. *Human Psychopharmacology, 28*(4), 289–307.

Poison Control. (2013). Inhaling alcohol is dangerous. Retrieved from http://www.poison.org/articles/2013-sep/inhaling-alcohol-is-dangerous

Poison Control (2017). Recognize a functioning addict. alcohol rehab. Retrieved from http://alcoholrehab.com/drug-addiction/recognize-a-functioning-addict/

Rogers, P., Heatherley, S., Mullings, E., & Smith, J. (2013). Faster but not smarter: effects of caffeine and caffeine withdrawal on alternates and performance. *Psychopharmacology 226*(2), 229–40.

Sacks, J., Gonzales, K., Bouchery, E., Tomedi, L., & Brewer, R. (2015). 2010 national and state costs of excessive alcohol consumption. *American Journal of Preventive Medicine 49*(5); e73–e79.

Sacerdote, P., Limiroli, E., & Gaspani, L. (2013). Experimental evidence of immunomodulatory effects of opioids. Retrieved from https://www.ncbi.nlm.nih.gov/books/NBK6402/

Sadoff, R. L., Drogin, E. Y., & Gurmu, A. S. (2015). Forensic implications of behavioral addictions. *The Behavioral Addictions*, 9–26.

Sansone, R., & Sansone, L. (2012). Hoarseness: A sign of self-induced vomiting? *Innovations in Clinical Neuroscience, 9*(10), 37–41.

Saunders, R., & Ascroft, R.E. (2012). Consumer genetics and addiction susceptibility testing—just what the consumer ordered. *Addiction. 107*(2). 2075–2076.

Scammell, T. (2015). Narcolepsy. *New England Journal of Medicine, 373* (27), 2654–2662.

Schuckit, M. A. (2014) "Recognition and management of withdrawal delirium (delirium tremens)." *The New England Journal of Medicine, 371*(22), 2109–2113.

Sharma, S. (2016). Latest trends in internet addiction disorder: Concepts, symptoms, theories, triggers and coping strategies. In S. Agawala, I. Das & K. Kumars (Eds.) Health Psychology. New Delhi: Allied Publishers Pvt. Ltd.

Shehab, N., Lovegrove, M.C., Geller, A.I., Rose, K.O., Weidle, N.J., & Budnitz, D.S. (2016). US Emergency Department Visits for Outpatient Adverse Drug Events, 2013–2014. *JAMA, 316*(20), 2115–2125.

Shippenberg, T., Chefer, V., & Thompson, A. (2009). Delta - opioid receptor antagonists prevent sensitization to the conditioned rewarding effects of morphine. Biological Psychiatry. Retrieved from https://www.ncbi.nlm.nih.gov/pmc/articles/PMC3832215/

Singer, L. T., Min, M. O., Lang, A., & Minnes, S. (2016). In *Utero Exposure to Nicotine, Cocaine, and Amphetamines*. In Pediatric Neurotoxicology (pp. 51–76). New York, NY: Springer International Publishing.

Singh, M. (2014). Mood, food, and obesity. Frontiers in Psychology, 5, 925. Retrieved from http://doi.org/10.3389/fpsyg.2014.00925

Smith, F., & Campbell, E. (2011). ADHD drugs used as an appetite suppressant. *Clinical Advisor. 14* (4), 95-95.

Spiller, H., Hays, H., & Aleguas, A. (2013). Overdose of drugs for attention-deficit hyperactivity disorder: Clinical presentation, mechanisms of toxicity, and management. *CNS Drugs, 27*(7), 531–543.

Steele, A., & Cunningham, P. (2016). Corrigendum to "a comparison of Suboxone and Clonidine treatment outcomes in opiate detoxification". *Archives of Psychiatric Nursing 30* (6), 818.

Stahlman, S., Javanbakht, M., Stirland, A., Guerry, S., & Gorbach, P. (2013). Methamphetamine use among women attending sexually transmitted disease clinics in Los Angeles county. *Sexually Transmitted Diseases, 40*(8), 632–638.

Substance Abuse and Mental Health Services Administration (SAMHSA). (2015a). Using prescription drug monitoring program data to support prevention planning. Retrieved from https://www.samhsa.gov/capt/sites/default/files/resources/pdmp-overview.pdf

Substance Abuse and Mental Health Services Administration (SAMHSA). (2015b). Methadone. Retrieved from https://www.samhsa.gov/medication-assisted-treatment/treatment/methadone

Substance Abuse and Mental Health Services Administration (SAMHSA). (2016).

American Indian and Alaska native: Tribal affairs. Retrieved from https://www.samhsa.gov/behavioral-health-equity/ai-an

Substance Abuse and Mental Health Services Administration (SAMHSA). (2016). Results from the 2015 national survey n drug use and health.

Detailed tables. Retrieved from https://www.samhsa.gov/data/sites/default/files/NS-DUH-DetTabs-2015/NSDUH-DetTabs-2015/NSDUH-DetTabs-2015.pdf

Substance Abuse and Mental Health Services Administration. (2010). Protracted Withdrawal. *Substance Abuse Treatment Advisory, 9*(1), 1–8.

Suissa, A. J. (2015). Cyber addictions: Toward a psychosocial perspective. *Addictive Behaviors 43*, 28–32.

The Economist. (2015). America's opioid epidemic is worsening. Retrieved from https://www.economist.com/blogs/graphicdetail/2017/03/daily-chart-3

University of Utah. (2017a). Genes and addiction. Retrieved from http://learn.genetics.utah.edu/content/addiction/genes/

University of Utah. (2017b) Drug delivery methods. Retrieved from http://learn.genetics.utah.edu/content/addiction/delivery/

U.S. Department of Health and Human Services. (2017). Nicotine addiction and your health. Retrieved from https://betobaccofree.hhs.gov/health-effects/nicotine-health/

U.S. Department of Justice. (2016). State prescription drug monitoring programs. Retrieved from https://www.deadiversion.usdoj.gov/faq/rx_monitor.htm

van Amsterdam, J., Nabben, T., & van den Brink, W. (2015) Recreational nitrous oxide use: Prevalence and risks. *Regulatory Toxicology and Pharmacology, 73*(3), 790–796.

Volkow, N. (2014). America's addiction to opioids: Heroin and prescription drug abuse. National Institute of Health. Retrieved from https://www.drugabuse.gov/about-nida/legislative-activities/testimony-to-congress/2016/americas-addiction-to-opioids-heroin-prescription-drug-abuse

Volkow, N., & McLellan, T. (2016). Opioid abuse in chronic pain—misconceptions and mitigation strategies. *The New England Journal of Medicine, 374*, 1253–1263.

Volkow, N., Swanson, J., Evins, A. E., DeLisi, L., Meier, M., Gonzalez, R., Bloomfield, M., Curran, H.V., & Baker, R. (2016). Effects of cannabis use on human behavior, including cognition, motivation, and psychosis: A review. *JAMA Psychiatry, 73*(3), 292–297.

Wardell, J.D., Quilty, L.C., & Hendershot, C.S. (2016). Impulsivity, working memory, and impaired control over alcohol: A latent variable analysis. *Psychology of Addictive Behaviors, 30*(5), 544–554.

Weaver, M, Hopper, J., & Gunderson, E. (2015). Designer drugs 2015: assessment and management. Addiction Science & Clinical Practice. 10(1); 8. Retrieved from https://www.ncbi.nlm.nih.gov/pmc/articles/PMC4422150/

Weathermon, R., & Crabb, D. W. (1999). Alcohol and medication interactions. *Alcohol, Research & Health. 23* (1), 40–54.

WebMD. (2016). Treating an addiction to painkillers. Retrieved from http://www.webmd.com/mental-health/addiction/breaking-an-addiction-to-painkillers-treatment-overvew#2

Wegsheider-Cruse, S. (1989). Another chance: Hope and help for the alcoholic family. Paulo Alto, CA: Science and Behavior Books.

Wegsheider-Cruse, S. (1976). The family trap. Bolder, CO: Johnson Institute.

Weintraub, S. (2017). Diazepam in the treatment of moderate to severe alcohol withdrawal. *CNS Drugs, 31*(2), 87–95.

West Virginia University (WVU). (2017). Behavioral roles of children of alcoholics. Retrieved from http://publichealth.hsc.wvu.edu/alcohol/effects-on-society/children-of-alcoholics/behavioral-roles-of-children-of-alcoholics/

White, N. D., & Noeun, J. (2016). Performance-Enhancing Drug Use in Adolescence. American Journal of Lifestyle Medicine, Retrieved from http://journals.sagepub.com/doi/pdf/10.1177/1559827616680593

Wiederhold, B. (2016). Low self-esteem and teens' internet addiction: What have we learned in the last 20 years? *Cyberpsychology, Behavior and Social Networking, 19*(6), 359–359.

Woititz, J. (1983) *Adult children of alcoholics.* Pompano Beach, FL: Health Communications.

World Health Organization. (Nov 2016) mhGAP Intervention Guide - Version 2.0. Retrieved from http://www.who.int/mental_health/mhgap/mhGAP_intervention_guide_02/en/

World Health Organization (WHO). (2014). Global Status Report on Alcohol and Health. p. XIII. 2014 ed. Retrieved from http://www.who.int/substance_abuse/publications/global_alcohol_report/msb_gsr_2014_1.pdf?ua=1.

Wright, P., Stewart, K., Fisher, E., Carlson, R., Falck, R., Wang, J., Leukefeld, C., & Booth, B. (2007). Behaviors among rural stimulant users: variations by gender and race/ethnicity. *AIDS Education and Prevention, 19*(2), 137–150.

Zawilska, J.B., & Andrzejczak, D. (2015). Next generation of novel psychoactive substance on the horizon—A complex problem to face. *Drug & Alcohol Dependence, 157*: 1–127.

## CHAPTER 14

# Infectious Diseases as a Population Health Issue

CHRISTINE RALYEA, DNP, MS-NP, MBA, NE-BC, CNL, OCN, CCRN
MARY A. BEMKER, PhD, PhyS, LADC, LPCC, CCFP, CCTP, CNE, RN
JENNIE PATTISON, DNP, RN

## Infectious Diseases as a Population Health Issue

INFECTIONS are on the rise worldwide, and this chapter will discuss many of the infections that are a population health issue and that are creating complex comorbidities in caring for many populations identified in this textbook. Epidemiology is the branch of medicine that deals with the incidence, distribution, and possible control of diseases and other factors relating to health (Centers for Disease Control and Prevention, 2017c). Often infections are studied using the epidemiologic principles of incidences and prevalence rates. It is important to understand the difference between these terms, which will be explained later in the chapter.

According to Anderson, Martin and Mate (2017), the Triple Aim and focus on population health must look to comprehensive prevention in the community of infections through rigorous preventative programs, including hand hygiene, safe food handling and processing, surveillance programs, antibiotic stewardship, and more. Looking at infections and infectious disease can cross over from population health management to public health service. Prevention is key and includes principles such as "monitoring the health status of the community, diagnosing and investigating health problems in the community, mobilization of community partnerships, development of policies, enforcement of laws and regulations that protect health, linking people to health resources, assuring a competent health workforce, and researching new insights and innovations to health problems" (Roach, 2014, p. 1). As part of today's population health strategy, communities must embrace disaster preparedness, the possibility of bioterrorism, and new infections such as EBOLA and the Zika virus.

## Governmental Influence

The government plays a vital role in regulation, control, and monitoring of infectious disease. "Infection prevention and health functions at the global, federal, state and local levels. The World Health Organization (WHO) functions under the United Nation's umbrella and collects information on the number of infectious diseases from countries. At the federal level, the executive order of the president provides the Secretary of Health and the Surgeon General with the authority to isolate and quarantine individuals suspected of having cholera, diphtheria, infectious tuberculosis, plague, smallpox, yellow fever, severe acute respiratory syndrome (SARS), influenza viruses causing or potentially causing a pandemic, and emerging multidrug-resistant microorganism" (Roach, 2014, p. 2). Then, the state level requires reporting for infectious diseases that are reported up to the Centers for Disease Control and Prevention (CDC).

## Prevention

The goal for infection prevention management is prevention in the population health arena. This includes surveillance programs, vaccination programs, screening (for example *Clostridium difficile* [C. diff] when treating a patient with watery stools), counseling, testing, education, and inspections in the community (e.g., monitoring for proper food handling and cooking temperatures at a restaurant).

### Primary Prevention

"Primary prevention is directed at avoiding disease and disability" (Roach, 2014, p. 4). Childhood vaccination programs are an example of primary prevention. Reaching 100% compliance with vaccinations for mumps, measles, and rubella (MMR) has been the goal since the late 1960s. In 1967, there were 186,000 cases of Mumps reported in the United States (U.S.) and District of Columbia (DC). Today there has been a 99% reduction in mumps. Between January 1 and March 25, 2017, there have been 1,965 cases of mumps reported in the same geographic region (Centers for Disease Control and Prevention, 2017c). Fostering and supporting vaccination programs serves as a primary prevention methodology with proven success. Primary prevention includes robust hand hygiene programs that are widespread in the community (e.g., restaurants, churches, airports, parks, theaters, grocery stores, and more). Starting at a very young age, it is never too early to teach children about persistent personal hand hygiene to prevent the spread of infections. Another example could be a routine screening for tuberculosis (TB) for all homeless patients who are admitted to the hospital with minor symptoms. Primary prevention also includes annual influenza vaccination programs. The goal of these campaigns is to obtain 100% engagement of teammates and healthcare workers to prevent Influenza infections and spread of these viruses throughout the communities.

*Secondary Prevention*

"Secondary prevention efforts focus in identifying or detecting existing health problems or conditions before they cause serious or long-term problems" (Roach, 2014, p. 4). An example of a secondary prevention is completing a TB screening on a healthcare worker who was exposed to a TB-positive patient during the time when the patient was pending a final diagnosis from their testing. Another example can be screening and cohorting hospitalized carbapenem-resistant Enterobacteriaceae (CRE) patients and following set protocols for protective equipment for teammates providing care.

*Tertiary Prevention*

Disease processes and infections that have already occurred require tertiary prevention measures. "Tertiary prevention activities aim to limit or reduce the condition's negative effects" (Roach, 2014, p. 4). When there is an outbreak of an infection, the provider focuses on decreasing the spread of the infection and minimizing the potentially harmful effects to the patient, with the goal of returning the patient to his or her prior state of health and functioning. Looking at that same cohort of CRE patients mentioned above, the advanced practice nurse (APN) will order appropriate antibiotics with sensitivity to the strain/organism, continue to mobilize the patient to avoid debilitation, address nutritional needs, and ensure hand hygiene education for the patient, family, and healthcare team. The APN will monitor for any clustering and spreading of organisms in the patient cohort.

### Incidence Versus Prevalence Rates

Now that an infection exists, it is essential to understand how infections are reported. "An incidence is a proportion. A measurement of new cases of disease within a population over a given period. The numerator is the number of new cases of the event being measured and the denominator is the initial population eligible or "at risk" to develop the condition or event. Also, known as cumulative incidence" (Lee *et al.*, 2004, p. 433). An example of an incidence rate is looking at the number of central-line associated blood stream infections (CLABSI) during the first quarter of the year. Calculating rates of infections is a more accurate measure than looking at raw numbers of infections. If the facility had three new infections from catheters (secondary line infections) as the numerator and the denominator looks at eligibility or at risk, which will be the total number of line days for the patient population, then an infection rate can be calculated. If a patient is in the hospital for six days and three of the days he or she had a central line placed for providing aggressive fluid management and medications, the denominator will be three. The risk is not one patient nor his or her entire length of stay—but the risk of the central line infection is associated with the six days stay will only support the catheter (line) days specifically for this patient example being three days. To restate the risk for the central line infection was three days. Calculating the incidence rate for the period of data/time will be number of infections, divided by the number of catheter days. This number is then multiplied by 1,000, as a standard for 1,000 line days in this case to establish a common unit of measure for all members (i.e. hospitals) in a comparison group. Simply restated the incidence rate is a measurement of the number of new individuals who contract a disease during a particular period of time.

*Prevalence Rate*

"Prevalence is a measurement of all individuals affected by the disease at a particular time, whereas incidence is a measurement of the number of new individuals who contract a disease during a particular period of time" (Centers for Disease Control and Prevention, 2017c). It is a snapshot of the disease at that one point of measurement. For example, looking at all ventilator patients on the first Friday of each month and reporting at a large tertiary trauma center, there was one ventilator associated hospital-acquired infection (numerator) out of the 95 mechanically ventilated patients (denominator) for the month being reported. This would be reported as a prevalence rate of 10.53 ventilator-associated infections on the first Friday of the month being reported. To show the calculations:

Calculating a ventilator-associated infection rate:

$$\frac{(1 \text{ ventilator infection})(1000 \text{ ventilator days})}{(95 \text{ ventilator days})} = 10.53 \text{ (infection rate)}$$

## Surveillance

Surveillance is defined by Lee *et al.* (2004) as "the ongoing, systematic collection, analysis, interpretation, and dissemination of data regarding a health-related event for use in public health action to reduce morbidity and mortality and to improve health. Surveillance, as part of infection prevention and control programs in healthcare facilities, contributes to meeting the program's overall goals, namely: (1) protect the patient; (2) protect the healthcare worker, visitors, and others in the healthcare environment; and (3) accomplish the previous two goals in a timely, efficient, and cost effective manner whenever possible" (p. 427). Infections occur and are on the rise, so the value of surveillance to protect patients, visitors/family members, and healthcare workers cannot be underestimated.

*Case Vignette (Lee et al., 2004, p. 429)*

Hospital A is a 1500-bed tertiary care medical center offering a wide range of inpatient and outpatient services. There are six critical care units (medical, surgical, coronary, neurosurgical, pediatrics, and neonatal). The open heart surgery program is one of the largest in the country. There is a large orthopedic surgery program and a predominant gynecology service as well. An analysis of surgical procedure data from the operating room database reveals that coronary artery bypass graft (CABG) procedures, orthopedic joint replacements, and hysterectomies are among the most commonly performed surgical procedures. Outpatient medical records indicate that primary care is available in the clinic setting, with large numbers of participants in both the pediatrics and geriatrics populations.

Hospital B is a 75-bed acute care hospital in a rural setting. Medical records show that most admissions are adult patients with a variety of acute medical diagnoses. General surgical procedures are performed by the two staff surgeons, with cholecystectomies, hysterectomies, and hernia repairs being the most frequently performed. Some nursing personnel have reported that many patients may have had indwelling urinary catheters longer than necessary or without a clear indication for use. One health problem noted by the local public health department is a recent increase in the incidence of TB.

A home health agency provides care to a wide range of patients, specializing in intravascular access/treatment with short-term and long-term central lines and with peripheral lines. There are also many patients with indwelling urinary catheters.

These are three very different scenarios. As the APN, what would be different considerations in each case for a robust infection prevention surveillance and control program?

## Basic Principles for Infection Prevention

Hand hygiene is a general term that applies to either handwashing, antiseptic hand wash, antiseptic hand rub, or surgical hand antisepsis handwashing per the Centers for Disease Control and Prevention (CDC) (2017 b). Stressing hand hygiene using friction, hand rubbing with both hands using soap and water is considered an antiseptic wash. "An alcohol-containing preparation designed for application to the hands for reducing the number of viable microorganisms on the hands. In the United States, such preparations usually contain 60–95% ethanol or isopropanol" (Boyce & Pittet, 2002, p. 5). Alcohol-based hand rubs are also effective and have become a common practice at many healthcare settings. As an APN, it is critical to understand hand hygiene principles and types of cleansing agents to be used to prevent infections and the spread of organisms. For example, a suspected C. diff patient will require the healthcare worker to use soap and water. Using the alcohol-based hand rub will not be effective to kill this organism.

The CDC developed a strong hand hygiene program in 2002. The Recommendations of the Healthcare Infection Control Practices Advisory Committee (HICPAC) and the HICPAC Hand Hygiene Task Force are available on the www.CDC.gov website. Per Boyce and Pittet (2002), ". . . normal human skin is colonized with bacteria; different areas of the body have varied total aerobic bacterial counts (e.g., $1 \times 10^6$ colony forming units (CFUs)/cm$^2$ on the scalp, $5 \times 10^5$ CFUs/cm$^2$ in the axilla, $4 \times 10^4$ CFUs/cm$^2$ on the abdomen, and $1 \times 10^4$ CFUs/cm$^2$ on the forearm). Total bacterial counts on the hands of medical personnel have ranged from $3.9 \times 10^4$ to $4.6 \times 10^6$. In 1938, bacteria recovered from the hands were divided into two categories: transient and resident. Transient flora, which colonize the superficial layers of the skin, are more amenable to removal by routine handwashing" (p. 4). It is alarming to learn the large volumes of bacteria on our skin pose such a high risk of infection for vulnerable patients and the community at large.

Many infections and identified organisms exist today, and this chapter will provide limited information to build an understanding of the infection, appropriate prevention measures, and what opportunities exist for the APN to implement primary, secondary and tertiary prevention principles. Primary prevention is the focus, but facing the challenges with the rise in infections will support practice guidelines and care of this patient population.

## Hepatitis

Hepatitis is a population health concern due to the chronic impact of the disease on individuals and the potential for spreading this disease to others. Contracted from a virus, the disease etiology can be linked back in part to drug use (licit or illicit), susceptibility related to certain medical conditions, and coming into contact with the virus via contaminated fluids. This section of the chapter will focus upon the etiology, symptomatology, prevention, and treatment of the three most prominent forms of this disease.

Viral Hepatitis, comprised of hepatitis A, hepatitis B, and hepatitis C, is distinct because of its specific impact noted on the liver. Although all three forms of this disease are similar in overall process, the way this process manifests differs according to viral type, and thus the treatment of each is unique.

## Hepatitis A

The hepatitis A virus (HAV) is found in the stool of infected individuals. It is highly contagious and is primarily spread from the fecal to oral route. Most notably, HAV is often connected to contaminated food or water. In addition, HAV can be transmitted by contact with an infected individual or through contact with contaminated material on an individual. HAV is rarely contracted through sexual encounters (Centers for Disease Control and Prevention, 2013). Although nearly 80% of adults who contract the disease experience some symptoms, children are typically unaware that they have this virus within their system. It is important to note that asymptomatic children infected with hepatitis A can still spread the disease (Centers for Disease Control and Prevention, 2015b).

The rate of known cases of hepatitis A has greatly been reduced. This is believed to be associated with the hepatitis A vaccination. Since the vaccination became available in 1995, incidents of hepatitis A have declined 95% in the United States. In 2014, the most recent year for which data are available, there were an estimated reported and projected unreported cases of 2,500 (Centers for Disease Control and Prevention, 2015b). (Between 1987 and 1997, an average of 28,000 cases of HAV were noted annually in the United States [Morbidity and Mortality Weekly Report [MMWR], 2011.)

The incubation period for HAV ranges from 15 to 50 days. HAV can live outside of the body for months, and the virus is killed when exposed to 185 degrees F for one minute. Water chlorination also prevents the spread of HAV. Both cooked food and treated water can spread HAV if the contamination occurs after preparation of food or if the water treatment is not sufficient to irradiate HAV (Centers for Disease Control and Prevention, 2015b).

*Case Vignettes*

Juan García loves to eat lunch at a local salad bar. He typically selects raw vegetables, apples, grapes, and strawberries to eat. When oysters on the half shell are on the menu, he is especially excited and loads his plate with this delicacy.

Monique Chen works in a parish daycare center. She works in the infant room, and she estimates that she changes at least 30 diapers a day. Monique is very busy, and she indicates she sometimes must go on to the next task before finishing up what she is doing completely.

Ernest James travels regularly for his work. He is currently heading to Pakistan and notes that there is a travel warning for that country as of 4/17. He is not sure for what reason the warning was issued by the U.S. Passports & International Travel (2017), and he notes he will be in that country for five days before returning home.

Consider what you have been presented with thus far in the segment on hepatitis.

Are any of the individuals in these vignettes at increased risk for contracting hepatitis A?

If you believe they are, for what reason did you make that deduction?

What advice would you provide Juan, Monique, and Ernest about prevention efforts against contracting hepatitis A?

Case Definition (Note: Developed by the CDC and Council of State and Territorial Epidemiologists as a means for uniform clinical and laboratory-testing criteria for nationally noted infectious diseases).

The case definition for acute viral hepatitis A is as follows (Centers for Disease Control and Prevention, 2015b):

Direct onset of symptoms:

* jaundice or
* elevated serum aminotransferase levels

Because symptoms for all three forms of viral hepatitis are the same, it is important that a patient has a positive serologic test for immunoglobulin M antibody for hepatitis A virus or that he or she exhibits the clinical case definition for one who resides with and/or has sexual contact with an individual who has been diagnosed with a laboratory confirmed case of hepatitis A (Centers for Disease Control and Prevention, 2015b).

Most individuals who contract hepatitis A recover within a span lasting a few weeks to six months. Symptoms are sometimes so mild that the individual may not even be aware of its presence. Liver damage is not noted as a permanent entity for most, and the disease tends to dissipate of its own accord. However, it has been noted that some who contract hepatitis A have died from liver failure; this is especially true in older adults (Centers for Disease Control and Prevention, 2015b).

**Hepatitis B**

Hepatitis B (HBV) can be contracted from blood, semen, and other bodily fluids produced by someone infected with hepatitis B. Transmission can occur when percutaneous or mucosal contact with infected blood or other bodily fluids occurs (Centers for Disease Control and Prevention, 2016e). Globally, nearly 2 billion individuals are infected with HBV, and it is estimated that 350 million individuals live with chronic HBV (Li *et al.*, 2016). In 2014, the last known reported data, 2,953 acute cases of HBV were reported in the United States.

Transmission of HBV can result when an individual has or does any of the following:

* has sexual contact with someone infected with HBV

- intravenous drug use when needles and other paraphernalia (e.g., drug preparation equipment) are shared
- is born to a mother that is HBV positive
- encounters open sores or blood from an infected individual
- needle sticks or exposure to sharp instruments sharing razors, toothbrushes, etc., with a person who has HBV (Centers for Disease Control and Prevention, 2016e)

HBV is NOT transmitted through casual contact such as hugging, kissing, sharing food and water, coughing, or sneezing. HBV can live outside of the body for seven days and still have the potential to cause an infection. Blood spills should be cleaned with 1:10 part household bleach to water ratio to ensure disinfecting exposed areas. Gloves should be used during cleaning (Centers for Disease Control and Prevention, 2016e).

*Case Vignette*

Les Wilkins, 15 years old, resides in a rural community in the Midwest. About 40 miles away, several cases of HBV had been noted and reported to the public health department. Les came in to speak with you because his girlfriend of 2 years resides in that town. He stated he is concerned that hugging and kissing his girlfriend could lead to his contracting HBV, and he wants to know if he needs to break up with her to prevent getting HBV.

- What additional information would you need to advise Les?
- What information would you share with him regarding transmission of HBV?

Since Les is the 10th young person to seek out similar information on HBV in your community, what could you do in partnering with the middle and high schools to educate young people about HBV?

**Incidence of Hepatitis B**

The number of cases in the United States has decreased notably (82%) since 1991. This decrease correlates to the time when routine vaccinations for children were instituted. It is estimated that 2.2 million Americans have chronic HBV, and an estimated 786,000 individuals die globally each year from chronic HBV (Centers for Disease Control and Prevention, 2016e; Lorano *et al.*, 2012).

The acute phase of this disease can range from a few weeks to several months. Many who are infected with this disease can become and remain virus-free after the acute stage. However, for some the virus remains, resulting in a chronic hepatitis B infection. This lifelong condition can promote more serious health concerns, such as cirrhosis, liver failure, and liver cancer. It can culminate in death (Lorano *et al.*, 2012).

During the acute stage of HBV, there is no known treatment. Symptoms can only be managed. During the chronic stages, treatment for liver failure and standards of care for the management of common liver diseases should be followed. For the most current information, please see the website for American Association for the Study of Liver Disease (AASLD, https://www.aasld.org/publications/practice-guidelines American Public Health, https://www.aasld.org/).

**Symptomatology**

During the acute phase of the disease, there may be no symptomatology. When symptoms are present, the symptomatology for hepatitis A, hepatitis B, and hepatitis C can be the same. These symptoms include the following (Centers for Disease Control and Prevention, 2016e):

- malaise
- nausea
- lack of appetite
- abdominal pain
- low grade fever
- jaundice
- dark urine
- clay-colored stool
- joint pain

HBV can be treated with antiviral medications (including Epivir, Hepsera, and Tyeka), interferon alfa-2b and, if progressed, a liver transplant (Mayo Clinic, 2014).

*Note*: When hepatitis B and hepatitis C become chronic, the individual may be asymptomatic for years. When symptoms occur, the liver may have already experienced damage.

**Hepatitis C**

Hepatitis C (HCV) is caused by a blood-borne pathogen and is generally contracted through shared needles or other equipment related to injection of drugs. However, symptoms may be absent for 70% to 85% of the individuals who have HCV, a chronic condition develops (Centers for Disease Control and Prevention, 2015b) that can lead to liver damage. As of 2014, the last year in which statistics are available, 2,194 cases of acute HCV were reported from 40 states. An estimated 2.7 to 3.9 million U.S. citizens are believed to have chronic HCV infections. It is believed that 15% to 25% of all persons infected with HCV will clear the virus without any treatment (Centers for Disease Control and Prevention, 2015c).

Those at risk for contracting HCV include the following (Centers for Disease Control and Prevention, 2015c):

- current and former intravenous drug users (one injection places a person at risk)
- those who received clotting factor concentrates prior to 1987
- individuals receiving hemodialysis on a regular basis
- persons with exposure to HCV (e.g., healthcare/community worker who had a needle stick associated with HCV + blood, recipients of blood or organs from an HCV+ donor)
- individuals born to a HCV+ mother
- sexual partner of a HCV+ individual
- recipient of blood, blood products, or organs prior to 1992
- sharing of items, such as a razor or toothbrush, with a person who has HCV+ participation in healthcare procedures that are invasive

**Vaccinations**

Vaccines have been developed for hepatitis A and hepatitis B. There currently is no vaccination for hepatitis C. When being vaccinated for HAV, an individual receives two full doses of the HAV vaccine. This vaccine has been deemed safe for individuals 12 months of age and older. An individual who contracted HAV and recovered from the disease does not need to be vaccinated (Centers for Disease Control and Prevention, 2015b).

HBV vaccination can be administered at birth. All children not previously vaccinated are recommended to receive the vaccination. Individuals deemed to be at risk for contracting HBV are encouraged to get vaccinated as an adult. Those with HIV infection, chronic liver disease, diabetes mellitus, and endstage renal disease, as well as anyone seeking protection from HBV, are suggested to get the HBV vaccination (Centers for Disease Control and Prevention, 2016a).

Immunoglobulin can be administered as a preventative measure for potential pre and postexposure to HAV. Protection is estimated to last approximately three months, and the desired administration time for maximum impact is 2 weeks (Centers for Disease Control and Prevention, 2015b). The most common side effects are redness, swelling, and pain at the injection site.

Although each vaccination series are set to a specific schedule, patients are encouraged to complete the series of vaccinations even if the desired window of administration has lapsed. Once the series of injections has begun, the completed injections do not have to be retaken for the series to be completed. Since developed, these vaccines are part of the traditional regimen for childhood immunization. The vaccine is not part of routine preventative intervention for adults. However, if an adult fits into one of the categories presented below, it would be advantageous to receive the vaccinations.

**Risk Factors**

Those at risk for hepatitis A include the following (Centers for Disease Control and Prevention, 2013, 2015b:

- those who come into contact with the hepatitis A virus due to employment
- anyone traveling, working in, or residing in areas where hepatitis A is widespread
- individuals treated with clotting-factor concentrates
- those with chronic liver disease
- those who partake in recreational drug use (Intravenous or not)
- men who have sex with men
- parents and children of individuals adopted from countries where hepatitis A is prevalent
- working with nonhuman primates

Those at risk for hepatitis B include the following (Centers for Disease Control and Prevention, 2013, 2016e):

- living with someone known to have hepatitis B
- anyone traveling, working in, or residing in areas where hepatitis B is widespread

- individuals whose work exposes them to blood
- individuals born to an infected mother
- those who undergo hemodialysis
- individuals who inject street drugs and/or share contaminated needles
- those with multiple sexual partners
- those who have contracted an STD
- men who have sexual encounters with men
- sexual partners of someone who has hepatitis B
- intravenous drug users
- residents and staff at facilities for developmentally disabled individuals
- parents and children of individuals adopted from countries where hepatitis B is prevalent

Combination vaccinations are available for administration and include the following (Centers for Disease Control and Prevention, 2016 e):

- PEDIARIX offers protection against HBV, diphtheria, tetanus, cellular pertussis, and polio. Administration age is between 6 weeks and 7 years.
- TWINRIX combines HAV and HBV protection. Recommended for those 18 years of age and older at risk for HAV and HBV.

Anyone providing care for a patient with hepatitis needs to be knowledgeable and current with all aspects of care associated with the specific hepatitis virus(s) the individual has. If uncomfortable with level of expertise, a specialist, such as an infectious disease physician, may be consulted (Centers for Disease Control and Prevention, 2015c). For a current list of treatments, consult Hepatitis C Online (2017). Regular data review is recommended for the most current program information related to hepatitis (Mezzo, Lamia, Schipani, Stokes, & Joacob-Ware, 2016).

Screening and vaccination need to be a part of regular practice, and cultural considerations need to be addressed as part of such. Knowing who to approach and how to approach individuals can be key to success, especially when an infected or potentially infected person feels well and believes he or she is not at risk (Li *et al.*, 2016).

*Case Vignette*

Misty Rogers is bringing her child in for his 4-year-old checkup. You notice the child has not been vaccinated against hepatitis viruses. What information could you provide to Misty about this?

After you share the information at hand, Misty lets you know that a friend from church had a next-door neighbor whose child is autistic. The minister told them it was God's will that children not be vaccinated and that is what caused the autism. How would you respond to this?

## HIV/AIDS

Human Immunodeficiency virus (HIV)/acquired immunodeficiency syndrome (AIDS) remains a global health concern that results in two million new HIV infections worldwide on an annual basis (Siemieniuk, 2015). As previously indicated, population health looks at the health and well-being of a subgroup within a population. Dynamics and major tenets within that group are identified, and the overall desired and actual outcomes are addressed. This dynamic is especially important when one looks at HIV and AIDS.

With the first identification of this population, there were many beliefs and values associated with those individuals being diagnosed with HIV/AIDS. Having individuals like Arthur Ashe (Finn, 1993), Ryan White (HRSA, 2016), and Elizabeth Glaser (Elizabeth Glaser Pediatric AIDS Foundation, 2017) die from this disease expanded the scope of insight and understanding about what was occurring. Although some may still hold unfounded beliefs regarding the "why" behind the disease, having the scientific knowledge about the etiology regarding HIV dispels much of what was originally believed about those who contracted AIDS.

The first AIDS cases were noted in the United States in 1981 (Centers for Disease Control and Prevention, 2001; Gallo & Montagneier, 2003). The report addressed five cases of *Pneumocystis carinii* pneumonia among five individuals in Los Angeles, CA, who previously had been healthy. After this, several other cases of young men exhibiting the same type of symptomatology were reported, and some physicians were calling for pentamidine to treat the symptoms expressed by these patients. By March 1983, the CDC, based on 18 months of research by epidemiologists, established recommendations for sexual, drug-related, and occupational transmission prevention standards (Centers for Disease Control and Prevention, 2001). From this base, understanding of this complex disease dynamic caused by a virus that attacks an individual's immune system has emerged. Known for making an individual susceptible to opportunistic infections that would not pose an imminent threat to a healthy individual, HIV/AIDS has been on the forefront of medical science investigation for over 35 years (AIDS.gov, 2017). In 2015, over 39,000 individuals were diagnosed with HIV (Centers for Disease Control and Prevention, n.d.b).

**Etiology**

The HIV virus is contracted through exposure to affected body fluids. Once in the bloodstream, the HIV virus seeks out and damages T-Helper lymphocytes, also known as T4 or CD4 cells. When this occurs, the T-cells are no longer able to signal for intervention by the antibody production specific for the HIV virus. If the CD4 count drops below 200 in relation to HIV, an individual is diagnosed as having AIDS (normal range for CD4 is 500 to 15,000) (U.S. Department of Veterans Affairs, 2017). The most common means of contracting HIV is via infected blood, semen, vaginal secretions, and breast milk. In some rare cases, cerebrospinal fluid, pericardial fluid, and other bodily fluids not general to contact may contain the HIV virus (Centers for Disease Control and Prevention, n.d.b). The latter are typically an issue only for healthcare professionals whose treatment of an individual would require them to come into contact with these bodily fluids.

The typical means of entry of the HIV virus is through skin that is not intact. This can occur through use of contaminated needles (e.g., needle sharing, unclean needles used in tattooing), unprotected sex, blood sharing activities (e.g., rites where individuals cut themselves and intermingle their blood), or sharing of items that might retain blood (e.g., razor or toothbrush) with an infected individual (Centers for Disease Control and Prevention, n.d.b).

Again, it is important to emphasize that the HIV virus is transmitted only if it is present. The acts themselves do not cause HIV to occur UNLESS the virus is already present. However, these activities may increase the probability of coming into contact with the HIV virus. Transmission of HIV is dependent upon two major criteria. These transmission routes are based on viability and virulence, and the HIV virus must be present at the time of the action. It is important to note, and share with the public, that HIV is NOT contracted through coughing, sneezing, or shaking hands or from food being prepared or served by an HIV-infected individual (Centers for Disease Control and Prevention, n.d.b).

## Probability of Transmission

The risk of contracting HIV varies depending upon the specific activities in which one is engaged, and not all forms of exposure carry the same level of risk. It is important to note that even small risks can compound over time and result in a much larger risk to that individual. In a sampling of information provided by the CDC, it is noted that receiving a blood transfusion with blood containing the HIV virus can result in a 9,250:10,000 chances of contracting HIV. Compare this to a needle stick that is a 23:10,000 chance of contracting HIV (Centers for Disease Control and Prevention, n.d. a). How is this information important in assessing patient risk factors and educating them to such?

### Case Vignette

Sally Strong is an 18-year-old female. She is in love for the first time, and even though she has been exposed to information regarding unprotected sex and the likelihood of contracting HIV, she decides to have unprotected sex with her partner. Her partner assures her that there is no cause for concern of contracting HIV or any STD. As far as she is aware, she and her partner have a monogamous relationship.

Sally is not aware that her partner is an IV drug user. The injection sites are in places that may not be obvious to an inexperienced individual like Sally. She does not, for example, look between her partner's toes or behind the knees. Although she loves this individual very much and she plans to make a life with them, Sally remains concerned about contracting HIV.

If you were manning an information booth that included information on HIV/AIDS, and Sally shared her story with you, what might you want to know further about the situation?

For example, would it be important to know if Sally's partner was male or female? After gathering information from Sally regarding the information you desire from Sally, what educational information would you provide Sally?

How could you do this without sounding as if you were judging her?

What actions would you recommend that Sally take?

How would you engage Sally in a discussion so that there was "buy in" by Sally?

What would you share specifically regarding repeated risky behavior?

## HIV/AIDS Progression

HIV Progression Research has shown specific dynamics and implications in the progression of HIV/AIDs. The following is a summation of such.

### Acute/Early HIV infection

This is the period when the HIV virus is establishing itself within the body. This time is denoted from when the HIV virus first enters the body to when antibodies are produced. It is estimated that this incubation period lasts from six to 12 weeks. Once the body responds to the HIV virus, a screening test can detect the presence of this virus in an individual. This early phase lasts approximately seven weeks, with the first three weeks being identified as acute, and the last four weeks being identified as early (AIDS.gov, 2017; Suthar et al., 2015).

### Clinical Latency/Asymptomatic

This period follows the acute stage of the infection. Although the individual may continue to look and feel healthy for extended periods, the virus is replicating and slowly destroying the CD4 cells. The disease can continue to be transmitted to others through sharing of body fluids. If a female is pregnant during this time, the HIV virus can be transmitted to the fetus in utero or to the baby during the birthing process. While technically not a stage in HIV progression, the "window period" of the disease needs to be considered when treating and educating about HIV. This period is the timeframe between initial infection and seroconversion where the HIV virus attaches the CD4 cells. During this period, the individual is infectious, yet he or she may not be aware of the HIV virus within his or her system. It is important to note that an individual can infect another without having enough antibodies to be detected by an HIV antibody test (Hunt & Powers, 2014; Lieshout-Krikke, Zaaijer, & van de Laar, 2015).

*Symptomatic Period*

This occurs when the individual begins to have noticeable physical symptoms linked to HIV. These may include the following:

- Low grade fever
- Pronounced weight loss without dieting
- Diarrhea that persists for one month or more
- Difficulty recovering from colds or the flu
- Response to a virus that is greater than what is typical
- Thrush
- Increased vaginal yeast infections (AIDS.gov, 2017; Gupta & Gupta, 2016).

Without antiretroviral therapy, it is estimated that an individual will live an average of 10 years from inception of this disease (Centers for Disease Control and Prevention, n.d.b). AIDS Indicators include a positive HIV test plus any one of the following (U.S. Department of Veterans Affairs, 2017):

- Candidiasis
- Cervical Cancer
- Cyrptodiodomycosis
- Cryptococcosis
- Cryptosporidiosis (with diarrhea > one month)
- Cytomegalovirus (with the exclusion of liver, spleen, or lymph nodes)
- Herpes simplex with mucosal ulcer lasting > one month or bronchitis, pneumonitis, or esophagitis
- HIV associated dementia
- HIV associated wasting
- Kaposi's sarcoma
- Lymphoma of the brain
- Tuberculosis

## Classification System

In 2014, the CDC updated their current classification system for HIV. This system is based upon CD4 count and clinical symptoms (CDC, 2014). The infections are classified into five groups and apply to individuals six years old and older (Selik *et al.*, 2014). The system is summarized as follows:

- *Stage 0*: the time between a negative or indeterminate HIV test followed less than 180 days by a positive test
- *Stage 1*: CD4 count > 500 cells/μL and no AIDS defining conditions
- *Stage 2*: CD4 count 200 to 500 cells/μL and no AIDS defining conditions
- *Stage 3*: CD4 count < 200 cells/μL or AIDS defining conditions
- *Unknown*: if insufficient information is available to make any of the above classifications

*Case Vignette*

Marvin Atkins, a 53-year-old male, came into the health clinic where you work. Marvin is complaining of an unexplained weight loss that is accompanied by diarrhea that has persisted for five weeks. Marvin states that he is too tired to work, and his employer is becoming impatient with him. Marvin is married and has two children in college. His wife works as a secretary for the metropolitan government where he resides.

Marvin insists that he is committed to his wife and had no sexual relationships outside of his marriage. Routine labs were run, and it was noted that Marvin did indeed have a major infection. He was treated and told to return in 10 days if the symptoms persisted.

Marvin returned to the clinic in five days. He stated that the symptoms had not improved and his employer was threatening to fire him if he did not return to work. Marvin states he is too ill to do so.

Additional labs were completed, including a screen for HIV. His CD4 count was 423. Based on the information that you have, is there a concern that Marvin has HIV?

In speaking with Marvin, he discloses that he has been on the "down low" for approximately three years. He reports multiple sexual encounters with partners he meets in clubs outside of the community. Marvin identifies his sexual orientation as bisexual. With this added information, what information do you share with Marvin?

What are your next steps in treating him?

In addition to possibility of having HIV, what other considerations might Marvin be concerned?

## HIV1 and HIV2

The HIV virus is categorized into two main types: HIV1 and HIV2. If no subtype is noted, it is generally HIV-1. HIV1 is the subtype that is noted worldwide. HIV-1 and HIV-2 have the same routes of transmission, and both can result in AIDS. It is important to note that HIV-2 needs to be differentiated from HIV-1, because the probability of developing AIDS from it is less likely than with HIV-1, and the modes of treatment differ. HIV-2 has a higher level of immune system activation and does not respond positively to some antiviral medications. HIV-2 cannot be determined from tests traditionally used for HIV1, because CD4 counts are higher in this strain (Brocail, 2015; Morbidity and Mortality Weekly Report 2011). Therefore, if tests for HIV-1 are inconclusive, inconsistent, or have a negative result in spite of symptomatology that reflects HIV presence, then testing for HIV-2 is warranted (Brocail, 2015; Morbidity and Mortality Weekly Report, 2011). The World Health Association estimates that the number of individuals with the prevalence of HIV was 36.7 million in 2015. In that same year, 1.1 million individuals died from AIDS-related illnesses. It is estimated that 0.8% of individuals 15 to 49 years old are living with AIDS, and the prevalence of AIDS throughout the world varies considerably. SubSaharan Africa is the most severely impacted, where nearly 1:25 adults have AIDS (World Health Organization, n.d.). By 2015, 1.2 million individuals in the United States had HIV. It is estimated that 1:8 are unaware of their condition. Nearly 40,000 individuals were newly diagnosed with HIV infections in the United States. The number of newly diagnosed individuals with HIV decreased 19% between 2005 and 2014. This decline is believed to be accurate with the stability with HIV testing noted (Centers for Disease Control and Prevention, 2016).

The following data are pertinent to HIV in the United States in 2015:

- Total number of individuals diagnosed with HIV infections: 39,513
- Gay and bisexual males account for 67% of all HIV diagnoses
- African American gay and bisexual men account for the largest number of HIV diagnoses. (White gay and bisexual males comprise the second largest group with HIV diagnoses.)
- Heterosexual men and women account for 24% of HIV diagnoses
- Heterosexual women account for 19% of HIV diagnoses (13% were linked to IV drug use).
- Heterosexual men account for 5% of HIV diagnoses (Centers for Disease Control and Prevention, 2016)

Ethnically, African Americans and Hispanics/Latinos are the two groups most disproportionately impacted by HIV. African Americans account for 45% of HIV cases, while comprising only 12% of the U.S. population. Hispanic/Latinos account for 24% of HIV diagnoses, while accounting for only 18% of the U.S. population (Centers for Disease Control and Prevention, 2016).

HIV and AIDs diagnoses by region in 2015 are as follows (Centers for Disease Control and Prevention, 2016):

- South (16.8:1000)
- Northeast (11.6:1000)
- West (9.8:1000)
- Midwest (7.6:1000)

It is imperative that the specific type of disease be detected/diagnosed for the patient to receive accurate, prompt initiation of treatment for the management of his or her HIV infection. The algorithm currently utilized by the CDC (U.S. Centers for Disease Control) is comprised of a combined screening immunoassay that can detect if the HIV virus is present and, if so, whether the virus is HIV-1 and/or HIV-2. It has been noted that HIV-2 is most common in India and West Africa; however, cases have been noted in other parts of the world including the United States. With the world "shrinking" because of extended travel, business ventures, migration, etc., the probability of HIV-2 cannot be eliminated without screening. The CDC recommends to first use a screening test to determine if the patient is reactive for the HIV-1/2/0 antibody and antigens. This test includes a nucleic acid test for HIV confirmation (Centers for Disease Control and Prevention, 2014). There is an issue with the potential of missing HIV-2 if the individual has both HIV-1 and HIV-2 (Zbinden, Durig, Shah, Boni, & Schupbach, 2016). In addition, there is evidence of a multi-drug resistant form of HIV. It is believed this mutation occurs from individuals who are taking antiretroviral medications and who transmit the HIV virus. Since the virus is believed to be treatable but not eradicated, the potential transmission by an HIVpositive individual receiving treatment has been noted (Knox, Anderson, Harrigan, & Tan, 2017).

*Preventative Behaviors*

Specific behaviors linked to the prevention of contracting HIV include the following (Calbrese & Underhill, 2015; Centers for Disease Control and Prevention, 2014):

- Sexual abstinence
- Monogamous relationships that are long lasting
- Limiting the number of sexual partners
- Safe sex practices (e.g., dental dams, use of latex condoms)
- Avoidance of sexual partners who have a history of multiple partners and/or use of injectable substances
- Participation in needle exchange programs if injecting illicit drugs
- Thorough cleaning of syringes and needles with bleach solution and a final rinse of water
- Seek out prescriptive pre-exposure prophylaxis prior to engaging in sexual behavior with someone who is HIV positive (male with male)
- Pre-exposure prophylaxis (PrEP)

*Organization Protocol*

Each healthcare facility needs an exposure control plan that provides employees with an understanding of their occupational potential for contracting the HIV virus. As a practitioner, it is key to know the risks for oneself and others in the workplace. In the public health setting, it is imperative that a risk assessment be done for the individuals who work in areas where the HIV virus might be transmitted so they will be protected. Protocols and procedures must be considered, including protective clothing, face shields, etc. Documentation of implementation of safety practices, inclusion of universal precautions and safer intervention practices (including practices that might be necessary for those administering first aid), and minimizing the exposure needed to be included in organizational infection prevention programs. These practices need to be updated yearly and whenever changes might occur that could impact exposure to the HIV virus. Treatments after a potential exposure for mucus membranes, needle sticks, bites and scratches, and vomit, urine, and feces that visibly contaminated with blood are a part of the APN role when caring for patients in all settings (Centers for Disease Control and Prevention, 2014).

*Testing for HIV*

Anyone who has potentially been exposed to the HIV virus should consider testing. Individuals can be tested at home, their local public health department, medical providers, or family planning clinics. Test results are confidential. Note: Concern regarding lack of test sensitivity and early false negatives increase potential for no further followup (Hunt & Powers, 2014).

Two such dynamics can be classified as negative results and indeterminable results. They are identified as the following:

- *Negative Results*: The person does not have the virus or the person has recently been infected and is still in the window period of the disease.
- *Indeterminable Results*: At times, someone may come back with an indeterminable result. This could mean that an individual has come into contact with the virus, but it is not at a high enough level to be verified accurately. The individual may still have HIV2, and testing for this type of HIV should then be obtained (Brocail, 2015; Morbidity and Mortality Weekly Report, 2011).

These results can also occur when there is a cross-reaction with other proteins (e.g., recent influenza vaccination, pregnancy). If an indeterminable result occurs, the individual should be provided with RNA testing (if behavior is high risk) or retested at one month out and three months out (if behavior is low risk) (Centers for Disease Control and Prevention, 2014; Wesolowski, Parker, Delaney, & Owen, 2017).

- *Positive Results*: When an individual has a CD4+ T-cell count below 200/mm$^3$ in the presence of HIV infection, this constitutes an AIDS diagnosis (Brocail, 2015; Morbidity and Mortality Weekly Report, 2011).

It is important for a diagnosis to be made early, to allow for earlier treatment and the possibility to maintain a healthy life for a longer period of time. Partner notification varies by state and, if done early, can prevent others from being infected with the HIV virus. Please note the regulations for reporting for the state in which you are practicing.

*Treatments*

Current treatments for the HIV virus are based on highly active antiretroviral therapy (HAART). These medications include protease inhibitors, nucleotide reverse transcriptase inhibitors, non-nucleotide reverse transcriptase inhibitors, entry inhibitors/fusion inhibitors, and integrate inhibitors (National Institute on Drug Abuse, 2012; National Institutes of Health, 2012). (Because medications are being approved and updated on a regular basis, please review the CDC and National Institutes of Health (NIH) websites for the most current related information.)

*Confounding Variables*

Many choose not to get tested due to the social stigma associated with HIV. In the past, much of this was linked to the "death sentence" mindset attributed to contracting this virus. Today there continue to be social and religious stigmas that are linked to this disease (Blumberg, 2014). When discussing this issue with a patient who is suspected to have or is diagnosed with HIV, listen to his or her concerns. What are his or her beliefs about this disease? What does his or her religious congregation and church leaders state about this? (For example, is it believed to be a result of not being a good person or living a sinful life in their opinion?) What support systems does the individual have if it is confirmed that he or she has HIV? How open is the individual to going to support groups and/or speaking to a counselor who specializes in dealing with individuals who have HIV? It is important that the provider or public health official does not make assumptions based on their own knowledge and values.

Even if an individual indicates he or she does not want the information, it is still important to provide it or offer direction as to how the information can be obtained. Denial, shame, fear, and a host of other emotions can emerge over the next few months (with a positive diagnosis or the potential for a positive diagnosis). Preaching, berating, fearbased commentary, or other negative messages directed toward the individual may only alienate him or her from the needed services. The patient needs to be met where he or she is, should be treated with dignity and respect, and should be provided access to education and supportive resources to successfully manage this disease process.

*Case Vignettes*

Antonio Garcia is a 15-year-old male who resides in a small farming community in the Midwest. Based on state laws, Antonio can drive the family truck if it is being used for farming purposes. About once a month, Antonio throws a few bales of hay in the back of the truck and heads to a metropolitan community near him. He socializes in the mall, at a church youth group, and at local coffee houses known for some drug distribution.

Antonio met a girl, Marcia, that he likes a few months ago. They kissed and shared food and drinks. He wants the relationship to go further sexually, but Marcia, his love interest, has been reluctant. This week he found out that Marcia had a sexual encounter with someone who has since told her that he is HIV positive.

Antonio has come to see you, the school nurse, and asks what his chances are that he has contracted HIV?

What would you say to Antonio?

Would you test him for HIV? (Please consider rationale.)

What additional information does he need to have?

D'shanya Jackson is a 78-year-old female who comes to the senior center where you provide health screening once a month. During her screening, D'shanya shares that she has a new love interest and they are sexually active. She states she doesn't worry about catching "anything" since they are both older. (Her sexual partner is 66 years old.)

What would you share with D'shanya about her assumption that she and her partner are too old to be concerned about HIV/AIDS?

## Sexually Transmitted Diseases

Sexually transmitted diseases (STDs) continue to impact healthcare outcomes at local, global, and national levels. The top three reported STDs in the United States in 2015 were chlamydia, gonorrhea, and syphilis (Centers for Disease Control and Prevention, 2016b). Healthcare workers must not only assess for potential risk of STDs and initiate prevention strategies, but also realize how STDs affect the health of individuals, communities, and overall populations. STDs can continue to spread rapidly through sexual contact before the onset of symptoms. Decreasing the spread of STDs both begins and ends with the education of individuals. The increased knowledge will lead to a decrease in risky behaviors, an increase in recognition of symptoms and, thus, a decrease in incidences.

Individuals diagnosed with an STD are at increased risk for other STDs. Multiple issues with potential complications and the contagious spread of these diseases make this a grave population concern. Thorough physical, behavioral, and social assessments are critical to strategize and provide much needed preventative education to the general population. Treatment of the individual and his or her sexual partner or partners, along with continued monitoring to ensure compliance of treatment regimens, are necessary interventions to counteract this growing problem within the population. The potential disastrous effects on individuals, pregnant woman, and unborn children make this a priority population health concern.

STD prevention, assessment, diagnosis, and treatment are complex and intricate. When an individual is diagnosed with an STD, assessment of sexual behaviors is necessary for all individuals diagnosed with an STD. Patient education regarding sexual behaviors and practices is aimed at safety and prevention strategies. Once an STD is diagnosed, all sexual partners need to be treated. Expedited partner therapy in which the partner is treated without an examination is a viable option for the partners of women diagnosed with chlamydia and gonorrhea (Centers for Disease Control and Prevention, 2017b). Co-existing sexually transmitted infections are common, which makes it imperative to test for other infections when an individual tests positive for one (Lowdermilk, Perry, Cashion, & Alden, 2016).

According to the CDC (2016d), STD screening is especially judicious for a pregnant woman, because serious complications can affect both the woman and her unborn child. The World Health Organization (WHO) (2017) reported that, in 2012, 39% of the 900,000 pregnant women globally had serious complications including stillbirths. Pregnant women should be screened for chlamydia, gonorrhea, syphilis, HIV, and both hepatitis B and C; initial screenings should be done on the first prenatal visit, with re-screenings occurring as necessary for any woman who exhibits high-risk behaviors (Centers for Disease Control and Prevention, 2016d).

Effective prevention efforts should combine counseling and behavioral modification practices, such as comprehensive sexual education programs that teach the use of condoms and other forms of barrier birth control methods for safety (World Health Organization, 2017). Routine screening and preventative education for STDs will increase awareness and decrease risky behaviors and, thus, assist to decrease incidences of STDs within the population. The goal of a behavioral approach is to attain self-efficacy in applying preventative interventions to one's own behavior.

## Human Papillomavirus (HPV) Infections

HPV, caused by the Condylomata acuminate virus, is the most commonly seen viral sexually transmitted infection (Lowdermilk *et al.*, 2016). According to the CDC (2017a), there are 79 million Americans infected with HPV and 14 million new infections diagnosed each year. HPV can cause genital warts and cervical cancer. It is imperative that parents and adolescents are properly educated regarding the prevention of HPV. HPV commonly exhibits no symptoms, making it hard to diagnose early (Lowdermilk *et al.*, 2016). The HPV vaccine is now recommended in two doses for all 11 to 12-year-old boys and girls (Centers for Disease Control and Prevention, 2017a). The HPV vaccine can be given to women up to age 26 years and men up to age 21 years, unless the man is homosexual, bisexual, or immunocompromised, in which the recommendation changes to 26 years old (Centers for Disease Control and Prevention, 2017a). The vaccine has been proven to be safe and effective in preventing HPV and its associated cancers (Centers for Disease Control and Prevention, 2017a). The CDC (2017a) also advises the use of condoms—although they are not 100% effective—combined with mutually exclusive sexual partners as a preventative means for HPV. Education regarding the safety and importance of the vaccine for patients, as well as the parents of young children, is crucial to increasing compliance for vaccination within the population.

### Chlamydia

Chlamydia, caused by *Chlamydia trachomatis*, is the most commonly reported sexually transmitted disease. In 2015, the CDC reported 1,526,658 cases in the United States alone, which is a 6% increase from the previous year (Centers for Disease Control and Prevention, 2016b). What makes chlamydia even more dangerous is the fact that there are often no symptoms. If left untreated, chlamydia can cause acute salpingitis or pelvic inflammatory disease (PID) and can increase the risk of HIV infection due to small openings that form within the cervix (Lowdermilk *et al.*, 2016). Untreated chlamydia can lead to infertility. According to the CDC (2015a), all sexually active woman under age 25 year need to be screened for chlamydia, especially given the fact that the majority of cases fall within the 15- to 24-year-old age group. The CDC (2015a) recommends treatment to include azithromycin or doxycycline. Screening recommendations for young men should be limited to populations with a high incidence of infection (Centers for Disease Control and Prevention, 2016b). The patient and all sexual partners need to be treated; education regarding risky behaviors is paramount and should include such behaviors as multiple partners and lack of a barrier birth control method (Lowdermilk *et al.*, 2016).

### Gonorrhea

The second most commonly reported STD is gonorrhea (Centers for Disease Control and Prevention, 2015a). Gonorrhea is caused by *Neis-*

*seria gonorrhoeae.* The CDC (2016a) reported 395,216 new cases in 2015, which is a 13% increase from the previous year. Gonorrhea is increasingly becoming resistant to penicillin-based drugs (Lowdermilk *et al.*, 2016), causing the CDC (2016a) to recommend a combination therapy of both a cephalosporin and azithromycin. As with chlamydia, gonorrhea infections often go undetected due to lack of symptoms. Most woman do not have symptoms until the complication of PID sets in. Men oftentimes will exhibit urethral infection symptoms, which will cause them to seek treatment, but spread of infection has most likely already occurred. The CDC (2016a) recommends annual screening for men and woman in the high-risk group of 15- to 24-year-olds. Screenings in other age groups should occur with high-risk behavior, such as multiple partners and lack of a barrier method of birth control. Education of individuals and communities regarding healthy sexual behaviors to prevent incidences and spread of gonorrhea remains an important preventative intervention.

### Syphilis

Syphilis is caused by *Treponema pallidum.* The CDC (2016c) reported 23,872 cases in 2015, which is a 19% increase when compared to the previous year. Syphilis presents in stages—primary, secondary, and tertiary—making it essential to diagnose this disease in the early stages to prevent the spread of the infection to others, complications, and death. Latent syphilis cases are those individuals who have a positive serology test but no symptoms. The recommended treatment regimen according to the CDC (2016c) is penicillin G given parentally. Longer courses of penicillin G are recommended for latent syphilis cases since it is difficult to determine length of infection (Centers for Disease Control and Prevention, 2016c). The CDC (2016d) recommendation is that all pregnant women are screened on their first prenatal visit, with retesting later in the pregnancy if the woman exhibits high risk behavior. Annual syphilis testing is recommended for all individuals with HIV and men who exhibit the high-risk behavior of having sex with men (Centers for Disease Control and Prevention, 2016c). Patient education remains critical regarding preventative behaviors, elimination of high-risk behaviors, and early recognition of symptoms.

Understanding specific populations in which an STD diagnosis commonly occurs will help to target identified behaviors of concern. Education plans can then be developed to modify behaviors in order to prevent STD occurrences.

*Case Vignette*

Sarah, a 20-year-old college student, arrives at the clinic asking for a pregnancy test.

Her last menstrual period was six weeks ago and she is experiencing some clear vaginal discharge.

What data should the advanced practice nurse (APN) collect during the health assessment interview?

When questioned regarding her sexual behavior, Sarah becomes very nervous and expresses that she is uncomfortable answering these types of questions.

What actions can the APN take to increase Sarah's comfort level?

Sarah admits to six sexual partners within the last two months. She uses condoms sporadically and only when her partner has them. Sarah denies drug use but admits to drinking vodka on the weekends.

The APN develops a plan to provide preventative health education. What key concepts are important for the APN to include?

The pregnancy test comes back positive. Sarah has no clue as to which of her partners is the father of the baby.

What other health screenings are essential for the APN to perform at this time and why?

Sarah's chlamydia culture comes back positive, and all other STD screenings are negative.

What is the recommended treatment for Sarah?

What, if any, adjustments will the APN make to the preventative health education plan?

*Case Vignette*

A 25-year-old male, Clyde, presents to the clinic for a third time with a sore throat. The past two throat cultures came back negative. Clyde denies other symptoms, except for some frequency of urination and pale green urethral discharge.

What health assessment questions are important for the APN to ask and why?

Clyde admits to bisexual practices since he was 18 years of age and has multiple partners of both sexes.

What diagnostic testing should be ordered at this time and why?

What should be included in the health education plan and why?

Clyde's throat culture comes back positive for gonorrhea.

What is the recommended treatment plan?

What changes, if any, will be made to the health education plan?

*Case Vignette*

A 73-year-old female client, Madelyn, presents to the clinic complaining of flu-like symptoms—muscle aches, headache and fever. Upon examination, a fine, red, rough rash is noticed on the soles of her feet and palms of her hand.

What questions should be added to the health assessment now and why?

Upon questioning, Madelyn comments on her monogamous relationship in the last six months. When asked if she had a sore such as a chancre sore within the last three months, she states that she did have a cold sore on her mouth, but it finally went away.

What diagnostic testing should be gathered at this time and why?

What should be included in the health education plan and why?

The VDRL comes back positive.

What treatment plan should be included at this time and why?

What, if any, adjustments should be made to the health education plan and why?

*Case Vignette*

A 12-year-old girl is at the clinic for a sports physical. The primary care provider prescribes the HPV vaccine. The mother adamantly refuses the vaccine for her daughter, stating that her daughter is a "good girl" and does not need the vaccine.

How will you educate the mother about HPV and the vaccine?

The mother responds that she feels that receiving the vaccine will send the wrong message to her daughter that sex is okay at her age.

How will you allay the mother's fears regarding this statement?

After the nurse has provided pamphlets and education materials, the mother still refuses the HPV vaccine.

What implications can this have to the general population?

How will the APN utilize this experience for future patient encounters?

## Respiratory Infections

"Acute Respiratory Infection (ARI) is consistently ranked among the top causes of morbidity and mortality worldwide. It has been referred to as a forgotten pandemic, which kills more than 4 million people each year globally" (Abubakar *et al.*, 2016, p. 514). "The International Health Regulations cite several acute respiratory illness (SARI) caused by common bacterial and viral pathogens, novel pathogens or those with the capacity to cause epidemics or pandemics that threaten international health security" (Abubakar *et al.*, 2016, p. 514) to explore respiratory infections. There are many viral and bacterial infections causing respiratory disease and illness. Several pathogens are the pneumococcal bacteria, respiratory syncytial virus, novel coronavirus, and the seasonal influenza.

According to Pisesky *et al.* (2016), respiratory syncytial virus (RSV) increases the cost of care and morbidity in young children. The incidence over time has showed no changes, lending to unsuccessful efforts for prevention. RSV can be the cause of an acute lower respiratory tract infection (ALRI), pneumonia, and bronchiolitis. "RSV, is a common respiratory virus that usually causes mild, cold-like symptoms. Most people recover in a week or two, but RSV can be serious, especially for infants and older adults. In fact, RSV is the most common cause of bronchiolitis (inflammation of the small airways in the lung) and pneumonia (infection of the lungs) in children younger than 1 year of age in the United States. It is also a significant cause of respiratory illness in older adults" (Centers for Disease Control and Prevention, 2017a).

The "novel coronavirus (nCoV) causing severe respiratory disease within some countries in the Middle East and in patients transferred from medical care in Europe" (Nicoll, 2013, p. S62). Severe acute respiratory syndrome (SARS) caused by nCoV requires aggressive treatment with mechanical ventilation and at times extra corporeal membrane oxygenation (ECMO). It is essential to reduce human-to-human transmission and treat the infection (Nicoll, 2013).

Respiratory infections can be prevented and significantly reduced by educating the community at large to cover their mouths when they cough, followed by hand washing and using paper tissues and disposal of tissues immediately as there is no need to reuse them and pass along their germs. Additionally, frequent hand washing is recommended when they are around infected individuals. Respiratory infections can be spread by droplets in the air that will sit on hard surfaces, so wiping the surfaces with an alcohol based wipes, clothes or most cleaning products will also reduce the spread of infections.

*Pandemic Influenza*

Human influenza A (H1N1), also called the pandemic influenza, has been referred to as the swine flu. It is pandemic because it has been identified in eight countries and has been associated with significant morbidity and mortality. H1N1 infection most commonly affects middle-aged persons and is community acquired. Establishing a strong surveillance program for the influenza infection in the community with flu vaccination programs has been shown to have the greatest impact on lowering influenza H1N1 infection rates.

Annual vaccination against Influenza is recommended for all patient populations. Respiratory viral infections are serious but pose an increased risk to those patients who are immunocompromised (Gupta, Capoor, Gupta, & Sachdeva, 2015). Healthcare workers are often strongly encouraged to receive the H1N1 flu vaccination as a preventative measure for Influenza. Yet adherence to vaccination rates varies, depending on policy implementation and consequences for noncompliance. "The PARiHS framework proposed that successful implementation of evidence into practice depends on three road factors (Evidence, Context, and Facilitation)" (Ullrich *et al.*, 2013). Utilizing the PARiHS framework can lend to greater compliance in H1N1 prevention guidelines that include the flu vaccination for patients and healthcare workers (HCWs). Providing the patients and HCWs with the evidence from previous years and research studies within the context of the flu prevention guidelines and how the flu vaccination (program) will be implemented can lend to greater compliance. For example, in your practice, you may offer a flu vaccination clinic during convenient hours for all potential participants. This may be a Saturday from 8:00 A.M. to 1:00 P.M. to support the working class. Prior to this clinic, you should provide information on any associated fees or seek opportunities to offer free vaccinations to support prevention and wellness. In the study by Ullrich *et al.* (2013), building a case for personal adherence added value. The patients' and healthcare workers' sense of staying well and not contracting the flu with potential days out of work, sickness with exacerbation of chronic illness, and the like contributed to adherence to flu prevention guideline compliance and vaccination. As an APN, it is critical to make correlations to personal wellness with patients; utilizing valid and accurate information showed stronger compliance flu vaccination rates and reduced influenza rates.

*Tuberculosis*

Tuberculosis is caused by a bacterium that typically affects the lungs as the primary site, but it can also affect the brain, spine, or kidneys. "Generally, persons at high risk for developing Tuberculosis (TB) disease fall into two categories: persons who have been recently infected with TB bacteria and persons with medical conditions that weaken the immune system" (Centers for Disease Control and Prevention, 2017a). "Persons who have been recently infected with TB bacteria include: close contacts of a person with infectious TB disease, persons who have immigrated from areas of the world with high rates of TB, children less than 5 years of age who have a positive TB test, groups with high rates of TB transmission, such as homeless persons, injection drug users, and persons with HIV infection, and persons who work or reside with people who are at high risk for TB in facilities or institutions such as hospitals, homeless shelters, correctional facilities, nursing homes, and residential homes for those with HIV" (Centers for Disease Control and Prevention, 2017a). TB is transmitted from person to person, through the air. An infected person can spread the disease to any person with whom they have frequent contact, such as a family member

Secondary prevention includes annual screenings for healthcare workers following an exposure to a patient with TB to monitor closely for development of the disease. "TB skin test (TST) and TB blood tests. A positive TB skin test or TB blood test only tells that a person has been infected with TB bacteria. It does not tell whether the person has latent TB infection (LTBI) or has progressed to TB". (https://www.cdc.gov/tb/topic/basics/tbinfectiondisease.htm). Other tests, such as a chest x-ray and a sample of sputum, are needed to see whether the person has TB disease" (Centers for Disease Control and Prevention, 2017 a, 20017 c). "A diagnosis of latent TB infection is made if a person has a positive TB test result and a medical evaluation does not indicate TB disease. The decision about treatment for latent TB infection will be based on a person's chances of developing TB disease by considering their risk factors" (https://www.cdc.gov/tb/topic/basics/risk.htm). The APN should screen high risk populations and develop programs that strengthen compliance with treatments and preventing spread of the TB bacteria.

## Methicillin-Resistant Staphylococcus aureus

The "emergence of antibiotic resistance in bacteria is becoming a widespread problem and a major health issue" (Fadheel, Perry, & Henderson, 2008, p. 4). Methicillin-resistant Staphylococcus Aureus (MRSA) rates are increasing in hospitals and in the community. There has been a rise in penicillin resistance for *Staphylococcus aureus* (S. aureus) to a rate of nearly 90% of the diagnosed cases. This progression of resistance was first seen the 1980s according to Fadheel *et al.* (2008) and is associated with a gene that is present on the bacteria. The "methicillin resistance gene (mecA) encodes a methicillin-resistant penicillin-binding protein (PBP2a) that is not present in susceptible strains and is believed to have been acquired from a distantly related species" (Fadheel *et al.*, 2008, p. 4). MRSA is found in the nasal passage and on the perineum. The hands are a common mode of transmission for MRSA, which leads to crosscontamination between patients. A nasal swab is the most common diagnostic test for MRSA and shows typically one of four strains of *S. aureus.* "In the general community, MRSA most often causes skin infections. In some cases, it causes pneumonia (lung infection) and other issues. If left untreated, MRSA infections can become severe and cause sepsis—a life-threatening reaction to severe infection in the body" (Centers for Disease Control and Prevention, 2017c). MRSA can also be associated with surgical site infections and CLABSIs in acute and longterm care facilities. According to the CDC (2017c), steps to reduce and prevent MRSA infections include the following: "maintain good hand and body hygiene. Wash hands often, and clean your body regularly, especially after exercise. Keep cuts, scrapes and wounds clean and covered until healed. Avoid sharing personal items such as towels and razors". Additionally, if you have a patient who thinks he or she has an infection, advise the patient to seek treatment early at the onset of symptoms, such as redness, soreness/pain, purulent drainage, and/or fever. Prevention of MRSA and other resistant infections is supported by antibiotic stewardship programs. These programs discourage the prescribing of antibiotics for symptoms without a confirmation of infection.

### Vancomycin-Resistant Enterococci (VRE)

Vancomycin-resistant enterococci (VRE) is an antibiotic-resistant bacteria seen in the community and healthcare facilities, much like MRSA. VRE is secondary to a vancomycin resistance. "An increased risk for VRE infection and colonization has been associated with previous vancomycin and/or multi-antimicrobial therapy, severe underlying disease or immunosuppression, and intraabdominal surgery. Because enterococci can be found in the normal gastrointestinal and female genital tracts, most enterococcal infections have been attributed to endogenous sources within the individual patient. However, recent reports of outbreaks and endemic infections caused by enterococci, including VRE, have indicated that patient-to-patient transmission of the microorganisms can occur either through direct contact or through indirect contact via (a) the hands of personnel or (b) contaminated patient-care equipment or environmental surfaces" (Centers for Disease Control and Prevention, 2017a).

"Guideline development should be part of the hospital's quality-improvement program and should involve participation from the hospital's pharmacy and therapeutics committee; hospital epidemiologist; and infection-control, infectious-disease, medical, and surgical staffs. The guidelines should include the following considerations:

1. Situations in which the use of vancomycin is appropriate or acceptable:
   - For treatment of serious infections caused by beta-lactam- resistant gram-positive microorganisms. Vancomycin may be less rapidly bactericidal than are beta-lactam agents for beta-lactam- susceptible staphylococci
   - For treatment of infections caused by gram-positive microorganisms in patients who have serious allergies to beta-lactam antimicrobials.
   - When antibiotic-associated colitis fails to respond to metronidazole therapy or is severe and potentially life-threatening.
   - Prophylaxis, as recommended by the American Heart Association, for endocarditis following certain procedures in patients at high risk for endocarditis
   - Prophylaxis for major surgical procedures involving implantation of prosthetic materials or devices (e.g., cardiac and vascular procedures and total hip replacement) at institutions that have a high rate of infections caused by MRSA or methicillin-resistant S. epidermidis. A single dose of vancomycin administered immediately before surgery is sufficient unless the procedure lasts greater than 6 hours, in which case the dose should be repeated. Prophylaxis should be discontinued after a maximum of two doses

2. Situations in which the use of vancomycin should be discouraged:
   - Routine surgical prophylaxis other than in a patient who has a life-threatening allergy to beta-lactam antibiotics
   - Empiric antimicrobial therapy for a febrile neutropenic patient, unless initial evidence indicates that the patient has an infection caused by gram-positive microorganisms (e.g., at an inflamed exit site of Hickman catheter) and the prevalence of infections caused by MRSA in the hospital is substantial
   - Treatment in response to a single blood culture positive for coagulase-negative staphylococcus, if other blood cultures taken during the same time frame are negative (i.e., if contamination of the

blood culture is likely). Because contamination of blood cultures with skin flora (e.g., *S. epidermidis*) could result in inappropriate administration of vancomycin, phlebotomists and other personnel who obtain blood cultures should be trained to minimize microbial contamination of specimens

- Continued empiric use for presumed infections in patients whose cultures are negative for beta-lactam-resistant gram-positive microorganisms

- Systemic or local (e.g., antibiotic lock) prophylaxis for infection or colonization of indwelling central or peripheral intravascular catheters

- Selective decontamination of the digestive tract.

- Eradication of MRSA colonization

- Primary treatment of antibiotic-associated colitis

- Routine prophylaxis for very low-birthweight infants (i.e., infants who weigh less than 1,500 g [3 lb 4 oz])

- Routine prophylaxis for patients on continuous ambulatory peritoneal dialysis or hemodialysis

- Treatment (chosen for dosing convenience) of infections caused by betalactam-sensitive gram-positive microorganisms in patients who have renal failure

- Use of vancomycin solution for topical application or irrigation.

3. Enhancing compliance with recommendations:

- Although several techniques may be useful, further study is required to determine the most effective methods for influencing the prescribing practices of physicians" (Centers for Disease Control and Prevention, 2017d, https://www.cdc.gov/mmwr/preview/ mmwrhtml/00039349.htm)

Following these recommendations can lead to primary prevention of VRE.

### Carbapenem-Resistant Enterobacteriaceae

Carbapenem-resistant *Enterobacteriaceae* (CRE) are multidrug-resistant gram-negative bacilli that can cause infections associated with high fatality rates and are emerging as epidemiologically important healthcare-associated pathogens in the United States (Elbadawi *et al.*, 2016, p. 906). "*Klebsiella* species and *Escherichia coli* (*E. coli*) are examples of Enterobacteriaceae" (Centers for Disease Control and Prevention, 2017) that progressively develop a resistance to a class of antibiotics called carbapenems. "Carbapenem resistance among Enterobacteriaceae is complex; unlike methicillin resistance among *Staphylococcus aureus* which, for the most part, represents one resistance mechanism in one species of bacteria, Enterobacteriaceae include more than 70 different genera and many different mechanisms can lead to carbapenem resistance. All carbapenem-resistant Enterobacteriaceae (CRE), regardless of the mechanism underlying the carbapenem resistance, are likely multidrug-resistant organisms for which interventions might be required in healthcare settings to prevent transmission. However, carbapenemase-producing CRE (CP-CRE) are currently believed to be primarily responsible for the increasing spread of CRE in the United States and have therefore been targeted for aggressive prevention" (Centers for Disease Control and Prevention, 2017 d, https://www.cdc.gov/hai/organisms/cre/definition.html )

Managing CRE relies on rapid identification, isolation, and proper antibiotic use. "The use of molecular technologies, including PCR testing, PFGE, and WGS, can lead to detection of transmission events and interruption of transmission by uncommon and multidrug-resistant organisms. Public health and other programs that include antibiotic stewardship and antimicrobial resistance monitoring might benefit from data generated by molecular testing of multidrug-resistant organisms to enhance detection of intra- and interfacility transmission events" (Elbadawi *et al.*, 2016, p. 909).

### Clostridium Difficile

*Clostridium difficile* (*C. diff*) comes from the use of antibiotics. The antibiotics kill normal flora in the gut and bowel, making the patient more susceptible to an overgrowth of the *C. diff* bacteria. Several preventative measures include instructing the patients and community to wash their hands before and after eating and to wash their hands before and after using the restroom. Instruct the patient to take their full course of prescribed antibiotics and do not interrupt the treatment. Additional education should be to report any episodes of diarrhea within 30 days of completing the antibiotic treatment. If a patient has diarrhea, encourage him or her to use a separate bathroom from the rest of the family, to avoid spread of potential *C. diff.* until a diagnosis is made (Centers for Disease Control and Prevention, 2017 c, https://www.cdc.gov/hai/organisms/cdiff/cdiff-patient.html).

For *C. diff*, primary prevention includes the education for hand hygiene. If the patient reports diarrhea and the APN screens for *C. diff* and educates the patient when the diarrhea starts to contact him or her and to use a separate bathroom, the APN is functioning at a secondary prevention level. Once the patient has a positive *C. diff* screening and is seeking fluid management in the acute care setting, when the APN places the patient on enteric precautions and engages the staff in use of soap and water for hand hygiene practices for *C. diff*, the APN is instituting tertiary prevention (minimizing the spread of the disease, treating the patient to support a return to a healthier well-being).

## Hospital Acquired Infections

Although patients seek care for surgery and/or illnesses, they run a high risk of acquiring hospital (or facility) care related infections. Hospital acquired Infections (HAI) have been monitored closely and have affected reimbursement for healthcare facilities since the early 2000s. The CDC (2017 c) reports reductions in infections between 2008 and 2014 for the following: CLABSI by 50%; surgical site infections (SSI) by 17% and between the years 2011 and 2014; and a 13% decrease in MRSA and a 3% decrease in *C. diff*. The CDC also reports that between 2009 and 2014, there has been no improvements in catheter associated urinary tract infections (CAUTI). Hospitals have developed many quality and process improvement projects, including nurse driven protocols, central line placement checklists, removing central lines as soon as possible, and more. Despite these efforts in 2014, 75,000 people still died from a hospital acquired infection (Centers for Disease Control and Prevention, 2017 c, https://www.cdc.gov/hai/surveillance/index.html). This is alarming and continued focus and efforts are needed.

### Ebola Virus

The Ebola Virus Disease (EVD) created a healthcare crisis in 2014, with spread from West Africa. According to Carroll *et al.* (2015), there have been "27,013 reported cases and 11,134 deaths...with the origin of the virus being a zoonotic transmission from a bat to a two-year-old boy in December 2013...spread by human-to-human contact throughout Guinea, Sierra Leone and Liberia" (p. 97). Being prepared for such an outbreak was led and supported by the World Health Organization (WHO). The typical incubation period is up to two weeks, generally following foreign travel. "The Centers for Disease Control and Prevention

(CDC) focus on measures which can be taken by the United States health system and extrapolated by others involved in preparedness and response. There are no short cuts to clinical preparedness for EVD" (Brett-Major *et al.*, 2015). HCWs must be trained to bundle care, minimizing exposure focused on safety and protection of self. "Care must be deliberate and vigilant . . . steps must be taken to ensure appropriate training and safe working conditions" (Brett-Major, 2015, p. 233). Patients typically present with hemorrhagic fever, gastrointestinal bleeding, myalgia, chest pain, abdominal pain, vomiting, nausea, and arthralgia. At the point of triage, a travel history is essential and initiating fluid replacement.

Care of the EVD patient includes use of standard contact and droplet precautions implemented by the HCWs and oral hydration, intravenous fluids, and electrolyte replenishing for the patients. The overall care environment must focus on HCW safety, including waste disposal and management, consideration for patient flow traffic patterns to minimize exposure of other patients and HCWs, water supply, and staffing mix looking at number of staff. Errors in any of these essential elements can increase harm and spread of infection to HCWs and the APN.

As the APN, you may find yourself in a public communication to alert the public about a positive Ebola case, active treatment, and potential impact to the community. It is important to communicate that the patient is in isolation, HCW safety practices are being maintained, and this serves as an opportunity for sharing safe foreign travel practices.

### Zika Virus Infections

New infections arise in other countries and with the number of businesses overseas to reduce labor expenses, foreign travel, and the like, infections have spread. For example, in 2015–2016, the outbreak of the Zika virus from the Flavivirid virus family, was spread by infected mosquitoes. This was noted in Brazil and spread to the Caribbean and Haiti (Journel *et al.*, 2017). Zika viral infections "were associated with adverse fetal outcomes and rare neurological complications in adults… leading to a Public Health Emergency of International Concern on February 1, 2016" (Journel *et al.*, 2017, p. 172). Infections were diagnosed by serum specimen viral testing. Adult patients had Guillain-Barre Syndrome (GBS) symptoms, including myalgia and headache, and additional symptoms commonly reported were maculopapular rash, fever, nonpurulent conjunctivitis, arthritis, and general pain. In the newborn and fetus (stillborn or miscarriage byproducts), commonly noted were microcephaly, spinal cord and limb deformities.

A commonality with diagnosis included foreign travel typically within a two-week period prior to the onset of symptoms. According to Journel *et al.* (2017), 29 Haitians have been infected with the Zika virus and there have been 3,036 suspected cases in the United States. The best practice when dealing with patients or the community is to remind them of safe travel tips, including use of mosquito repellent containing diethyltoluamide (DEET), use of net beds if sleeping or resting at any time outdoors, wearing long sleeves and pants covering and preventing skin exposure, hand hygiene, maintaining a clean environment, and keeping your drinking water containers covered. Information can be shared with patients who are traveling from the Pan-American Health Organization and The WHO.

One example of a public health concern related to the Zika virus is noted in the state of South Carolina. In fear of the virus transmitted by the *Aedes aegypti* mosquitoes, the State sprayed Naled to destroy the potential virus-carrying mosquitos, with a negative impact on the honeybees. Two and a half million bees were killed (Raines, 2016), and the impact on crosspollination of crops, honey, and other natural sources is devastating. This has increased the price of homegrown foods in the SouthEastern region and will lend to additional population health issues.

## Conclusion

Infections have become a large population health issue. This chapter is the tip of the iceberg. Many other infections, such as Lyme disease, malaria, Dengue, foodborne illnesses (*Salmonella, Eschericia coli* [*E. coli*], *Listeria*), meningitis, and more could have been identified. The common theme is prevention. Good hand hygiene programs that are consistent in the community and in healthcare settings are a mandate. Educating the public and making every effort to support preventative practices such as vaccination programs should be the goal of any population health intervention to decrease infection risks and disease prevalence rates. Early treatment can also reduce the spread of the active disease. As APNs, every effort must be made to reduce infections, increase infectious treatment compliance, and reduce the alarming mortality rate from hospital acquired infections.

## Tool Kit and Resources

American Association for the Study of Liver Disease (AASLD). (2017)

Retrieved from https://www.aasld.org/publications/practice-guide-lines and https://www.aasld.org/

American Public Health Association www.apha.org

Centers for Disease Control and Prevention (CDC) www.cdc.gov
- Can search any infectious disease for signs/symptoms, treatment, diagnosis and testing, data and statistics, prevention, transmission, healthcare providers, educational materials, frequently asked questions, and more

CDC National Prevention Information Network (NPIN), P.O. Box 6003, Rockville, MD 20849-6003, E-mail: npin-info@cdc.gov

Centers for Disease Control and Prevention CDC (2017). www.cdc.gov/
- Multiple topics including hand hygiene programs, travel guidelines, vaccination requirements (as examples)

Center for Disease Control and Prevention CDC Viral Hepatitis Serology Training. Retrieved from http://www.cdc.gov/hepatitis/resources/professionals/training/serology/ training.htm

*Hepatitis*

Hepatitis B Foundation Support Groups. Retrieved from http://www.hepb.org/resources-and-support/online-support-groups/

Viral Hepatitis—Liver inflammation linked to a virus. Incidents can be acute or chronic. The most common types are Hepatitis A (HAV), Hepatitis B (HBV) and Hepatitis C (HCV).

*Morbidity and Mortality Weekly Report* (MMWR), www.cdc.gov/mmwr

National HPV and Cervical Cancer Prevention Resource Center American Sexual Health Association (ASHA), P. O. Box 13827, Research Triangle Park, NC, 27709-3827, 1-800-783-9877

TABLE 14.1. Types of Hepatitis.

|  | HAV | HBV | HCV |
|---|---|---|---|
| Transmission | Enteral | Parenteral | Parenteral |
| Classification | Picornavirus | Orthohepadnavirus | Hepacivirus |
| Genome | +ssRNA | DsDNA-RT | +ssRNA |
| Incubation | 20–40 days | 45–160 days | 15–150 days |
| Severity | Mild/acute | Severe-chhronic | Subclinical-chronic |

(CDC, 2013; CDC, 2015a; CDC, 2015 c; CDC, 2016 b)

World Health Organization (WHO) (2017). Sexually transmitted infections (STIs). http://www.who.int/mediacentre/factsheets/fs110/en/

*HIV*

CDC Provider Resources. Retrieved from https://www.cdc.gov/actagainstaids/campaigns/hssc/providerresources.html?gclid=CNeC_q3F4NMCFRSewAodqLcEJw

Foundation Support Groups. Retrieved from http://www.hepb.org/resources-and-support/online-support-groups HIV/AIDS.

HIV risk reduction tool. Retrieved from https://wwwn.cdc.gov/hivrisk/ Centers for Disease Control and Prevention CDC

HIV-transmission. Retrieved from https://t.cdc.gov/synd.aspx?js=0&rid=cs_3605&url=http://t.cdc.gov/VIK Centers for Disease Control and Prevention CDC

Morbidity and Mortality Weekly Report (MMWR). Retrieved from www.cdc.gov/mmwr

Opportunistic infections and their relationship to HIV/AIDS. Retrieved from https://www.aids.gov/hiv-aids-basics/staying-healthy-with-hiv-aids/potential-related-health-problems/opportunistic-infections American Association for the Study of Liver Disease (AASLD). (2017) Retrieved from https://www.aasld.org/publications/practice-guidelines American Public Health and https://www.aasld.org/

Screening. Standard Care. Resources for Primary Care. Retrieved from Providers.https://www.cdc.gov/actagainstaids/campaigns/hssc/providerresources.html?gclid=CjwKEAjwz9HHBRDbopLGh-afzB-4SJABY52oFrM4ZC2nAPcr76iQK7-swO3J3YW3NVH4CBf_I_F4EDRoCmI_w_wcB

U.S. Department of Veterans Affairs. Retrieved from https://www.hiv.va.gov/index.aspHIV

*Definitions*

*Epidemiology*—the branch of medicine that deals with the incidence, distribution, and possible control of diseases and other factors relating to health.

*Expedited Partner Therapy*—the automatic prescribing of medication to sexual partners of a patient who is diagnosed with a sexually transmitted disease in lieu of an examination.

*Hospital Acquired Infections* (HAI)—occur during and/or within 30

days of hospitalization/hospital stay and are associated with the acute care stay.

*Incidence Rate*—calculating the incidence rate for the period of data/ time will be number of infections, divided by the number of catheter days. This number is then multiplied by 1,000, as a standard for 1,000 line days in this case to establish a common unit of measure for all members (i.e., hospitals) in a compare group.

*Prevalence Rate*—this is a measurement of all individuals affected by the disease at a particular time, whereas incidence is a measurement of the number of new individuals who contract a disease during a particular period of time.

*Prevention*

*Primary Prevention*—Directed at avoiding disease and disability

*Secondary Prevention*—Efforts focus on identifying or detecting existing health problems or conditions before they cause serious or long-term problems.

*Tertiary Prevention*—Activities aim to limit or reduce the condition's negative effects.

*Syphilis*

*Primary Syphilis*—The first stage of syphilis in which a painless chancre sore is the main symptom.

*Secondary Syphilis*—The second stage of syphilis occurring 6 weeks to 6 months after the primary stage, in which general malaise symptoms and rash appear.

*Tertiary Syphilis*—This occurs when syphilis is untreated and the infection affects the cardiovascular, musculoskeletal, and neurological system.

*Latent Syphilis*—There are no symptoms of syphilis, but the serum blood test is positive.

*Surveillance*—ongoing, systematic collection, analysis, interpretation, and dissemination of data regarding a health-related event for use in public health action to reduce morbidity and mortality and to improve health.

*Definitions for HIV*

*Negative Results*—The person does not have the virus or the person has recently been infected and is still in the window period of the disease.

*Indeterminable Results*—At times, someone may come back with an indeterminable result. This could mean that an individual has come into contact with the virus, but it is not at a high enough level to be verified accurately. The individual might have HIV2, and testing for this should follow.

*Vigilant*—Keep a continued watch over patient for possible complication or disease progression.

*Vulnerable*—Have increased susceptibility to a disease or situation.

### Discussion Questions

Have students develop a manual for identifying and treating individuals who are susceptible to the hepatitis virus. Include similarities and differences between the three most common forms of virus (HAV, HBV, and HCV).

Have students do a community assessment that includes risks, resources, and potential prevention interventions related to hepatitis. Make the information age-specific (child, adolescent, adult, older adult). Share information on a social media site such as Pinterest.

### Case Study 1

Mrs. Smith is a 28-year-old, recently married woman who traveled to Africa for her honeymoon. She and her husband had a great time and went on a safari ride. One week after she returned, she complained of general fatigue and myalgia. She continued to go to work the next day, knowing she had just returned from being off for two weeks. While at work, she frequented the restroom and by mid-day she had bloody stool. Within an hour, she reports having six trips to the restroom, each time with bloody stool. She now mentions to her coworker that she feels flushed, lightheaded, and dizzy and has been to the restroom multiple times. The friend offers to drive her to the local hospital emergency room (ER).

As the APN doing an history and physical in the ER:

- What are important history questions needed to gather accurate information for the assessment of Mrs. Smith?
- What test will you order to diagnosis Mrs. Smith?
- The differential diagnosis includes EVD based on her recent travel and her current symptoms. What will be your communication with Mrs. Smith's peer/coworker who brought her to the ER?

- What will be your plan to share information for her admission to the hospital to support HCW and environmental readiness to care for Mrs. Smith?

## References

Abudakar, A., Malik, M., Pebody, R.G., Elkoly, A.A., Khan, W., Bellos, A., & Mala, P. (2016). Burden of acute respiratory disease of epidemic and pandemic potential in the WHO Eastern Mediterranean region: A literature review. *WHO Regional Office for the Eastern Mediterranean—Eastern Mediterranean Health Journal*, 513–526.

AIDS.gov. (2017). Opportunistic infections and their relationship to HIV/AIDS. Retrieved from https://www.aids.gov/hiv-aids-basics/staying-healthy-with-hiv-aids/potential-related-health-problems/opportunistic-infections/

American Association for the Study of Liver Disease (AASLD). (2017). Retrieved from https://www.aasld.org/publications/practice-guidelines-0

Blumberg, A. (2014). Fourteen percent of Americans believe AIDS might be God's punishment: Survey. The Huffington Post. Retrieved from https://www.drugabuse.gov/sites/default/files/rrhiv.pdf

Boyce, J. & Pittet, D. (2002). Recommendations of the Healthcare Infection Control Practices Advisory Committee and the HICPAC/SHEA/APIC/IDSA Hand Hygiene Task Force. *MMWR 51*(16), 1–56.

Brett-Major, D., Jacob, S., Jacquerioz, F., Risi, G., Fischer, W., Kato, Y., & Fletcher, T. (2015). Perspective Piece: Being Ready to Treat Ebola Virus Disease Patients. *Am J. Trop Med Hyg. 92*(2), 233–237.

Brocail, M. (2015). The differences between HIV-1 and HIV-2. Retrieved from https://www.stdcheck.com/blog/the-differences-between-hiv-1-and-hiv-2/

Calabrese, S.K., & Underhill, K. (2015). Hostigma surrounding the use of HIV pre-exposure prophylaxis undermines prevention and Pleasure: A call to destigmatize "Truvada whores". *American Journal of Public Health, 105*(10), 1960-4. Retrieved from https://www.ncbi.nlm.nih.gov/pubmed/26270298

Carroll, M., Matthews, D., Hiscox, J., Elmore, M., Pollakis, G., Rambaut, A., Gunther, S. (2015). Temporal and Spatial Analysis of the 2014–2015 Ebola Virus Outbreak in West Africa. *Nature 524* (6), 97–105.

Centers for Disease Control and Prevention. (n.d.a). HIV risk behaviors. Retrieved from https://www.cdc.gov/hiv/risk/estimates/riskbehaviors.html

Centers for Disease Control and Prevention. (n.d.b). HIV-transmission. Retrieved from https://t.cdc.gov/synd.aspx?js=0&rid=cs_3605&url=http://t.cdc.gov/VIK

Centers for Disease Control and Prevention, (CDC). (2001). Morbidity and Mortality Weekly Report. Retrieved from https://www.cdc.gov/mmwr/pdf/wk/mm5021.pdf

Center for Disease Control and Prevention. (2013). Hepatitis A. Retrieved from https://wwwnc.cdc.gov/travel/diseases/hepatitis-a

Centers for Disease Control and Prevention. (2014). Laboratory testing for the diagnosis of HIV infection: updated recommendations. Retrieved from https://stacks.cdc.gov/view/cdc/23447

Centers for Disease Control and Prevention, (CDC). (April 11, 2014). "Revised surveil-lance case definition for HIV infection—United States, 2014.". *MMWR. Recommen-dations and reports: Morbidity and mortality weekly report. Recommendations and reports / Centers for Disease Control. 63* (RR-03):1–10.

Centers for Disease Control and Prevention. (2016). HIV in the United States: At a glance. Retrieved from https://www.cdc.gov/hiv/statistics/overview/ataglance.html

Centers for Disease Control and Prevention (CDC). (2015 a). Chlamydia infections: Chlamydial infections in adolescents and adults. Retrieved from https://www.cdc.gov/std/tg2015/chlamydia.htm

Center for Disease Control and Prevention (CDC). (2015 b). Viral hepatitis. Hepatitis A FAQs for Health Professionals. Retrieved from https://www.cdc.gov/hepatitis/HAV/index.htm

Center for Disease Control and Prevention (CDC). (2015 c). Viral hepatitis. Hepatitis C. Retrieved from https://www.cdc.gov/hepatitis/hcv/index.htm

Centers for Disease Control and Prevention (CDC). (2016 a). 2015 sexually transmit-ted diseases treatment guidelines: Gonococcal infections in adolescents and adults. Retrieved from https://www.cdc.gov/std/tg2015/gonorrhea.htm

Centers for Disease Control and Prevention (CDC). (2016 b). 2015 sexually transmitted diseases treatment guidelines: Screening recommendations and considerations ref-erenced in treatment guidelines and original sources. Retrieved from https://www.cdc.gov/std/tg2015/screening-recommendations.htm

Centers for Disease Control and Prevention (CDC). (2016 c). 2015 sexually transmit-ted diseases treatment guidelines: Syphilis. Retrieved from https://www.cdc.gov/std/tg2015/syphilis.htm

Centers for Disease Control and Prevention (CDC). (2016 d). STDs during pregnancy: CDC fact sheet (detailed). https://www.cdc.gov/std/pregnancy/stdfact-pregnancy-detailed.htm

Center for Disease Control and Prevention (CDC). (2016 e). Viral hepatitis. Hepatitis B FAQs for Health Professionals. Retrieved from https://www.cdc.gov/hepatitis/hbv/hbvfaq.htm#overview

Centers for Disease Control and Prevention (CDC). (2017 a). Genital HPV infection-fact sheet. Retrieved from https://www.cdc.gov/std/hpv/stdfact-hpv.htm

Centers for Disease Control and Prevention (CDC). (2017 b). Sexually transmitted dis-eases (STDs): Expedited Partner Therapy. Retrieved from https://www.cdc.gov/std/ept/default.htm

Centers for Disease Control and Prevention CDC (2017 c). Mumps cases and rates, Retrieved from https://www.cdc.gov/mumps/outbreaks.html

Centers for Disease Control and Prevention (CDC) (2017 d). Recommendations for Preventing the spread of vancomycin resistance recommendations of the Hospital Infection Control Practices Advisory Committee (HICPAC). Retrieved from https://www.cdc.gov/mmwr/preview/mmwrhtml/00039349.htm

Elbadawi, L., Borlaug, G., Gundlach, K., Monson, T., Warshauer, D., Walters, M., Davis, J. (2016). Carbapenem-resistant enterobacteriaceae transmission in health care facilities- Wisconsin, February-May 2015. *MMWR 65*(34), 906–909.

Elizabeth Glaser Pediatric AIDS Foundation (2017). Retrieved from http://www.ped-aids.org/

Fadheel, Z., Perry, H., & Henderson, R. (2008). Comparison of methicillin-resistant staphylococcus sureus (MRSA) carriage rate in the general population with the health-worker population. *New Zealand Journal Medical Laboratory Science, 62*, 4-6.

Finn, R. (1993). Arthur Ashe, tennis star, is dead at 49. New York Times. Retrieved from http://www.nytimes.com/learning/general/onthisday/bday/0710.html

Gallo, R.C., & Montagneier, L. (2003). The discovery of HIV and the cause of AIDS. *New England Journal of Medicine, 349*, 2283–2285.

Gupta, A., Capoor, M., Gupta, S. & Sachdeva. H. (2015). Concomitant infections of influenza a H1N1 and disseminated cryptococcosis in an HIV seropositive patient. *Journal of Laboratory Physicians, 7*(2), 134–136.

Gupta, R. & Gupta, P. (2016). Opportunistic bacterial infections. *Pathology of opportunistic infections, 5*, 5–16.

Hepatitis C Online. (2017). Hepatitis C treatments. Retrieved from http://www.hepatitisc.uw.edu/page/treatment/drugs

HRSA. (2016). Who was Ryan White? Ryan White and Global HIV/AIDS programs. Retrieved from https://hab.hrsa.gov/about-ryan-white-hivaids-program/who-was-ryan-white

Hunt, C. & Powers, K. (2014). Self-testing for HIV and its impact on public health. HHS Public Access. Retrieved from https://www.ncbi.nlm.nih.gov/pmc/articles/PMC4005336/

Journel, M, Andrecy, L., Metellus, D., Pierre, J., Faublas, R., Juin, S., Adrien, P. (2017). Transmission of zika virus- Haiti, October 12, 2015-Septemer 10, 2016. *MMWR US Department of Health and Human Services/Center for Disease Control and Prevention* (66)6, 172–176.

Knox, D., Anderson, P., Harrigan, P., & Tan, D. (2017). Multidrug-resistant HIV-1 infection despite preexposure prophylaxis. *The New England Journal of Medicine, 376*, 501–502.

Lee, T., Montgomery, O., Marx, J., Olmsted, R. & Scheckler, W. (2007). Recommended practices for surveillance: Association for Professionals in Infection Control and Epidemiology (APIC), Inc. *American Journal of Infection Control, 35*, 427–440. Doi:10.1016/j.ajic.2007.07.002

Li, S., Lee, L., Pollack, H., Wyatt, L., Trinh-Shevrin, C., Pong, P., & Kwon, S. (2016). Hepatitis B screening & vaccination behaviors in a community-based sample of Chinese & Korean Americans in New York City. *American Journal of Human Behavior, 41*(2), 204–214.

Lieshout- Krikke, R., Zaaijer, H., & van de Laar, T. (2015). Predonation screening of candidate donors and prevention of window period donations. *Transfusion, 55*(2), 373–378.

Lowdermilk, D. L., Perry, S. E., Cashion, K., & Alden K. R. (2016). *Maternity and women's health care* (11th ed.). St. Louis, MO: Elsevier

Lozano, R., Naghavi, M., Foreman, K. Lim, S., Shibuya, K., Aboyans, S...Murray, C.

(2012). Global and regional mortality from 235 causes of death for 20 age groups in 1990 and 2010: a systematic analysis for the Global Burden of Disease Study 2010. *The Lancet, 380*, 2095–2128.

Mayo Clinic. (2014). Hepatitis B. Retrieved from www.mayoclinic.org/diseases-

Mezzo, J., Lamia, T., Schipani, A., Stokes, S., & Jacobs-Ware, E. (2016). The hepatitis testing and linkage-to-care data review process: An approach to ensuring the quality of program data. *Public Health Methodology, 131*, 44–48.

Morbidity and Mortality Weekly Report (MMWR). (2011). HIV-2 infections surveillance—United States, 1987–2009. Retrieved from https://www.ncbi.nlm.nih.gov/pubmed/21796096

National Institute on Drug Abuse. (2012). Research report series. Drug abuse and HIV. Retrieved from https://www.drugabuse.gov/sites/default/files/rrhiv.pdf

National Institute for Health (NIH). (2012). What is HAART? Retrieved from https://www.drugabuse.gov/publications/research-reports/hivaids/what-haart

Nicoll, A. (2013). Public Health Investigations Required for Protecting the Population Against Novel Coronaviruses. *European Centre for Disease Prevention and Control*, S61–S63.

Pisesky, A, Benchimol, E., Wong, C., Hui, C., Crowe, M., Belair, M. McNally, J. (2016). Incidence of Hospitalization for Respiratory Syncytial Virus Infection Amongst Children in Ontario, Canada: A Population-Based Study Using Validated Health Administrative Data. *PLOS ONE, 10*(137), 1–13.

Raines, K. (2016). Spraying in South Carolina to combat zika virus kills millions of honeybees, *Scholar. Google*, Retrieved at http://insider.foxnews.com/2016/09/02/millions-honeybees-killed-anti-zika-spraying-sc

Roach, R. (2014). APIC Text of Infection Control and Epidemiology. Retrieved from http://insider.foxnews.com/2016/09/02/millions-honeybees-killed-anti-zika-spraying-sc

Selik, R., Mokotoff, E., Branson, B., Owen, S., Whitmore, S., & Hall, H. (2014). Revised surveillance case definition for HIV infection—United States, 2014. CDC. Morbidity and Mortality Weekly Report. Retrieved from https://www.cdc.gov/mmwR/preview/mmwrhtml/rr6303a1.htm

Suther, A., Granich, R., Kato, M., Nsanzimana, S., Montaner, J., & Williams, B. (2015). Programmatic implications of acute and early HIV infection. *Journal of Infectious Diseases, 212*(9), 1351–1360.

Ullrich, P., Lavela, S., Evans, C., Miskevics, S., Weaver, F., & Goldstein, B. (2013). Association between perception of evidence and adoption of H1N1 influenza infection prevention strategies among healthcare workers providing care to persons with spinal cord injury. *Journal of Advanced Nursing: Informing Practice and Policy Worldwide Through Research and Scholarship*, 1793–1800.

U.S. Department of Veterans Affairs. (2017). CD4- count (or T-count). Retrieved from https://www.hiv.va.gov/patient/diagnosis/labs-CD4-count.asp

U.S. Passports & International Travel. (2017). Alerts and Warning. Retrieved from https://travel.state.gov/content/passports/en/alertswarnings.html

Wesolowski, L., Parker, M., Delaney, K., & Owen, S. (2017). Highlights from the 2016.

HIV diagnostics conference: The new landscape of HIV testing in laboratories, public health programs and clinical practice. *Journal of Clinical Virology.* Retrieved from http://www.sciencedirect.com/science/article/pii/S1386653217300240

World Health Organization (WHO). Global health observatory. HIV/AIDS. Retrieved from http://www.who.int/gho/hiv/en/

Zbinden, A., Durig, R., Shah, C., Boni, J., & Schupbach, J. (2016) Importance of an early antibody differentiation Immunoassay for detection of dual infection with HIV-1 and HIV-2. *PLOS one, 11*(6): e0157690. doi: 10.1371/journal.pone.0157690.

World Health Organization (WHO) (2017). Sexually transmitted infections (STIs). Retrieved from http://www.who.int/mediacentre/factsheets/fs110/en/

# Section 3

# Tools for Managing Population Health Issues

## CHAPTER 15

# Health Coaching

SANDRA M. OLGUIN, DNP, MSN, RN

## Health Coaching

H EALTHCARE PROVIDERS (HCPs) are obligated to teach clients how to promote health and wellness, prevent disease and infection, and reduce the risk of injury or harm. Nurses have always helped clients by managing, directing, leading, and providing patient care through education, advocacy, and application skills. Advanced practice nurses (APNs) understand, value, and integrate the nursing process into their practice. They assess, diagnose, develop goals, implement evidence-based interventions, evaluate progress and, when necessary, reformulate the plan of care. In today's world, APNs are advancing evidence-based research, implementing research into practice, and leading and driving healthcare policy and change. The nursing profession is integral to healthcare and the delivery of safe, competent, and compassionate care. This chapter discusses the nurse as a health coach, highlighting what is a health coach, the benefits of health coaching, guiding theories and models for behavioral change, health coaching skills, how to integrate health coaching into nursing practice, and future considerations.

Health coaching is an approach to support the health and wellness of people across the life-span in any population. This process works with patients and clients, in the community, and with healthcare providers. Through the application of Motivational Interviewing and other therapeutic techniques used as a health coach, APNs are equipped with tools

441

to support desired behavior change for persons experiencing a condition that is not conducive to his or her optimal health. By understanding the APN's role as a health coach and integrating the coaching practices, the APN will impact the health of the population.

This strategic intervention works especially well when one is addressing chronic health dynamics. When working with each of these populations, their overall health and well-being has the potential to be positively impacted, and lasting healthy practices emerge. Not specific to any one grouping, this strategic intervention is directed by the individual's needs and potential desired outcomes. Therefore, it is appropriate to use with any population health grouping.

### Background

Historically, nurses have been charged to solve problems and have all the answers to every client question. Nurses' first reaction to clients' problems is to fix them and provide clients with information through education. Often, after a detailed explanation and list of instructions from the nurse, the client is discharged home with the assumption that all the information provided will be embraced and followed. However, when the client, suffering from a chronic disease, returns due to "noncompliance," the nurse may be abhorrently surprised and show signs of disappointment, because the client did not adhere to the plan of care, created collaboratively or by their nurse. The client may feel frustrated, ashamed, embarrassed, and angry toward themselves and others. The cycle of teaching followed by readmissions and disappointment continue and the client's condition gets progressively worse. Nurses may struggle with guiding clients through behavioral change. Because of previous negative experiences with educating clients, nurses may choose to avoid or minimize the opportunity for instruction. Often, there appears to be a gap between what patients say and what patients do. Patients' desires to please the nurse, an authoritative figure, during healthcare education to avoid confrontation or embarrassment may influence the gap. Patients may have experienced threatening statements such as "If you don't manage your diabetes, you can die" and "You should stop smoking; it's not good for you and the people you love." As a result, patients may disengage completely, with a sequel leading to more severe complications.

In a survey conducted by Y & R's BAV Consulting for Xerox, Mack (2016) reveals incongruence between healthcare providers' and clients' perceptions of who takes responsibility for the client's health. Although 50% of healthcare consumers believe they "take complete responsibility for their health," "less than six percent of healthcare professionals agree" (Mack, 2016). The healthcare provider educates and encourages clients to behavioral change. However, in the study, clients identified that although they do not need encouragement from the healthcare provider; "more than 63 percent polled desire a connection with healthcare providers and payer in their personal care" (Mack, 2016).

Nurses may feel they do not have the time, tools, or confidence to help clients be successful in managing their care and making behavioral changes. When nurses partner with clients in developing their plans of care, compliance increases and positive effects on healthcare ensue. Nurses who engage client-centered care in encouraging behavioral change decrease the gap between what the client says and what the client does. Nurses who acquire and apply health coaching skills move from an authoritative figure to a partner in the clients' healthcare. By incorporating the role as a health coach, nurses will influence nursing practice and patient outcomes, as well as experience personal growth and satisfaction.

## What Is a Health Coach?

First, the health coach this chapter discusses is not a nurse who provides fitness and sports coaching or develops physical activity plans for clients. The health coach this chapter highlights assists the client through clear and unobstructed effective communication to enhance his or her well-being as defined by the client. The health coach engages the client to own his or her healthcare, provides the client with education to make healthy decisions, recognizes the positive steps toward self-determination, and guides the conversation to behavioral change. According to Hall (2013), health coaching "is a conversation or series of conversations with the aim of helping people learn, grow and fulfill their potential" (p. 17).

The nurse, as a health coach, ensures the client has all the necessary information to make informed decisions. Client-centered care is provided, with the client and his or her healthcare needs central to the interaction. Although what has led up to the interaction is important, the focus of the conversation is in the present moment working toward a better today and tomorrow. The primary function of a healthcare coach is to assist in cultivating a healthier lifestyle. Examples include the following:

- Establishing a trusting, therapeutic, and professional relationship.
- Assessing the current health condition of the client.
- Integrating mindfulness into the interaction.
- Finding out what the client knows about his or her health condition and situation.
- Assisting the client with setting health goals.
- Utilizing therapeutic and nonjudgmental communication.
- Documenting a client's progress and sharing it with the client.
- Conducting behavioral health screenings.
- Collaborating with the client to develop a treatment plan.
- Providing feedback and guidance.

The conscientious health coach integrates awareness in his or her coaching. The practice in mindfulness-based stress reduction (MBSR) founder, Jon Kabot Zinn (1994), identifies the practice as "paying attention in a particular way: on purpose, in the present moment and nonjudgmentally" (p. 4). Hall (2013) identifies the resiliency attributed from mindfulness and suggests that it helps with "work-life balance; stress management; decision-making; coping with ambiguity; dealing with crises; employee engagement; heightening focus and clarity; communication; increasing presence; and improved listening."

## Benefits to Integrating Health Coaching into Advanced Nursing Practice

*What Does the Evidence-based Literature Say?*

According to the Centers for Disease Control and Prevention (CDC, 2016), seven out of 10 deaths are attributed to chronic diseases. Chronic diseases and conditions, such as heart disease, chronic obstructive pulmonary disorder, type 2 diabetes, arthritis, and stroke, are very costly to the United States (U.S.). The CDC (2016) asserts 86% of the healthcare costs are spent on treating people diagnosed with a chronic disease.

Focusing on empowering people to make healthy choices requires nurses to ensure the population has the "knowledge, ability, resources, and motivation" to make healthy choices and live a healthy life (National Prevention Council, 2014). The federal government supports research and programs that lead people to make healthy decisions. Two of the four recommendations from the National Prevention Strategy to empower people include "providing people with tools and information to make healthy choices" and creating positive social interactions that support healthy decision making (National Prevention Council, 2014). Behavioral change consists of a client leading the process while the nurse is assisting, supporting, guiding, and occasionally directing.

## Health and Wellness Coaching Utilizing Motivational Interviewing

### *What is Motivational Interviewing?*

According to Kaplan & Sadock's Synopsis of Psychiatry: Behavioral Sciences Clinical Psychiatry, motivational interviewing is an interviewing "technique used to motivate the patient to change his or her maladaptive behavior" (Sadock, Sadock, and Ruiz, 2014, p. 208). Kennedy and Blair (2014) assert motivational interviewing helps identify "the patient's current stage of change as well as motivate him or her to make changes" (p 328). Motivational interviewing is a patient-centered counseling style designed to address the common problem of ambivalence about behavioral change (Miller and Rollnick, 2013). The technique is not a way to manipulate someone into doing something they do not wish to do, but to explore what it is the client wants to change and support them in the process. The essence or "spirit" of motivational interviewing is the culmination of several characteristics including "collaborative, evocative, and honoring of patient autonomy" (Rollnick, Miller, and Butler, 2008, p 6).

### *What are the Client Outcomes Related to Motivational Interviewing?*

Using motivational interviewing as a health coach has the potential to improve client outcomes, increase client and nurse satisfaction, and reduce healthcare costs. Sadock *et al.* (2014) discuss the application of motivational interviewing with clients who have mental disorders and the effectiveness in altering behavior with persons dealing with addiction.

In a study incorporating 10 healthcare practices, Pollak (2011) found that, at the end of three months, the healthcare providers who integrated motivational interviewing techniques into their practices saw a significant weight loss in their patients who were either overweight or obese. Even when nonprofessionals use motivational interviewing, Graff Low, Giasson, Connors, Freeman, and Weiss (2012) found motivational interviewing a useful tool in weight loss in female patients with heart disease.

At Kaiser Permanente, Northern California, clients who received health coaching through telephonics were asked to describe their perception of health coaching (Adams *et al.*, 2013). The results revealed a high satisfaction rate with the program, a perception of success due to health coaching, and recommendation to continue integrating health coaching.

*Who Benefits from Health and Wellness Coaching?*

Through health coaching, the client is empowered to identify what is important to him or her, make decisions related to behavioral choices, and decide what he or she wants to pursue and how to do it. The client is heard and feels supported. The nurse naturally promotes wellness, prevents disease, and reduces the risk of complications caused by chronic diseases, such as congestive heart failure, diabetes, and COPD/ Asthma. By integrating health coaching, the responsibility shifts. The nurse is responsible for delivering competent, current, and relevant education, developing a safe environment, and providing support, guidance, and occasional direction. When nurses empower the clients to be leaders of their healthcare, they become less burdened by owning the client's health disease and condition. The outcome of health coaching impacts the relationship between the coach and the client as a consumer of health. The client, as a consumer of health, chooses to be in control of their health and to partner with providers who treat them with respect and dignity.

*Which Professional Practices Can Utilize Health Coaching?*

All healthcare professionals are recommended to incorporate health coaching into their practice. Many therapists, counselors, and other healthcare providers are experts in therapeutic communication; however, motivational interviewing has not mainstreamed into curricula and many professionals take extra classes to acquire the tools. Imagine healthcare with the therapists, counselors, social workers, dieticians, physical therapists, physicians, educators, dentists, physician assistants, nurses, and other professions, who empower clients to be leaders in their health.

### Theories and Theoretical Model for Change

Orem's theoretical framework guides the nursing practice as a health coach. Orem's Theory of Self-Care Deficit consists of three associated theories including Self-Care, Self-Care Deficit, and Theory of Nursing Systems (Tomey & Alligood, 2006). Major concepts and definitions delineated by Orem focus on the person's ability and willingness to perform self-care behaviors. The belief is people want to manage their chronic diseases to prevent further complications and costs. There are three phases of Orem's Self-Care, according to Tomey and Alligood (2006): investigative, judgmental, and decision-making stages. Health coaching provides nurses with a tool to assist clients diagnosed with a chronic disease or illness in goal setting and in adopting ways to perform self-management. Orem's framework (Self-Care) mirrors this behavioral change.

> Intrinsic motivational factors consist of doing something because it feels good and is the right thing to do. It is an innate desire or pleasure of doing that motivates the person. No one needs to be looking, and rewards and recognition are not the driving forces. Values, beliefs, and emotions satisfies the need and desire to push forward and move toward achieving the goal. Ryan and Deci (2000), identify several types of extrinxic motivational factors. For the purpose of this chapter, extrinsic motivational factors include rewards or recogonitions and avoiding punishment, embarrassment, or shame. Outcomes are the same, even when what motivates individuals to reach the same outcome may be vastly different. For example, a nurse working overtime to cover a co-worker's day off request, may be motivated by covering a peer's shift because it feels good to be of service or he/she enjoys taking care of patients. This same person may be motivated by the financial gain, recognition from leadership, or the dept the peer will owe in the future.

Intrinsic motivation is the desire to do something for the pleasure of doing it. The person is moved by gaining knowledge, accomplishing something great, enjoyment, and stimulation. Intrinsic motivation can be instinctive and or learned through an environment that promotes the behaviors as natural and fun. In a study conducted by Ryan and Connell (1989), students were observed completing homework. When the external regulation was implemented, the students demonstrated less "interest, value, or effort, and the more they indicated a tendency to blame others, such as the teacher, for negative outcomes" (Ryan & Deci, 2000, p. 63). Contrary to external regulation, students who were exposed to intrinsic motivation, behaved differently and appeared to be interested and demonstrate enjoyment, competence, and positive coping.

The conceptual framework is a "group of concepts that are broadly defined and systematically organized to provide a focus, rationale, and tool for the integration and interpretation of information" (Moran, Burson, and Conrad, 2014, p. 127). It is utilized as a visual aid for mapping and connecting relevant project concepts to support project planning, implementing, and evaluation (Moran *et al.*, 2014). The Transtheoretical Model (TTM) of change compliments Orem's Theory of Self-Care Deficit and provides insight into the strategic process of change. The TTM, as stated by Prochaska, DiClemente, & Norcross (1992), "is an integrative, biopsychosocial model to conceptualize the process of intentional behavior change." The TMM identifies seven stages in which a person progresses or regresses through precontemplation, contemplation, preparation, action, maintenance, termination, and relapse (Bastable, 2014; Prochaska *et al.*, 1992). Utilizing this model is valuable to help nurses identify contemplation where the motivational interviewing is most effective in influencing behavioral change (Miller & Rollnick, 2013). Integrating this information into a teaching lesson assists the nurse in assessing patient readiness to learn and create desired behavioral changes.

## Becoming a Health Coach

### What Education is Required to be a Health Coach?

Current practices do not require a degree or certification to becoming a health coach; however, some institutions require certification or the agreement to obtain certification upon being hired. Nurses are health coaches. They have many roles, including educators, advocates, leaders, researchers, counselors, policy makers, change agents, and healthcare providers, managers, and partners. Nurses utilize many of the concepts of health coaching by establishing trusting relationships, using their expertise, and supporting clients through change. They make excellent health coaches; however, education, training, and practice are necessary to increase the nurse's confidence to integrate health coaching into practice and effectiveness as a coach.

Certifications and degrees offered throughout the internet and organized institutions should be scrutinized. Several organizations offering online certification require the completion of a personal data sheet prior to previewing the curriculum and courses and do not have an address or phone number. However, the School of Nursing at Vanderbilt University (2016) and The Osher for Integrative Medicine at Vanderbilt, an accredited institution and program, offer a Health Coach Certificate Program open to qualified applicants who are licensed in the healthcare field. The program is fully disclosed on their website and openly accepts into their program professionals who are medical doctors, physical therapists, occupational therapists, psychologists, counselors, social workers, and other healthcare providers. As of August 19, 2016, the cost of the 6-month long program was $4,800.00 if paid in full by the due date.

Established by Rollnick and Miller (2008), the Motivational Interviewing Network of Trainers (MINT) training elucidates extensive and valuable resources to develop and integrate motivational interviewing into practice. The calendar found on the website displays the courses available by date, location, and instructor. Each instructor is an independent practitioner and not an employee of MINT. As of November 1, 2016, the basic three-day motivational interviewing introductory course costs $350.00, the one-day intermediate course costs $120.00, and the two-day advanced course costs $599.00 in England and $379 in San Diego, California.

## Health Coach Using Motivational Interviewing in Practice

The nurse as a health coach creates a safe and therapeutic environment for collaboration and uses his or her nursing knowledge along with health coaching skills to support the client in creating and embracing change to promote health and wellness. Integrating motivational interviewing as a health coach takes time and effort. Miller and Rollnick (2013) describe several motivational interviewing considerations.

1. Establish rapport.
2. Determine the client's desire, ability, reason, and need for change.
3. Guide the client to clearly delineated concrete and measurable goals.
4. Engage the client in the planning process.
5. Summarize and evaluate.

The first steps to coaching include providing a safe environment and maintaining a professional relationship. Within the environment, the coach exudes a calm and attentive demeanor by listening to understand with an empathetic and nonjudgmental ear. A professional relationship is developed and professional boundaries are adhered.

After determining the client's desire, ability, reason, and need for change, the health coach begins the assessment process as early as the introduction to the client. Both subjective, what the client says, and objective, what the coach observes, give the coach valuable information outside of just knowing the health condition. Asking the client what he or she knows about his or her health status and situation not only engages the client, but also allows the coach to assess the client's desire, ability, reason, and need for change.

Traditionally, healthcare professionals want to see patients make behavioral changes; therefore, the provider, rather than the client, identifies the behavior to be changed, suggests approaches for change, and makes recommendations for goal setting (Kennedy & Blair, 2014). Developing client health goals is the client's responsibility; however, the coach, through active listening, guidance, and occasional direction, helps the client develop health goals based on the client's values, confidence, and feasibility. The client-created goals may take time and effort; therefore, the health coach needs to remain patient and supportive. When the client appears stuck, the health coach may ask permission to interject and offer advice or counsel.

The planning process helps the client to identify what works for him or her. Dant (2011) delineates that the nurse's role is to utilize therapeutic and nonjudgmental communication, document client's progress, and share it with the client, identify behavioral health needs, collaborate and partner with the client to develop a plan, and provide honest and respectful feedback and guidance. Occasionally, barriers arise during coaching and Dant (2011) explains the importance of understanding the barriers to create and maintain a therapeutic relationship and conversation. Several "traps" of motivational interviewing, according to Dant (2011) include the following: repetitive questions and answers, being for or against their views, giving the client a reason to advocate for the unhealthy behavior, labeling, assuming the focus of the conversation before eliciting it from the client, and placing blame on the client. Along with the "traps," Rollnick *et al.* (2008), Dant (2011), and Miller and Rollnick (2013) delineate six barriers that may inhibit effective motivational interviewing. The barriers include resistance, ambivalence, change talk (desire, ability, reasons, needs, commitment, taking steps), personal values, lack of commitment, and communication skills. Nurses who are effective communicators maintain self-awareness of both their verbal and nonverbal communication and are comfortable with silence. Silence sends the message to the client that what he or she has to say is important and he or she has time to finish and express his or her thoughts.

Summarizing what the client has said and committed to doing gives the client the opportunity to accept, reject, or clarify their thoughts and position. The evaluation of the conversation raises the client's awareness of the behavioral change and the progress produced by the health coaching experience.

*Health Coaching Examples*

A.B., a 44-year-old client, married with two children, was discharged from the hospital and requested to follow-up with the nurse practitioner due to experiencing severe fatigue, elevated blood sugar level, and recent hospitalization. A.B.'s vital signs in the office include the following: B/P: 150/89, Pulse: 95, Temp: 97.7, R: 20, O2Sat: 98% Room Air, BMI: 3 42, 0/10 Pain level. Client has a diagnosis of hypertension and early signs of diabetes.

Nurse: Hello, A.B. My name is Chris. Why are you here today?

A.B. I'm here because the hospitalist at the hospital told me I'm probably diabetic and said to follow-up with my nurse practitioner.

Nurse: You think you have diabetes? Did you know some forms of diabetes are preventable? Does it run in your family?

A.B. Look, I know I'm heavy and that's why I probably have diabetes. What should I do?

Nurse: If you eat healthy and exercise, you will be healthier. Diabetes can lead to many other life-altering consequences, even death.

A.B. I know I need to eat healthier and exercise. Do I need to start taking insulin?

Nurse: I can refer you to a trainer and a dietician. Hopefully, you won't need insulin and you can start eating better and exercising. Here is the trainer's business card.

A.B. A trainer is expensive.

Nurse: You can do exercises at home. Just go to the internet, find workout videos on YouTube, and do them. That won't cost as much money as a gym membership and trainer. Also, since you can do this at home, you won't have to spend money on gas. Sounds like a good idea to me. What do you think?

A.B. Yea, OK.

Nurse: Great! If you exercise and eat healthy, you may not end up with diabetes. Right now, you are in the prediabetic stage and we are worried about you. You are taking the right steps to address it now, before it's too late.

A.B. Um, OK. Thanks.

While reviewing the previous dialogue, one may identify many conversation pitfalls. Asking "Why are you here today?" puts the client on the defensive and may be guarded during the rest of the conversation. After the client answers the initial question, the nurse asks several questions abruptly, with the expectation that the client is following along. The questions are closed; therefore, the client is unable to express himself or herself freely. Closed-ended questions may be helpful when used to seek clarification; however, the questioning the nurse is using is for the nurse's intent to clarify his or her assumptions about the client rather than being helpful to the patient. Once the problem has been identified, the nurse tells the client how to solve the problem rather than soliciting solutions from the client. The previous example is a strained healthcare encounter, leaving the client and the nurse dissatisfied, frustrated, and exhausted.

The following exemplar integrates several components of motivational interviewing as demonstrated by Miller and Rollnick (2013).

Nurse: Hello A.B. It's a pleasure to meet you. (Shake hands) My name is Chris, your nurse practitioner. I have read your chart; however, I'd like to ask you a few questions, if that's OK with you?

A.B. Sure.

Nurse: What brings you in today?

A.B. I'm here because the hospitalist at the hospital told me I'm probably diabetic and said to follow-up with my nurse practitioner.

Nurse: Thank you for being here and letting me know what brought you in. There is concern about your blood sugar level being high and other risk factors. It looks like the news came as a shock to you.

A.B. Yes it did!

Nurse: Would it be OK if we talk about why the hospitalist referred you?

A.B. That's fine. I hate thinking that I'm diabetic! I know I'm heavy and should lose some weight. It's easier said than done though!

Nurse: On one hand, you want to lose weight but feel it is too difficult to do so.

A.B. That's right! I want to fit into my clothes again and stop wearing sweats all the time, but I can't lose weight.

Nurse: What else will you gain by losing weight?

A.B. If I lost weight, I wouldn't have to worry about all the health problems that come from being unhealthy. I wouldn't have to be talking to you right now, no offense. I would have a better life, for sure.

Nurse: Those are excellent reasons for getting fit. Are there any other benefits to losing weight besides fitting into your clothes and not having any health problems?

A.B. I think I would just feel better about myself and have better relationships with my family and co-workers.

Nurse: A.B., you have mentioned many wonderful benefits to losing weight. You mentioned how you will look and feel better and have better relationships. On a scale of 1, not important, to 10, very important, how important is losing weight to you?

A.B. About a 7.

Nurse: What makes the importance of losing weight a 7 to you and not a 5?

A.B. I think it's pretty important. I mean, it's my health that we're really talking about. Five is in the middle of the road, take it or leave it attitude.

Nurse: Losing weight is one way of being healthy, which is important to you.

A.B. That's right!

Nurse: What do you think may happen if you decide to make other healthy changes in your life?

A.B. I would probably have a better life, be able to do things, maybe live longer.

Nurse: There are many ways you can create a healthier life-style, and it sounds like you have already been thinking about it.

A.B. Yes, I have tried diets and walking, but it's been a challenge.

Nurse: I know a little about healthy habits; however, would you be interested in talking to a dietitian and a fitness trainer?

A.B. I'll talk with the dietitian, but I'm not ready for a fitness trainer.

Nurse: Eating healthier is your main concern. I have the name and number right here. When should they expect your call?

A.B. I will do it after we're finished. Thank you for listening to me.

Nurse: My pleasure. Sometimes things get in the way and steer us off track. What barriers do you face moving forward with your plan to eat healthy?

A.B. Well fast food is convenient and not very expensive if I get two tacos for $1.00! I'm going to have to take a different route home so I stop my habit of getting fast food after work.

Nurse: Removing the choice is a wise decision.

A.B. I'm hopeful the dietitian will help me find foods that taste good and fill me up.

Nurse: On a scale of 1, being not very confident, and 10 being very confident, what is your confidence level to eat healthy?

A.B. With the help of a dietician, an 8. I know if I believe in myself, I can do anything.

Nurse: In the past, it was challenging for you to integrate healthy habits, however now that you have a plan to avoid the convenience store and collaborate with the dietician, you believe you will be successful with reaching your goals. Are there any other comments, thoughts or ideas before we set up your next appointment?

## The Future of Health Coaching

With the growing population of persons diagnosed with multiple chronic diseases and the baby boomers reaching retirement, there will be a greater need for healthcare providers, particularly nurses. There will be an increased emphasis on disease prevention and health and wellness promotion. Who better to serve the community than a nurse who integrates health coaching into his or her practice?

Today, healthcare organizations and institutions utilize health coaches in the clinical setting and outpatient services. The practice settings may include medical offices, integrative medicine practices, private practices, health departments, hospitals, universities, insurance agencies, community-based clinics, and home health.

In an advertisement for a full-time Health Coach position, Hansen Family Hospital describes the role and responsibility of the Health Coach as follows:

"The Health Coach will work collaboratively with physicians, providers, staff, other healthcare professionals, and community resources to provide care coordination across the healthcare continuum for targeted patients within the community. He/she is an integral member of the healthcare team who works to ensure safety, best practice and high quality standards of care are maintained across the continuum. Responsible for coordinating a wide range of self-management support and disease registry activities for the targeted patient population. In conjunction with the Population Manager (the coach is) also responsible for overall operations of department including creation of operating plans, policies, and procedures departmental goals. Site implementation and ongoing daily flow would be the responsibility of the health coach. Success will be measured by the results of the process and outcome performance measures of the populations of patient in populations served and achievement of department operational goals and plans. The Health Coach must be a RN with an active license in Iowa. The selected candidate must be currently certified as a Health Coach or willing to obtain this certification."

## Conclusion

The significance of nurses as health coaches is demonstrated by improving patient outcomes, reducing costs associated with chronic disease, increasing client and nurse satisfaction, and providing nurses an evidence-based method to help promote behavioral change for persons battling a chronic disease. When individuals suffer from chronic disease and are unable to be successful in behavioral changes, adverse consequences affecting their health, work, relationships, community, and finances ensue. The APN meeting the needs of our society is relational to our commitment to providing safe, competent, and compassionate care. Hamric, Spross, and Hanson (2009) discuss the APN leader of today needing "to use the tools of empowerment and motivation to mentor future leaders who can lead with creativity, innovation, and caring" (p. 277). The tools of empowerment and motivation should also be used to mentor peers as well as clients to create a healthy life. It is our ethical and professional obligation to understand and incorporate best-practice methods to enhance client outcomes.

### Tool Kit and Resources

### Case Study

Monica is the oldest daughter of a patient you have been caring for over the last three weeks. She has stayed at the hospital around the clock and does not want to leave and take meals. Although her other brothers and sisters are in and out during visiting hours, Monica believes, as the family matriarch, it is her responsibility to remain at her parent's side. In the last few days, you notice that Monica is tearful. When you ask what has changed for her, Monica indicates that she realizes the situation with her parent is hopeless. She believes she can't make a difference, and she feels compelled to remain because of family tradition. Monica shares that she has focused on her parents most of her life, and she does not know what to do to correct this situation. She says she started to not feel anything anymore, and she dreads what the day will bring for her. After screening for potential suicidal ideation, what would you as the healthcare provider do in response to what Monica has shared with you?

- What has Monica shared with you that leads you to believe she might need some sort of intervention?
- What else would you need to know in order to be successful in your determination of the exact issues facing Monica?
- What are the potential consequences if Monica continues with her beliefs and continuing to place her parent before herself when it comes to care?
- How can you support Monica at this point in the process?
- What potential options and outcomes might Monica focus?
- What are expected barriers that Monica might present (or that you might ask her to consider if she does not bring them forth)?
- How might Monica overcome these barriers?

**Case Study**

The Emergency Department (ED) in a major trauma center requires all nurses to have ACLS certification and to be licensed as an APRN. This has left the ED with a shortage of nurses to cover the shifts as they are assigned. As a result, four APRNs are continually required to rotate as relief for the ED. These nurses are not offered any additional compensation, and the overall culture supports nurses doing what is needed in order for coverage to be maintained. One of the APRNs was physically assaulted by a patient's family member, and there has been pressure on this nurse to return to the ED "as soon as you can move". The other three APRNs are having to pick up additional shifts to cover for the injured nurse until she returns. All of the APRN relief team members are in committed relationships and have at least one child. Prior to the nurse getting hurt, it was difficult at best to plan when each APRN would be off and could attend family events. The ED manager continually talks about the need to be committed to the job and how "professional nurses" put the job above all else. As a means of support, the manager has offered the APRNs the opportunity to sleep when they are between shifts or if there is any downtime on their shifts.

The injured nurse attempts to explain to her orthopedic specialist why she needs to return to her work prior to the projected release date. The other APRNs are becoming resentful and do not want to go in to work. They are complaining about stress, headaches, and lack of energy. They are short with patients, and none of them want to deal with patient's families. All have been looking for another job, but they feel like they are betraying the other nurses who are on their shift rotation.

- Working with these four nurses as a group, what would be the focus of the first session?
- What will happen if these behaviors do not change for these nurses?
- How will you support these nurses as they work through the process of deciding what to do about the work situation?
- What consideration will these nurses need to make in relation to their needs as opposed to the organization, family or other nurses?
- What barriers do you emerging, and what potential options could be considered in relation to these?

## References

Adams, S. R., Goler, N. C., Sanna, R. S., Boccio, M., Bellamy, D. J., Brown, S. D. Schmittdiel, J. A. (2013). Patient satisfaction and perceived success with a telephonic health coaching program: The natural experiments for translation in diabetes (NEXT-D) study, Northern California, 2011. *Preventing Chronic Disease 10*, 1–12. DOI: http://dx.doi.org/10.5888/pcd10.130116

Bastable, S. (2014). *Nurse as educator: Principles of teaching and learning for nursing practice*. Burlington, MA: Jones & Bartlett Learning.

Centers for Disease Control and Prevention (2016). Chronic disease prevention and health promotion. Retrieved from http://www.cdc.gov/chronicdisease/index.htm

Dant, M. A. (2011). *Motivational interviewing in nursing practice: Empowering the patient*. Sudbury, MA: Jones and Bartlett Publishers

Graff Low, K., Giasson, H., Connors, S., Freeman, D., Weiss, R. (2012). Testing the effectiveness of motivational interviewing as a weight reduction strategy for obese cardiac patients: A pilot study. *International Society of Behavioral Medicine, 20*, 77–81. DOI 10.1007/s12529-011-9219-9

Hall, L. (2013). *Mindful coaching: How mindfulness can transform coaching practice.* London: Kogan.

Hamric, A. B., Spross, J. A., & Hanson, C. M. (2009). *Advanced practice nursing: 1 An integrative approach.* (4th ed.). St. Louis, Missouri: Saunders, an imprint of Elsevier Inc.

Hansen Family Hospital (2017) RN, health coach. https://emhia.applicantpro.com/jobs/568220.html

Kennedy, A. B., & Blair, S. N. (2014). Motivating people to exercise. *American Journal of Lifestyle Medicine, 8*(5), 324–329.

Kabat-Zinn, J. (1994). *Wherever you go, there you are.* New York: Hyperion.

Kennedy, A. B., & Blair, S. N. (2014). Motivating people to exercise. *American Journal of Lifestyle Medicine, 8*(5), 324–329.

Mack, H. (2016). Study finds patients, healthcare professionals differ on perception of who takes control of care. Retrieved from http://mobihealthnews.com/content/study-finds-patients-healthcare-professionals-differ-perception-who-takes-control-care

Miller, W.R. & Rollnick, S. (2013). *Motivational interviewing: Helping people change.* New York, New York: The Guilford Press.

Moran, K., Burson, R., & Conrad, D. (2014). *The doctor of nursing practice scholarly project: A framework for success.* Burlington, MA: Jones & Barlett Learning

National Prevention Council (2014). National prevention strategy: Empowered people. Retrieved from http://www.surgeongeneral.gov/priorities/prevention/strategy/empowered-people.pdf

Pollak, K. (2011). How can I help patients change unhealthy behaviors? Medscape. Retrieved from http://www.medscape.com/viewarticle/740155

Prochaska, J.O., DiClemente, C.C., & Norcross, J.C. (1992). In search of how people change: Applications to the addictive behaviors. *American Psychologist, 47,* 1102–1114. PMID: 1329589.

Rollnick, S., Miller, W. R., & Butler, C. C. (2008). *Motivational interviewing in health care: Helping patients change behavior.* New York, New York: The Guilford Press.

Ryan, R. M., & Connell, J. P. (1989). Perceived locus of causality and internalization: Examining reasons for acting in two domains. *Journal of Personality and Social Psychology, 57,* 749–761.

Ryan, R.M., & Deci, E. L. (2000). Intrinsic and extrinsic motivations: Classic definitions and new directions. *Contemporary Education Psychology, 25,* 54-67. Retrieved from http://selfdeterminationtheory.org/SDT/documents/2000_RyanDeci_IntExtDefs.pdf

Sadock, B.J., Sadock, V. A., & Ruiz, P. (2014). *Kaplan & Sadock's synopsis of psychiatry: Behavioral sciences/clinical psychiatry.* (11 Ed.). Lippincott: Williams & Wilkins

Tomey, A. M. & Alligood, M. R. (2006). *Nursing theorists and their work.* St Louis, Missouri: Mosby, Inc.

Vanderbilt University School of Nursing (2016). Health coaching certificate program. Retrieved from https://nursing.vanderbilt.edu/certificate_programs/health_coaching/index.php

## CHAPTER 16

# Care for Self: Compassion Fatigue and Burnout

MARY BIDDLE, DNP, RN, CNE, CCFP

MARY A. BEMKER, PhD, PhyS, LADC, LPCC, CCFP, CCTP, CNE, RN

## Care for Self: Compassion Fatigue and Burnout

**T**HE purpose of this chapter is to address the holistic needs of an individual as it relates to population health. Within this framework, that individual might be a patient or it might be ourselves. Chronic health issues and responses to being exposed to secondary stress from health issues of others, impact the entire individual. Until these issues are addressed, health problems will arise. As nurses, we tend to focus on others to the exclusion of our own needs. This is not only an unhealthy perspective for nurses, but it also impacts those for whom we care. We cannot adequately care for others if we ourselves are not healthy, and the mind-body-spirit connection is one that needs to be maintained and nourished for health to ensue.

## Compassion Fatigue and Burnout

Nursing is a caring profession. As nurses, we empathize and are impacted by the lives of the patients for whom we care, their families, and those with whom we work. Compassion is one of the central emotional responses nurses enact that impact their professional practice. Therefore, it is important for us to discuss in a book on population health for advanced practice nurses (APNs), the phenomena of compassion fatigue. Nursing is a vulnerable population. This is due in part to the nature of the work that nurses are exposed on a consistent basis. This applies to many caring professions, such as veterinarians, first respond-ers, physicians, occupational therapists, physical therapists, physician's assistants, and others that work on a continued basis with patients who suffer. Knowing this, how does compassion fatigue related to APRNs and others in the health profession?

## Compassion Fatigue

What is compassion fatigue? Why are advanced practice nurses more prone to compassion fatigue as compared to the general population? Nurses are a unique, caring population with distinctive self-care needs. During job performance, traumatic events are observed and reported to the nurse, nurse practitioner, and others in healthcare, thus exposing them to compassion fatigue.

The nursing profession lends itself to compassion fatigue because of a unique and psychologically internal skill set. Empathy allows nurs-es to absorb the pain patients and clients experience as they enter the healthcare environment due to illness. Empathy is felt for the physical, mental, and spiritual pain of the patient and their loved ones, for whom nurses administer care during practice. Empathy is an excellent skill in the helping profession allowing nurses to anticipate the needs for those whom they care, but this same dynamic can also be detrimental to the nurses. Empathy is not something nurses, or other individuals for that matter, innately know how to switch on and off (van der Wath, van Wyk, & van Rensburg, 2013). It is not something left at office or hospital at the end of the shift. The empathetic pain remnants ex-perienced at work are carried home in the body and soul of the care-giver. It is for this reason compassion fatigue is included in this text. The emphasis noted within this chapter will be recognition of Com-passion Fatigue etiology, prevention dynamics, and a means to care for the self and others.

Sympathy and empathy are mainstays for a person of a caring nature. Sympathy is a feeling of sadness, sorrow, and grief for another's mis-ery or despair (Merriam-Webster, 2017). Empathy, however, is having an emotional and spiritual connection to their pain (Merriam-Webster, 2017). As nurses, we relate to these feelings as we are continually ex-posed to these traumatic and painful experiences (Lombardo & Eyre, 2011). Repeated empathetic episodes can increase susceptibility to compassion fatigue by eroding the personal defenses and the resiliency of the nurse. Eliminating and decreasing the effects of compassion fatigue in nursing is why tools to build personal resiliency and compassion satisfaction should be taught to all in caring professions.

Not only does the personality traits of compassion and caring lend itself to compassion fatigue, but also the societal and cultural expectations of the nursing role. Nursing and healthcare has a culture of its own. The traditional role of Angel of Mercy in nursing lends itself to the development of compassion fatigue in those that serve in the profession (Harris & Griffin, 2015). Societal roles for women, and nursing historically being a female profession, have also contributed to the traditional nursing role expectations that lend itself to compassion fatigue (Minority Nurse Staff, 2013). In conclusion, any circumstance or role that puts others before the self can create an environment for the development of compassion fatigue.

Like those working in the Emergency Department (ED), the repetitive dynamics of caring for those in pain can have a lasting impact (Emergency Department Association [ENA], 2014), which is similar to dealing with a few patients over time. Noting the characteristics of compassion fatigue and knowing what to do when they occur can assist anyone in the helping profession repeatedly exposed to the trauma of pain and anguish of others.

Since nursing, as a caring profession, lends its participants to compassion fatigue, it is important to learn about the origins and research related to such. Compassion fatigue was first linked to nursing by Carol Joinson, RN (1992). Charles Figley (1995) expanded recognition of compassion fatigue in 1980's, comparing it to secondary post-traumatic stress disorder. Compassion fatigue is defined by Figley (1995) as a caregiver experiencing the traumatic event through their compassion and empathy for the person whom they are treating. This vicarious trauma (or empathetic trauma) can result from events or client histories taken that occur during management of healthcare services (McCann & Pearlman, 1990). Figley (1995) hypothesizes that the level of empathy experienced by nurses that is generated by the traumatized patient or family member, is significant in this transference relationship.

In the last 20 years, compassion fatigue has intensified in discussion among healthcare professionals, and this topic has been expounded upon in the professional literature (Durkin, Smith, Powell, Howarth, & Carson, 2013; Sabin, 2013; Severn, Searchfield, & Huggard, 2012). Much of the literature correlates organization setting types to compassion fatigue. Of specific notice are the areas of hospice, critical care, and emergency care. However, one study by Hooper, Craig, Janvrin, Wetsel, & Reimels, (2010), demonstrated this was not always the case. No correlation in occurrence of compassion fatigue was found within the different types of nursing practice, as evidenced among nurses working in nephrology, intensive care, the emergency department, and oncology. As healthcare professionals, it is more important to be aware of the signs and symptoms of compassion fatigue as opposed to determining relevance of a specific area of care and practice. The only requirement for being affected by compassion fatigue is that the professional identifies with the pain and suffering of the patient, client, or family (Figley, 1995; Hunsaker, Chen, & Heaston, 2015; Seagar, 2014).

Compassion fatigue not only impacts advanced practice nurses and others in healthcare, it also impacts the healthcare institution. This is noted by a lack of productivity, high level of staff turnover (costly for faculty and staff), and overall quality of healthcare given at the facility (Frampton & Goodrich, 2014; Iles, 2014; Markaki, 2014). Therefore, it is important to understand what compassion fatigue is, what causes it, and how to bolster resiliency. Otherwise, how can advanced practice nurses provide optimal care when not functioning at peak performance?

## Signs and Symptoms of Compassion Fatigue

The signs and symptoms of compassion fatigue are holistic and multifactorial. They can be physical, psychological, social, spiritual, and professional work manifestations. Physical symptoms can be vague and include somatic complaints like a headache and gastrointestinal distress (Lombardo & Eyre, 2011). Physical manifestations resulting from compassion fatigue can also be noted as a general malaise and fatigue. These physical symptoms may also exhibit as being nervous or upset, and they can create changes in sleep patterns (Lombardo & Eyre, 2011). These disturbed sleep patterns may include insomnia, excessive sleeping, decreased quality of sleep, or other sleep disorders (Gentry, 2013).

Psychologically we can be worn down and lose cognitive and emotional resilience. Forgetfulness, brain fog, and similar processes have been noted with compassion fatigue (Kearney *et al.*, 2009). These psychological symptoms can include emotional problems. The emotional manifestations can vary from rage, irritation, or impatience. The symptoms can vacillate across the spectrum depending on the individual. Sometimes memory and judgment can be impaired (Kearney *et al.*, 2009; Gentry, 2013). Other psychological manifestations may appear as substance use disorders that can range from mild to severe as described in the *Diagnostic and Statistical Manual of Mental Disorders, Fifth Edition* (DSM-5) (American Psychiatric Association, 2013) if the individual tries to self-medicate.

Social manifestations can include disinterest in life, difficulty tolerating others, and distancing self from social situations (Boyle, 2011). Disinterest in life can impact the self-care of the individual nurse, and in a like manner, the quality care of the patient or client for whom they are responsible. Together, with difficulty tolerating others, this disinterest can impact healthcare team dynamics and decrease the quality of healthcare service provided. Similarly, distancing self from social situations can impact self-care by alienating the social supports needed to foster emotional strength and resiliency (Gentry, 2013). As discussed above, these social manifestations of compassion fatigue can impact the nurse or other healthcare professional, patient, and healthcare environment.

Spiritual manifestations may also be impacted when the provider is not at their best. Compassion fatigue can lead to a decrease in spiritual self-expression and practices (Boyle, 2011). Spiritually, we may question our existence and our Higher Power's care for us and others.

Spiritual practices can bolster resilience and help individuals to accept and overcome coping difficulties. If spirituality has been a previous coping strategy and is now abandoned, the individual could experience difficulty resolving emotional and psychological issues related to their professional life. It is important to assess and realize the importance of the spiritual self-expression and practices, especially if spirituality is minimized because of the pain of compassion fatigue. Ultimately, this loss will have to be considered and not overlooked.

Professional manifestations include reduced interest in job performance and issues. Another key point is decreased job performance resulting in decreased quality of patient care (Boyle, 2011). Ethical practice may be impaired with decreased interest and ability for job performance (Lachman, 2016). In healthcare, ethical actions and attitudes must be maintained at all times.

Human beings are a process. When we feel physical, emotional, or spiritual pain, and/or social isolation, it impacts our whole self. We then do not interact with others at the same level or efficiency as when we are healthy. With this in mind, diminished interaction or quality interaction is important to consider when responsible for the care of others. Because of these potential dynamics, it is important to realize the symptoms and individual reactions to such as a system's response to compassion fatigue. It is easy to determine that self-evaluation and recognition are important to establishing self-care. All things considered, a behavioral system model of nursing such as the one developed by Dorothy Johnson (Petiprin, 2016), Calista Roy (Mitchell, 2007) or Neuman (Verberk & Fawcett, 2017) can help to view and synthesize the dynamics of compassion fatigue in nursing and help establish behavioral changes for life balance.

### Neuman's Healthcare Systems Model

The Neuman's Healthcare Systems Model centers around the client as a dynamic, open system (Lawson, 2017). This conceptualization provides a nursing framework to consider the impact of compassion fatigue and what can be done to prevent and address such. The conceptualization of individual needs is fluid, and the overall process is based on exploring the relationship between and within a system, such as an individual, community, nation, or world. This fluid exchange of energy is a healthy dynamic, and when it is closed due to addressing an overflow of stressors, health consequences emerge.

Neuman defines the client as an open system that interacts with the environment through behavioral adjustments, or the environment adapts to meet their personal needs (Bemker, 1997; Neuman & Fawcett, 2002). Client may be a person, group, family, community or another grouping. When elements are continuously exchanging energy and information between and within an organization, the system is said to be open (Bemker, 1997; Neuman & Fawcett, 2002).

Stress and reactivity to stress is a part of an open system, and does not necessarily delineate unhealthy dynamics. Without some stress, as an example, we would not get out of bed, eat meals, or care for ourselves in other ways. It is when stress overloads the system that problems become a reality (Bemker, 1997; Neuman & Fawcett, 2002). With compassion fatigue, however, an unhealthy response pattern is noted. This pattern can be demonstrated through physiological problems within the individual associated with health. Specifically, symptomatology from compassion fatigue can be seen as sleep disturbances, GI disorders, headaches, and other somatic manifestations.

Being a system, emotional and spiritual response patterns will also be impacted. Irritability; disassociation and apathy, depression, lowered self-esteem, pessimistic attitude, hopelessness and helplessness, lack of interest in activities, consumed by thought related to nursing care, and anger toward employers, peers, clients and others, are but a few of the unhealthy emotional responses noted with compassion fatigue. Loss of spirituality and decreased spiritual connection can be seen in many cases (Gentry, 2013). Connected to the physical attributes mentioned above, this holistic response pattern results in chronic, negative dynamics that lead to an unbalanced life.

When stress is generated, the client experiences changes within the physiological, psychological, sociocultural, developmental, and spiritual realms. The relationship between these various parts, facilitate a unique set of survival factors within the client that convey values within a range of options noted within most individuals (Gentry, 2013).

Cognitive response patterns can also be influenced by compassion fatigue. Difficulty with judgement and decision making, slowing of cognitive processing, and lack of connection to outcomes may be a result (Gentry, 2013). Knowing when this is occurring and caring about such may also have a disconnect when compassion fatigue is evidenced.

When a plethora of individuals within the healthcare organization experience compassion fatigue, the organization, as a client, becomes unhealthy. Cynicism and lack of connection to patient and employee needs are but two dynamics associated with an unhealthy work environment (Frampton & Goodrich, 2014; Iles, 2014; Markaki, 2014). Often, when this occurs, those who are not as impacted by unhealthy choices leave, and the system becomes unhealthier. It is during this state, that frequent lack of judgement within the system, errors, and other negative consequences can be noted.

A client's basic *structure* is protected by internal *lines of resistance* (resource factors that aid clients in defending their core against stressors) (Bemker, 1997; Neuman & Fawcett, 2002). With compassion fatigue, this could be noted as an individual shutting down their emotions and becoming apathetic. When overloaded with secondary stressors, the key process is for survival. While this can work in the short term, there are problems that will emerge when utilized for a terminal response. The amount of resistance is influenced by the interrelationship of the dynamics noted within the various parts of the client system. Balance between these parts aid in establishing state of adaptation that is known as a normal line of defense within Neuman's Model (Neuman & Fawcett, 2002).

When a client is in a stable state, a normal line of defense ensues (Bemker, 1997; Neuman & Fawcett, 2002). This is the standard that determines what the normal is for an individual. From that point forward, the client uses the normal line of defense to evaluate any deviations from wellness (Neuman & Fawcett, 2002). Coping patterns, work-life balance, and mental status are all evaluated from such. An enhanced state of wellness is evidenced when the normal line of defense is expanded (Neuman & Fawcett, 2002). Constriction of this line of defense conversely indicates a diminished state of health.

When an individual experiences stress, there is a system reaction that is followed by adaptation in an attempt for the client to return to a state of wellness. Interventions are needed when the flexible line of defense no longer can protect against a stressor(s). When this occurs, the stressor(s) breaches the normal line of defense, resulting in the lines of resistance around the central core of the client attempting to restore balance. This disequilibrium is the individual's way of coping, and restoring order and protection within the client. The circumstances that creates the stressors and imbalance within the client can vary between individuals, communities and organizations; these dynamics are dependent upon the spiritual, socio-cultural, developmental, physiological, and psychological condition within the client (Neuman & Fawcett, 2002).

**Framework**

Neuman and Fawsett (2002) describes the degree of reaction of an individual to a stressor as the amount of system instability occurring in response to being exposed to the stressor. This reaction is determined by natural and learned resistance, and it is evidenced by the strength of the lines of resistance and by the normal and flexible lines of defense. The amount of each individual's reaction to a stressor is based upon timing, type, and strength of the stimuli. An individual's core structure, experiences and energy resources also play a part in the overall impact, as does the individual's perception of the stressor. To adapt, the individual may try to cope by returning to and maintaining system stability. Through this reconstruction, a person may place themselves in a higher or lower state of wellness.

Noting this, it is easy to visualize the dynamic processes with compassion fatigue (Bemker, 2015). As an individual continually is impacted by stressors in response to others trauma and pain, additional instability occurs. Innate and learned response patterns to other's pain are applied and the normal line of defense is constricted. If the individual has enough healthy dynamics available, he or she will be able to ward off stress. However, once the system is worn down, disequilibrium results. At this point, ability to respond to additional stressors becomes more rigid.

*Case Vignette*

Ruth Rubenstein, a nurse educator in a master's program in advanced nursing practice, teaches the first course in the program. Ruth listens to the student's difficulty and negative feelings experienced in acclimating to the new program. While Ruth does not talk about the administration, faculty, or the program, she attempts to help students develop appropriate plans of action to be successful in their new environment. Over the last few years, she has realized the suggested interventions have produced little or no positive outcomes. She commiserates with students rather than offering viable options for their concerns.

Known for her empathy, students also bring personal issues or traumatic events to her. Thus, Ruth spends much of her personal and professional time thinking about these problems. She finds it even interferes with her sleep and she has illicit nightmares at times. Ruth feels emotionally depleted and unable to care as she used to. Think about some examples that need to be in healthcare outside of nursing.

Points to consider:

- Do you believe this case study typifies compassion fatigue?
- What criteria support this being considered compassion fatigue?
- Do you identify with this example?
- If you were in Ruth's position, how do you believe you would handle this?
- What would your top three priorities be for change?

## Compassion Fatigue versus Burnout

The terms compassion fatigue and burnout are often confused. However, each has their specific dynamics. While compassion fatigue reflects the response to others pain, burnout is a result of situational stress or personal stressor dynamics enacting upon the individual (Gentry, 2013). Burnout has been defined since the 1990's as a prolonged reaction to continuous emotional and interpersonal negative stimuli at a place of employment (Maslach, Jackson, & Leiter, 2010). Burnout exhibits itself as emotional exhaustion and fatigue. In healthcare, the individual can exhibit emotional disassociation from patients and clients, and decreased completion and satisfaction of professional duties or functions. Emotional, physical, and mental exhaustion is a hallmark of burnout. Burnout is a consequence generated from long-term exhaustion and distress that leads to diminished interest in daily life and results in physical, mental, and emotional exhaustion (Portnoy, 2011).

### Signs and Symptoms of Burnout

Common signs and symptoms of burnout include lack of motivation, cynicism, or criticism of work or employer, or difficulty starting tasks at work, irritability or impatience with management, coworkers and patients and families. Lack of productivity and overall satisfaction at work, disenchanted with employment and professional achievement. Abuse of drugs, alcohol, food, or other substances or actions to mask feelings. Changes in appetite or sleep patterns, unexplained physical manifestations such as headaches, general malaise or back pain (Mayo Clinic, 2017). Burnout can be a consequence of various dynamics including the feelings of mismatched professional values and the organizational culture, feeling little or no control over decisions; for example, employers demand versus individual choice. Related working conditions, such as staffing, resources, and workload. Blurry and ever changing job expectations, incivility, and negative dynamics, poor suitability of job match, lack of work life balance, lack of social, and professional supports. Burnout tends to focus on conflict and occurs over time, whereas compassion fatigue focuses more on emotional responses and can appear more quickly (Boyle, 2011). In conclusion, burnout focuses more on response to the organizational and external stressors.

### Case Vignette

Juan Ortega is a nurse practitioner that has worked in an emergency department in a large metropolitan medical center for four years. Juan works 12-hour shifts where he sees an average of 50 patients daily. He is often called into work early several days a week and has yet to get off work on time. The hospital has instituted a new mandatory overtime policy that extends to nurse practitioners requiring them to schedule at least one extra shift per week until further notice. Juan already feels that he has no social life and has lost contact with friends and family due to the high demands of his employment. Juan has learned to disassociate from his patients and coworkers to manage this demanding workload.

Even though Juan was originally hired to care for the emergency care walk-in clinic, he finds he is pulled to the trauma side of the emergency department intermittently where the majority of his patients have life-threatening illnesses. In addition, Juan is the part of the acute care team that is called upon to treat medical problems on the psychiatric floor. His employer is urging all nurse practitioners to complete their Doctorate Nursing Practice (DNP) within the next 18 months. To do this, Juan must go to an accelerated program that he does not feel he can be successful with at this time. One of his personal and professional goals is to obtain his DNP. His request to work part-time in order to be successful in this goal has gone unheeded by administration. The administration keeps promising to consider this when more nurse practitioners are hired. However, the medical center is unable to attract and retain new nurse practitioners. Juan does not have the energy to seek a new position. On rare days off, Juan feels exhausted and depressed and chooses to spend most of his time vegetating in front of the television or sleeping. Juan is dissatisfied with his health choices. He does not have time to go to the gym or fix healthy meals. Instead, he chooses fast food or convenient food from the grocery. Juan feels at the end of his rope. He believes all nurse practitioner positions are alike and going to another facility might not change anything. He contemplates leaving the profession altogether.

Points to consider:

- Do you believe this case study typifies burnout?
- What criteria supports the scenario being burnout? What does not?
- Do you identify with this example?
- If you were in Juan's position, how do you believe you would handle this?
- What would be your top 3 priorities for change?
- Most importantly, as an advanced practice nurse, what could you do to positively impact this work condition?

## How are Compassion Fatigue and Burnout Similar?

Compassion fatigue and burnout are similar in signs, symptoms, and manifestations. Burnout occurs over time and increases the effects of compassion fatigue (Craig & Sprang, 2010). Compassion fatigue, also known as secondary traumatic stress disorder develops over time because of working with patients and families experiencing trauma

(Figley, 1995a). Compassion fatigue like burnout has been associated with depersonalization of others, squelching of feelings and less than optimal patient care. Burnout is caused by long-term exposure to multifactorial stressors that results in physical, emotional, and mental exhaustion (Maslach, 1982). Burnout as a syndrome originated from psychologist Herbert Freudenberger (Freudenberger, 1977). Compassion fatigue is sometimes compared with burnout, but the causes are different. Another apt description to help one understand Compassion Fatigue is Compassion Exhaustion.

Consider the two previous case vignettes, how was Ruth's experience similar to and different than Juan's?

## Occupational Hazards

Characteristics of an unhealthy work environment create occupational hazards that contribute to the development of compassion fatigue. Occupational hazards, such as a professional and/or organizational culture that does not support a healthy lifestyle at work, can create compassion fatigue. Extended and/or irregular work hours, coupled with patients and clients with more aggressive or severe symptoms, are being noted in many healthcare environments. This in turn, supports an environment where Compassion Fatigue can flourish. An organizational culture that promotes depersonalization of a patient, and healthcare providers focusing on performing instead of providing compassionate care, also compound this dynamic (Patterson et al., 2011). Another environmental hazard that creates an unhealthy work culture is not being fully staffed. This can lead to increased work hours and exposure to secondary trauma. Couple this with shift changes, additional days being added to a work schedule and other work changes, and individual stress can increase. These variables added together do not offer a situation where an individual can address work dynamics in a healthy manner.

In addition, having a workforce that is relatively new (or at least new to that department), issues of lateral violence, not being able to attend functions that are important to the nurse or those significant in the nurse's life, all add up to increased stress and may be perceived as lack of organizational support. When this occurs over a short period, one can handle these changes. However, when they are repeatedly the norm, work-life balance becomes masque and the possibility of compassion fatigue increases.

## Compassion Satisfaction

Compassion Satisfaction is the positive emotions obtained from help-ing those we care for (Sacco, Ciurzynski, Harvey, & Ingersoll, 2015). Compassion Satisfaction can also be measured in the ProQOL 5, a tool developed by Beth Stamm, which includes questions about satisfaction derived from the work one does helping others (Professional Quality of Life Elements Theory and Measurement, 2015). In a study of criti-cal care nurses, Compassion Satisfaction results varied by age, educa-tion, and unit acuity (Sacco *et al.*, 2015). Compassion Satisfaction and Compassion Fatigue have demonstrated to inversely affect each other (Yoder, 2010). Thus, it can be deduced that increasing Compassion Satisfaction by individualizing interventions decreases Compassion Fatigue. One method, developed by Eric Gentry, includes developing mindfulness, education, and reducing stress (International Association of Trauma Professional [IATP], n.d.) to increase Compassion Satisfac-tion and develop a balance between Compassion Satisfaction and Com-passion Fatigue.

## Interventions to Decrease Compassion Fatigue

The identification and recognition of compassion fatigue symptoms are utmost in self-care revolving around compassion fatigue. A compas-sion fatigue measurement tool was developed by Beth Stamm called the Professional Quality of Life Elements Theory and Measurement Ver-sion 5 (ProQOL5) (Professional Quality of Life Elements Theory and Measurement, 2015). The ProQOL5 is a measurement tool for compas-sion satisfaction and compassion fatigue. In this tool, Stamm combines burnout and secondary traumatic stress as two integral parts of compas-sion fatigue. The tool has a self-grading key to allow the participant to complete and review the tool in privacy. This tool can provide the individual with insight to begin to recognize and take action to decrease compassion fatigue.

Knowing what is occurring within oneself allows for a clear under-standing of where one is in the overall process. Considering where one wants to be allows for developing a plan of action. This is the premise behind 5-year plans in career management. Once a clear goal is deter-mined, then specific actions to meet that goal can be developed. Short and long term goals can both support healthy change.

Interventions that can be performed to specifically decrease compassion fatigue include increasing or maintaining physical exercise. Physical exercise is considered one of the best ways to deal with stress as it relates to compassion fatigue (International Association of Trauma Professional [IATP], n.d.). Find something enjoyable to do. Make sure the activity does not feel like work (Cameron, 2016).

Another suggestion is to find a spiritual connection and expression through religion, meditation, and communing with nature (Berger, 2006). Determine what activities speak to you. Consider trying something new and incorporate that into your life. Include reading a motivational passage every day, as an example, can be a routine that supports positive thinking and recharges the spirit. Doing yoga for 15–30 minutes every evening can support in relaxing and preparing for sleep.

Think about what you would like to do and try it. For some, painting is a relaxing way to spend time and recharge. It is a means of being creative and provides an outlet for self-expression. For others, this is an anxiety producing experience that can cause more stress than what it might relieve. If the focus is on doing everything perfectly or feeling as if one has failed at the activity, choose something else to do for fun! There is no right or wrong here, other than what is right or wrong for you.

Nursing focuses on outcomes rather than the process. While we may be able to attain two or three small goals, we may not be able to accomplish all the goals set out for us. Therefore, as nurses, we may feel like failures if patient and nurse alike cannot achieve all the desired goals. An example of this could be a nurse practitioner without autonomous practice rights unable to contact the physician. Not being able to manage the pain of a patient, having little luck with known interventions, and not being able to consult with the primary physician can be frustrating at best. This scenario may appear to be insurmountable when looked at. What strategy might be utilized to make a small impact on the situation? Who else can serve as a resource in this situation? Is there something that can be done regarding the "thinking" of the patient rather than the physical dynamics that appear to be out of control? Is this a pattern with the physician or a onetime occurrence?

By looking at the process from a perspective where something might be accomplished (both long and short term), the overall process could be focusing on hope instead of hopelessness. Also, the development of focus on what can be accomplished instead of what is not able to be achieved is a proactive rather than a reactive dynamic (Professional Quality of Life Elements Theory and Measurement, 2015).

Maintain or develop social supports through family or family of choice. Encourage team building and professional peer support. Develop or maintain interests and relationships outside of work. Put an emphasis on developing work-life balance. Focus on positive aspects and outcomes in which your choices and actions make a difference at work and outside of work. Look at or perform focused solutions instead of just looking at problems.

Work on developing stress reducing strategies, such as joining support groups at work, journaling clubs to increase knowledge, and help build techniques to bolster resiliency. Mindfulness therapy, yoga therapy, art therapy, music therapy, and gardening, are all creative outlets that can be incorporated into the nurse's routines to reduce and minimize stress. Sleep and rest can decrease stress symptoms. Sleep disturbances are considered internal stressors that contribute to development of compassion fatigue (Beaumont & Hollins-Martin, 2016). Measures can be taken to increase rest and sleep benefits. These include making the sleeping area more conducive to restfulness. Interventions, such as removing or silencing electronics, like tablets, smart watches, and phones, adjusting the temperature and light in the sleeping room to individual sleeping preference, and considering some holistic alternatives (such as lavender therapy). Other actions to take would be to avoid heavy meals, caffeine and alcohol before bedtime (Carter, Dyer, & Mikan, 2013). Developing and following an individual sleep hygiene program can increase the quality and quantity of sleep and decrease stress (Miller, Shattuck, & Matsangas, 2011). Given these points, mindfully creating an internal and external, comfortable, and healthy sleeping environment, would be conducive to getting the quality and quantity of sleep needed to replenish the body and spirit.

## Interventions from the Advanced Practice Nurse to Decrease Compassion Fatigue

As advanced practice nurses, one can effect change on an institutional level using professional knowledge and leadership skills. As an advanced practice nurse, you are in a prime position to recognize and facilitate education about Compassion Fatigue. Compassion Fatigue education could be included in annual training like sexual harassment and other institutional policies. Compassion Fatigue self-evaluation, peer, and management evaluation, could be implemented in an attempt to recognize and eliminate or decrease Compassion Fatigue.

Nurse leaders are in a perfect position to decrease compassion fatigue and its ramifications (Romano, Trotta & Rich, 2013). Stress relieving modalities, such as Zumba, massage chairs, yoga, Pilates, Tai Chi, meditation, mindfulness training, nutrition, and wellness classes, can all be encouraged and facilitated immediately before or after work. These interventions can improve overall health and well-being, support work-life balance, and interject fun and relaxation into the nurse's life. In order to facilitate participation in these events, multiple offerings that are sensitive to nurses' schedules and accommodate all shifts need to be provided.

Also, structured activities, such as nurse huddles and journal clubs, can be used to promote team building, personal expression and group support. This, in turn, can facilitate a healthy work culture for all involved. Nurse huddles afford participants a quick, ongoing forum, where they can share stressors and traumatic events that may have occurred during their shift. In addition, this allows others to hear about what other nurses are experiencing and helps promote peer to peer support. By encouraging such sharing, acknowledgment of work stressors, and continuous debriefing are realized.

Journal clubs provide a venue for education and peer support. These clubs can be conducted face to face or in an asynchronous, online format. Relevant topics related to nursing and compassion fatigue can be included in this exchange. Knowledge related to prevention, intervention, and sources of compassion fatigue are but a few of the topics that can be considered in this format. Acknowledgment and acceptance that compassion fatigue can be a part of a nurse's life is key to attitudinal changes while addressing prevention and intervention processes.

Nurses need a quiet place for physical and emotional relaxation. This room needs to be separate from a break room and in an area, free from interruptions. In the literature, it has been called a healing room or renewal room (Romano, Trotta, & Rich, 2013). This room should include comfort measures that can be individualized to the needs of staff. Rules need to be established for this room to promote its purpose. This room needs to be free from stress and promote rejuvenation of mind, body, and spirit. Included in this room are such things as aroma therapy, reclining chairs, massage chairs, relaxing music or calming white noise, and lowering of lights. Headphones, partitions, and other means of separation can be provided so multiple participants can utilize the room without interruption. Décor should be simplistic and calming.

Healthcare facilities may not be able to provide all the amenities at first. However, the nurse leader should not allow this to prevent the start of this project. A few items can be included in a room at first, and additional resources can be added as budget allows. Having staff input is important, and promoting staff support as far as fundraising and continued development allows all to feel part of this important addition.

Many have utilized natural relaxation in areas already present on the campus grounds. Simply adding a bench in an area apart from the main entrances of the healthcare organization can provide an area of respite for staff. Like the room described above, this external site can begin small and be expanded as available. It will be important, however, that this area is specific for staff and strict rules for use be imposed so that the tranquil nature desired can be supported.

Labyrinths have been used as a means for meditation and contemplation. Permanent or temporary, labyrinths can be set up outside or inside and can be simple or elaborate. Examples of labyrinths used include a walking path painted on a large, durable fabric; paths cut into tall grasses; can be built of a hedge, and painted or tiled on wood or concrete.

Cumulative stress debriefings and support rounds (Griner, Shirk, Brown, & Hain, 2017) are peer-driven programs that leaders can implement and support. This style of debriefing validates the experiences of nurses with whom the leader works. By using scheduled periodic and as-needed debriefings, this structured intervention can provide and support healthy coping with stresses found in the healthcare setting.

Support rounds allow nurses to know that the leader is there and is interested in what the individual nurse is experiencing. Acting as a sounding board, resource, and advocate, a leader can use support rounds to check the overall needs and status of nurses under their direction. Additional understanding of work stressors, compassion fatigue dynamics, and other potential variables that could undermine the nurse's ability to provide safe and quality care, can also be assessed.

One of the most important roles of a nurse leader is to foster a culture of safety and a healthy work environment. Without this, the quality and care of nursing is put in jeopardy. In addition to impacting the patient directly, patient safety can be indirectly influenced by compassion fatigue dynamics. These may result from stressors noted in nurses responding to patients' reactions to their disease, prognosis, and overall environment in which they find themselves.

Whenever possible, best practices support work-life balance for nursing staff (Compassion Fatigue Awareness Project, 2015). If a nurse's life is primarily focused on work, it is much easier for compassion fatigue to develop. Having additional interests and life experiences can place what occurs at work to be a part of a nurse's life, not their entire life.

Conclusion thoughts include further research, using education, and coaching to decrease Compassion Fatigue. Also, increasing and disseminating knowledge about Compassion Fatigue to raise awareness and decrease the impact on caregivers will be important for a healthy ongoing resolution and management of Compassion Fatigue as it affects nursing.

**Tool Kit and Resources**

*Coping and Prevention of Compassion Fatigue*
This is a resource tool kit to help to provide education about Compassion Fatigue. It does not replace the care of your healthcare provider for any of your medical or psychological needs. Use for a ready reference and ideas for self and patients/clients.

*Fun Stuff for Relaxation*
This website suggests 29 Ways to Boost Your Mood When You Are Feeling Low HYPERLINK "http://diply.com/lessons/mental-health-tips-boost-your-mood-happy/155425/5" http://diply.com/lessons/mental-health-tips-boost-your-mood-happy/155425/5

*Printable Fall Bucket List* (from "http://www.avirtuouswoman.org/" www.avirtuouswoman.org) that includes activities like drinking apple cider and going on a nature walk. "https://app.box.com/s/w6b-fzgp66vsqfkhzhy98" https://app.box.com/s/w6bfzgp66vsqfkhzhy98

Relaxation for natural pain relief. This website offers insights into natural things that can assist with stress and pain. http://www.webmd.com/pain-management/guide/stress-relief-for-painUniversity of Maryland Medical Center Relaxation Techniques that are simple and easy to do.http://www.umm.edu/health/medical/altmed/treatment/relaxation-techniques" An example of a website where you can find quotes about joy, courage, and peace "http://www.heartsandminds.org/quotes/quotes.htm" http://www.heartsandminds.org/quotes/quotes.htm 35 positive affirmations that can brighten your dayhttp://www.huffington-post.com/dr-carmen-harra/affirmations_b_3527028.html

Exercise Choose something you like to get physical . . . walk in the park or go dancing. (Remember to check with your healthcare provider before starting an exercise program.)

*You Tube Videos*

Compassion Fatigue video for nurses created by Angela Synder. This is an animated video that discusses the main points in an easily understood format. https://www.youtube.com/watch?v=u6oiFIyhnUo

There are lots of YouTube videos on fun stuff to do. Did you always want to learn how to crochet or play a guitar? What about dancing and learning a new perspective through TED talks? Have some fun!

*Journal Articles*

This article discusses Compassion Fatigue and support from a Christian point of view. One of the points of interest in this article is the workplace ideas to decrease and address compassion fatigue. This article in the Journal of Christian Nursing can be read and completed as a Continuing Education (CE) of 2.5 contact hours for nurses until June 30, 2017. The CE has a fee. Harris, C., & Griffin, Q. T. (2015). Nursing on empty: Compassion fatigue signs, symptoms, and system interventions. *Journal of Christian Nursing, 32*(2), 80–87.

This article discusses ideas to promote a healthy work environment. One concept discussed is the correlation of increasing compassion satisfaction with decreased compassion fatigue. Harr, C. (2013). Promoting workplace health by diminishing the negative impact of compassion fatigue and increasing compassion satisfaction. *Social Work and Christianity, 40*(1), 71–88. http://dx.doi.org/

Figley in 1995(a) studied Compassion Fatigue and called it Secondary Traumatic Stress Disorder because the caregiver only experienced the stress as a secondary exposure. This book is a more technical read but does discuss some of the early discussions on Compassion Fatigue. This is included in the resource kit because many of the early thoughts started with Figley. Figley, C. R. (1995). Compassion Fatigue: Coping with Secondary Traumatic Stress Disorder In those who treat the traumatized (1st ed.). New York, NY: Routledge.Here is a workbook on the topic by Figley as well:http://www.figleyinstitute.com/documents/Workbook_AMEDD_SanAntonio_2012July20_RevAugust2013.pdf

This is a resource on Compassion Fatigue that can be completed for certification and continuing education credit for nurses and other healthcare professions. The CE is available at a cost through PESI Continuing Education. It is more technical in nature but comprehensive if more study on Compassion Fatigue or if continuing education credits is desired. PESI continuing education information can be found here: http://

www.pesihealthcare.com/ Gentry, E. (2013). Certified compassion fatigue professional training: Tools for hope [CD-ROM]. Eau Claire, Wisconsin: Premier Publishing and Media.

This article discusses compassion fatigue and compassion satisfaction. The article points out that compassion fatigue can be decreased by compassion satisfaction. A correlation in patient satisfaction is seen also when the caregivers have more satisfaction. Strategies to increase compassion satisfaction are also discussed. Burton, P. L., & Stichler, J. F. (2010). Nursing work environment and nurse caring: relationship among motivational factors. *Journal of Advanced Nursing, 66,* 1819–1830. http://dx.doi.org/doi: 10.1111/j.1365-2648.2010.05336.x

This article by Houck discusses coping techniques to handle compassion fatigue and grief. The target audience discussed is oncology nursing which is applicable to Hosparus nursing. Houck, D. (2014, August). Helping nurses cope with grief and compassion fatigue: An educational intervention. *Clinical Journal of Oncology Nursing, 18*(4), 454–458. http://dx.doi.org/10.1188/14.CJON.454-458

This article by Joinson is older, but it is one of the first articles specifically addressing compassion fatigue in the nursing profession. Although different groups can experience compassion fatigue, nursing and primary care givers are unique in intimate and sustained contact. Joinson, C. (1992). Coping with Compassion Fatigue. *Nursing, 22*(4), 116, 118–9, 121. Retrieved from http://www.lwwonline.com/pt/re/lwwonline

This article discusses the effects of death and Compassion Fatigue tendencies. Melvin, C. S. (2012, December 18). Professional compassion fatigue: What is the true cost of nurses caring for the dying? *International Journal of Palliative Nursing, 18*(12), 606–611. Retrieved from http://www.magonlinelibrary.com/toc/ijpn/current

The Ohio Nurses Association (2012) has a brief and easy to read article on Compassion Fatigue and caregivers. Ohio Nurses Association (2012, May, June, July). I've fallen and I can't get up: Compassion Fatigue in nurses and nonprofessional caregivers. Indiana State Nurses Association Bulletin, 5–9. Retrieved from

Walton and Alvarez (2010) discuss Compassion Fatigue training for nurses. The article addresses the need to educate caregivers on Compassion Fatigue interventions. This is a great perspective to help reduce the incidence or severity in caregivers. Walton, A. M., & Alvarez, M. (2010). Imagine: Compassion fatigue training for nurses. *Clinical Journal of Oncology Nursing, 14*(4), 399–400. http://dx.doi.org/10.1188/10.

CJON.399-400

This article discussed Hospice caregivers specifically and some of the challenges and interventions to help them. Boundary setting is important to decrease the effects of Compassion Fatigue in helping professions and situations. This article discusses specifically setting professional boundaries to help the caregiver to cope in a healthier manner.

Anewalt, P. (2009). Fired up or burned out? Understanding the importance of professional boundaries in home healthcare hospice. *Home Healthcare Nurse, 27*(10), 591–597.

*Other Information of Interest*

Naomi Rachel Remen quote, "The expectation that we can be immersed in suffering and loss daily and not be touched by it is as unrealistic as expecting to be able to walk through water without getting wet." Her website can be found here. http://www.rachelremen.com/The website lists her books that are available; for example Kitchen Table Wisdom: Stories that Heal. The site also has a sample of her writings with self-care ideas including journaling about healing yourself. Other examples of self-care included on her site include yoga: Remember the heart: A 90 second heart yoga. http://www.rachelremen.com/learn/self-care/Rachel Naomi Remen MD: Remembering your power to heal. (2012). http://www.rachelremen.com/

The website Proquol.org contains resource links on compassion fatigue and a pocket handout on self-care that can be laminated for use. A self-scoring questionnaire on compassion fatigue developed by Beth Stamm is available at this website with other supportive resources. Professional Quality of Life Elements Theory and Measurement. (2015). http://www.proqol.org/Home_Page.php

> *"Happiness can be found in even the darkest times,*
> *if only one remembers to turn on the light"*
> —J.K. Rowling

*Definitions*

*Compassion Fatigue, aka Secondary Traumatic Stress* (Valent, 1995)—
The consequences from caring for others who are experiencing trauma or pain, and is usually coupled with burnout. The caring connection may be with a small group of individuals over an extended period of time, or they may be multiple experiences with a short duration.

*Compassion Satisfaction*—Feelings generated when hope is a part of an individual's interaction with others - individually, family, community, etc.

*Coping Skills*—Conscious effort to provide personal strategies and interventions that reduce the potential for anxiety and stress.

*Hopelessness*—Feeling that no matter what is done, the situation will not change for the better.

*Self-care*—Integrating thoughts and experiences into one's life that nourishes the spirit and soul of the individual. Activities, such as stress and anxiety reduction, are examples of self-care. (Valent, 1995)

*Discussion Questions*

1. Have students develop an area for healthcare professionals that can rejuvenate them at work. The area needs to have at least five components to it, and there needs to be a rationale for the inclusion of items or events. For example, an outside area away from most could be developed for rejuvenation. A labyrinth could be cut in the grass for contemplative time. Picnic tables could be painted with chalkboard material, and various colors of chalk could be located at the site. An outside reading library with short stories, meditations, etc., could be available for employee breaks. An area could be mowed where Tai Chi, yoga, and other relaxation activities could be done individually and as a group.

2. Explain the rationale behind nurses and other healthcare providers being more susceptible to CF that the general population. What specific actions can advanced practice nurses take to prevent such from occurring?

3. Work life balance is key to a healthy lifestyle. Develop three objectives for advanced practice nurses related to such. Link specific activities to these objectives. Identify actions as easy to attain, moderate to attain, or difficult to attain. Provide rationale.

4. Develop a one year plan that integrates self-care into it. Make certain the plan includes a work component, a personal component, and a leisure component to it. Explain why you believe this plan will foster healthy life choices and serve to prevent CF.

5. As an APRN you are a leader in the community and at your employment. As a leader, it is important to foster health and support our colleagues. What are some signs that you would look for to identify CF in others who work with you? If you noticed these

signs, how would you address the situation? (Be specific and provide rationale)

6. Develop a YouTube video individually or in groups. The video needs to focus on one of the following:

   • Signs and Symptoms of CF among healthcare professionals
   • Recipe for healthy living—Compassion Satisfaction
   • A day in the life—typical dynamics in a healthcare professional's work time and dynamics linked to a work-life balance (e.g., sitting down for a meal!)
   • Any topic pre-approved by instructor and linked to this CF. Figley, C. R. (1995b)

## Case Study 1

*Compassion Fatigue*

Andrea Garcia, a 42-year-old circulating nurse in the Operating Room, has been feeling lethargic and dreading going to work. She has shared with her fellow nurses that she can't sleep at night unless she has a few drinks. She was previously known for being the peacemaker in the OR, and in the last six months several instances have been noted where she has snapped at surgeons, other nurses, and techs. She complains that all her previous interests outside of work are just too draining, and she tells her nurses that she tends to work and go home and try to sleep.

Andrea feels as if she can never do anything right anymore. Her room does not have the items she needs for each case, and she has been described as turning into *Robo Nurse*. Her affect is flat, and she just focuses on the task.

Andrea has thought about getting a physical checkup. She reports she is forgetful and she wishes that patients would come in already anesthetized so she did not have to interact with them. While she was originally the nurse that spoke the longest and was the most reassuring in the OR, she is tired of hearing about their pain and does not connect any longer when patients talk about their concerns regarding the operation's outcomes. She shared with the Chief Nurses Anesthetist that she believes these patients are just faking it all, and that they are not in as much pain as they used to be. Despite what Andrea states, she finds that she often thinks about the cases and what patients have said on her drive home and many times while she is trying to get to sleep. To try and deal with this, Andrea no longer looks at her assignments for the next day. If she does, she focuses on what the day will be like, all the "horror and drama" that will be surrounding these cases, and her lack of control over these instances. All of this makes Andrea feel hopeless.

Shifts were changed without nurses in the OR being consulted. The new hours are longer, and nurses are expected to work swing shifts to cover all shifts. Pay will remain the same. This is causing major problems for Andrea, since she will no longer be able to work a part time job at a local surgical clinic. She and her spouse are already disagreeing about the finances, and this is just one more variable that is creating problems for her at home.

- Based upon this scenario, is Andrea experiencing Compassion Fatigue?
- What criteria did you use to make this determination?
- Should she speak to her manager about her concerns?
- How could she use the other nurses as a support system?
- Should she seek outside help?
- What do you consider her most pressing issue as presented here?
- Should any of these issues be brought forth in staff meetings so that other nurses can chime in?
- Contribution by Camille McNicholas PhD, APRN, CRNA

**Case Study 2**

Nicholas Jenkins is a 36-year-old nurse who has worked for Hospice for 10 years. He is reluctant to go into work because of all the infighting and incivility that he sees at his workplace. He is being asked to work an additional 10 hours a week, and that brings his total workload to 50 hours. He states that he enjoys working with the patients and providing them comfort.

- Do you believe that Nicholas is demonstrating compassion fatigue?
- What additional information would you like to have to make a clear determination?
- What strategies would you provide Nicholas in addressing the issues he presents here?

**Case Study 3**

Geri Falcon has worked in the Emergency Department for 25 years. She manages the department and gets along well with others. Recently

Geri has been moved to the 7 pm to 7 am shift. She reports difficulty sleeping for long periods when she gets home, and she complains of nightmares.

The ED where Geri works is very busy so her shift goes by quickly. Her ED is part of a major trauma center and they are busy all night long. Geri complains that she is always tired of hearing other nurses cry if a patient is lost. She believes that nurses need to buck up and be brave when dealing with these situations. She stated she learned a long time ago that having "sappy feelings" gets in the way of things.

- If you were assessing Geri for possible compassion fatigue, what would be the indicators that she might have this problem in her life?
- What else would you want to know about Geri's situation to make a more accurate determination?
- If Geri did have compassion fatigue, what would you recommend she do to support compassion satisfaction in her life?

## References

American Psychiatric Association. (2013). Diagnostic and statistical manual of mental disorders (5th ed). Washington, DC: American Psychiatric Association.

Beaumont, E. & Hollins-Martin, C. J. (2016). *British Journal of Midwifery, 26*(11), 777–786. Retrieved from http://dx.doi.org/10.12968/bjom.2016.24.11.777

Bemker, M. (2015). Compassion fatigue. *Nevada Information. 25*(1), 16.

Bemker, M.A. (1997). Adolescent female substance abuse: Risk and resiliency factors. *Dissertation Abstracts International, 57,* 75446B.

Berger, R. M. (2006). Prayer: It does a body good. *Sojourners Magazine, 35*(17). Retrieved from https://sojo.net/

Billings, D. M. & Halstead, J. A. (Eds.). (2012). Creating interactive learning environments using media and digital media. *Teaching in Nursing: A guide for faculty* (4th ed., pp. 369–385). St Louis, MO: Elsevier.

Boyle, D. A. (2011). Countering compassion fatigue: A requisite nursing agenda. *The Online Journal of Issues in Nursing, 16*(1). Retrieved from http://dx.doi.org/10.3912/OJIN.Vol16No01Man02

Cameron, J. (2016). *The artist's way: A spiritual path to higher creativity* (25th Anniversary ed.). New York, NY: Tarcher Perigee.

Carter, P. A., Dyer, K. A., & Mikan, S.Q. (2013). Sleep disturbance, chronic stress, and depression in Hospice nurses: Testing the feasibility of an intervention. *Oncology Nursing Forum, 40*(5), 368–373. Retrieved from http://dx.doi.org/10.1188/13.ONF.E368-E373

Compassion Fatigue Awareness Project. (2015). Retrieved from http://www.compassionfatigue.org/index.html

Craig, C. D. & Sprang, G. (2010, May). Compassion satisfaction, compassion fatigue, and burnout in a national sample of trauma treatment therapists. *Anxiety, Stress, & Coping, 23*(3), 319–339. Retrieved from http://dx.doi.org/10.1080/10615800903085818

Durkin, M., Smith, J., Powell, M., Howarth, & Carson, J. (2013). Wellbeing, compassion fatigue and burnout in APs. *British Journal of Healthcare Assistants, 7*(9), 456–459.

Empathy. (n.d.). In Merriam-Webster.com. Retrieved from https://www.merriam-webster.com/dictionary/empathy

Emergency Department Association (ENA). (2014). Compassion fatigue. Retrieved from https://www.ena.org/practice-research/Practice/Documents/CompassionFatigue.pdf

Figley, C. R. (1995). *Compassion Fatigue: Coping with Secondary Traumatic Stress Disorder In those who treat the traumatized* (1st ed.). New York, NY: Routledge.

Frampton, S. & Goodrich, J. (2014). Current initiatives for transforming organizational cultures and improving the patient experience. In Shea, S., Wynyard. R., & Lionis, C. (Eds). (pp.197–213). Providing Compassionate Healthcare: Challenges in Policy and Practice. New York: Routledge.

Freudenberger, H. J. (1977). Burnout: Occupational hazard of the child care worker. *Child and Youth Care Forum, 6*, 90–99.

Gentry, E. (2013). Certified compassion fatigue professional training: Tools for hope [CD-ROM]. Eau Claire, Wisconsin: Premier Publishing and Media.

Griner, T. E., Shirk, M., Brown, G., & Hain, P. (2017). Cumulative stress debriefings: Support for clinicians and nurse leaders. *Nurse Leader, 15*(1), 53–55.

Harris, C., & Griffin, M. (2015). Nursing on empty: compassion fatigue signs, symptoms, and system interventions. *Journal of Christian Nursing, 32* (2), 80–87.

Hooper, C., Craig, J., Janvrin, D. R., Wetsel, M. A., & Reimels, E. (2010, September). Compassion Satisfaction, Burnout, and Compassion Fatigue among Emergency Nurses compared with nurses in other selected inpatient specialties. *Journal of Emergency Nursing, 36*(5), 420–427. Retrieved from http://dx.doi.org/10.1016/j.jen.2009.11.027

Hunsaker, S., Chen, H., & Heaston, S. (2015). Factors that influence the development of compassion fatigue, burnout, and compassion satisfaction in emergency department nurses. *Journal of Nursing Scholarship, 37*(2), 186–194. http://dx.doi.org/doi:10.1111/jnu.12122

Iles, V. (2014). How good people can offer bad care: understanding the wider factors in society that encourage non-compassionate care. In Shea, S., Wynyard, R., & Lionis, C. (Eds). (pp. 183–196). Providing Compassionate Healthcare: Challenges in Policy and Practice. New York: Routledge.

International Association of Trauma Professional. (n.d.). *Certified Compassion Fatigue Professional*. Retrieved from traumapro.net

Joinson, C. (1992). *Coping with Compassion Fatigue. Nursing, 22*(4), 116, 118–9, 121. Retrieved from http://www.lwwonline.com/pt/re/lwwonline

Kearney, M., Weininger, R., Harrison, R., Mount, B., Kearney, M., Weininger, R., Vachon, M., Harrison, R., & Mount, B. (2009). Self-care of physicians caring for patients at the end of life: "Being connected... a key to my survival". *JAMA, 301*(11), 1155-E1.

Lachman, V. D. (2016). Ethics, law, and policy. Compassion fatigue as a threat to ethical practice: Identification, personal and workplace prevention/management strategies. *MEDSURG Nursing, 25*, 275–278. Retrieved from http://www.medsurgnursing.net

Lawson, T. (2017). Betty Neuman: Systems model. In Allgood, M. (Ed.) *Nursing Theorists and Their Work*. (281–302). St. Louis, MO: Elsevier.

Lombardo, B. & Eyre, C. (2011). Compassion fatigue: A nurse's primer. *The Online Journal of Issues in Nursing, 16*(1). Retrieved from http://dx.doi.org/10.3912/OJIN.Vol16No01Man03

Markaki, A. (2014) In Shea, S., Wynyard, R., & Lionis, C. (Eds). Understanding and protecting against compassion fatigue. (pp. 214–232). Providing Compassionate Healthcare: Challenges in Policy and Practice. New York: Routledge.

Maslach, C. (1982). *Burnout: The cost of caring*. Englewood Cliffs: NJ: Spectrum.

Maslach, C., Jackson, S. E., & Leiter, M. P. (2010). *Maslach burnout inventory manual* (3rd ed.). Menlo Park, CA: Mind Garden.

Mayo Clinic. (2017). Job burnout: How to spot it and take action. Retrieved from https://www.mayoclinic.org/healthy-lifestyle/adult-health/in-depth/art-20046642?p=1

McCann, L. & Pearlman, L. A. (1990). Vicarious traumatization: A framework for understanding the psychological effects of working with victims. *Journal of Traumatic Stress, 3*(1), 131–149. Retrieved from http://dx.doi.org/10.1007/BF00975140

Miller, N. L., Shattuck, L. G., & Matsangas, P. (2011). Sleep and fatigue issues and continuous operations: A survey of U.S. Army officers. *Behavioral Sleep Medicine, 9*, 53–68.

Minority Nurse. (2013, March 30). Rethinking gender stereotypes in nursing. Minority Nurse. Retrieved from http://minoritynurse.com/rethinking-gender-stereotypes-in-nursing/

Mitchell, G. (2007). Picturing the nurse-person/family/community process in the year 2050. *Nursing Science Quarterly, 20*(1), 43–44.

Neuman B. & Fawcett J. (2002). *The Neuman Systems Model* (4th ed.). Upper Saddle River, NJ: Prentice Hall.

Patterson, M., Nolan, M., Rick, J., Brown, J., Adams, R., & Musson, G. (2011). *From metrics to meaning: Culture change and quality of acute hospital care for older people*. Retrieved from http://www.nihr.ac.uk/

Peery, A. (2010). Caring and burnout in registered nurses: What's the connection? *International Journal for Human Caring, 14*(2), 53–60.

Petiprin, A. (2016). *Health behavioral theory*. Retrieved from http://www.nursing-theory.org/theories-and-models/johnson-behavior-system-model.php

Portnoy, D. (2011, July/August). Burnout and compassion fatigue: Watch for the signs. *Health Progress*. Retrieved from Health progress.pdf

Professional Quality of Life Elements Theory and Measurement. (2015). http://www.proqol.org/Home_Page.php

Romano, J., Trotta, R., & Rich, V. (2013). Combating Compassion Fatigue: An exemplar of an approach to nursing renewal. *Nursing Administration Quarterly, 37*(4), 333–336. Retrieved from http://dx.doi.org/10.1097/NAQ.0b013e3182a2f9ff

Sabin, K. (2013). Compassion fatigue in liver and kidney transplant nurse coordinators: A descriptive research study. *Progress in Transplantation, 23*(4), 329–335.

Sacco, T. L., Ciurzynski, S. M., Harvey, M. E., & Ingersoll, G. L. (2015). Compassion Satisfaction and Compassion Fatigue among Critical Care Nurses. *Critical Care Nurse, 35*(4), 32–42. Retrieved from http://dx.doi.org/10.4037/ccn2015392

Seager, M. (2014) Who cares for the carers? Keeping compassion alive in care systems, cultures and environments. In S. Shea, R. Wynyard, &C. Lionis (Eds.) *Providing Compassionate Helathcare: Challenges in Policy and Practice.* NewYork, NY: Routledge.

Severn, M., Searchfield, G., & Huggard, P. (2012). Occupational stress amongst audiologists: Compassion satisfaction, compassion fatigue, and burnout. *International Journal of Audiology, 51*(1), 3–9.

"Sympathy." Merriam-Webster.com. Merriam-Webster, n.d. Web. 30 Apr. 2017.

Valent, P. (1995). Survival Strategies: A Framework for Understanding Secondary Traumatic Stress and Coping in Helpers. In C. R. Figley (Ed.) *Compassion fatigue: Coping with secondary traumatic stress disorder in those who treat the traumatized.* NY: Brunner/Mazel. pp. 21–50. ISBN 9780876307595.

van der Wath, A., van Wyk, N. & van Rensburg, E. (2013). Emergency nurses' experiences of caring for survivors of intimate partner violence. *Journal of Advanced Nursing, 69* (10), 2242–2252.

Verberk, F., & Fawcett, J. (2017). Thoughts about created environment: A Neuman Systems Model Concept. *Nursing Science Quarterly, 30*(2), 181–183.

Yoder, E. A. (2010). Caring too much: Compassion Fatigue in Nursing. *Applied Nursing Research, 23*(4), 191–197. Retrieved from http://www.appliednursingresearch.org/

## CHAPTER 17

# The Use of Social Marketing in Population Health Nursing

NANCYRUTH LEIBOLD, EdD, RN, PHN, CNE

LAURA M. SCHWARZ, DNP, RN, CNE

## The Use of Social Marketing in Population Health Nursing

SOCIAL MARKETING (SOCMRKT) is a strategy that can reach populations with health messages to improve the quality of life. As advanced practice nurses (APNs), the value and role of social marketing and use of social media cannot be underestimated. Sometimes social media are a medium in social marketing campaigns. Much like a television advertisement, social media is one means to the SOCMRKT project. This chapter is an exploration of the concept of SOCMRKT and mediums of SOCMRKT, such as social media, as well as other marketing mediums and their relevance to population health. The process of SOCMRKT, including the 8 Ps (Weinreich, 2011), theories, examples, evidence, and how nurses can use SOCMRKT to target populations with healthy messages, is the focus on this chapter.

## Social Media

Social media and social marketing (SOCMRKT) are not the same thing. Social media are techniques within the application of SOCMRKT. Social media are online social software that allows individuals to interact with each other, such as twitter and Facebook (Affinito & Mack, 2016). Through social media, people can communicate, share information, and collaborate (Fung, Tse, & Fu, 2015). Social media allows public health officials and providers to communicate health messages to populations (Kass-Hout & Alhinnawi, 2013). Additionally, health papers are often tweeted (Haustein, Peters, Sugimoto, Thelwall, & Lariviere, 2014), alerting the information to others in population health. The use of social media is an emerging area in public health surveillance (Fung *et al.*, 2015; Eggleston & Weitzman, 2014; Eke, 2011). One use is epidemiologic monitoring for information to detect for disease outbreaks, and estimate the forecasts of disease incidences (Fung *et al.*, 2015). During disasters, social media helps families and friends track each other, as well as alert where help is essential.

SOCMRKT campaigns engage populations by using social media. Lister et al. (2015) describe the use of The Laugh Model. The Laugh Model is a framework of using social media and technology to transmit health messages designed to change behaviors in the online forum (Lister *et al.*, 2015). The Laugh Model engages populations in two-way communication about healthy messages in a low-budget forum (cost per person reached reported as 0.2 cents). A business-like approach to market public health messages by public health organizations promotes health information campaigns. Lister *et al.* (2015) describe a SOCMRKT campaign in Utah to promote healthy family meals through social media using Facebook, Twitter, Pinterest, and Instagram.

Huesch, Galstyan, Ong, and Doctor (2016) studied the use of social media, online social networks, and internet searches, as mediums for public health interventions. Specifically, the targeted populations were women and the area of maternity care. The researchers wanted to know if the target population would use social media to access health information. Public health maternity messages to influence the behavior of the target population were posted using Twitter, Facebook, and Google. The researchers report that over 140,000 consumers each day accessed Twitter, Facebook, and Google searches in Los Angeles for health information. It was concluded that the social media platforms were used by the population daily. The cost for the number of people reached was reported by Huesch *et al.* (2016) as low at about $1 per targeted consumer. This is a low-cost intervention strategy.

Not all social media is SOCMRKT. Communications on social media may be social with no mention of health. Some social media does not include a plan with a healthy message or even have intended products for a target population. Not all SOCMRKT includes social media. The medium used, or the place and promotion (as discussed in a future section of this chapter) may not be social media. Social media may not be the best choice for all target populations. For example, some elderly may not use social media, so this would not be an effective way to reach this population. As time passes, more elderly people are connected to social media. APNs can find data on populations by age groups (as well as education levels, income levels, and rural/urban/suburban dwellers) at the Pew Research Center website. According to Greenwood, Perrin, and Duggan (2016), 62% of adults over the age of 65 years use Facebook, whereas only 8% use Instagram, and 10% use Twitter. APNs should consider data on populations when planning SOCMRKT campaigns to best match the medium to the target audience.

Other limitations of social media include the need for electronic equipment, internet, and the unwanted consequences of some communications. Some people may engage in unwanted and unhealthy behaviors after social media interactions. One pitfall of social media relates to suicide risk, which may increase in some vulnerable groups after using social media (Luxton, June, & Fairall, 2012). In a research review by McCreanor *et al.* (2013), one concern was that in the young adult population, pro-alcohol drinking behaviors may be exhibited on social media by telling pro-drinking stories that over glorify drinking on social media. These unwanted consequences of social media are important for advanced practice nurses to consider when designing SOCMRKT campaigns.

## Social Marketing (SOCMRKT)

Social media (Snapchat, Twitter, Facebook, etc.) are common electronic mediums for delivering messages (see Figure 17.1), but SOCMRKT is the utilization of the best marketing practices to employ social media and other forms of communication. SOCMRKT uses marketing principles aimed at changing knowledge levels, attitudes, values, beliefs, behaviors, and practices of the intended population (Keller, Strohschein, Lia-Hoagberg & Schaffer, 2004).

According to Harvey (1999), SOCMRKT started in India during the 1960s to promote family planning education. Since then, it has spread to use across the world to promote a variety of health messages. In the 1970s, SOCMRKT became a discipline (Weinreich, 2011). SOCMRKT varies from commercial marketing in that the purpose of SOCMRKT is not to make profits, but to change behaviors (Sharma, 2017). According to Weinreich (2011), some common examples of issues used in SOCMRKT campaigns are breastfeeding, breast cancer, condom use, high

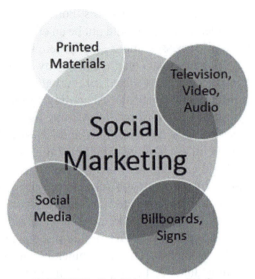

*FIGURE 17.1.  Social Marketing and Mediums*

blood pressure, violence, HIV/AIDS, immunizations, physical activity, and recycling.

An approach to tackling a frustrated or concerned consumer by developing a creative solution is interwove with the notion of SOC-MRKT. For example, a consumer who wants to know about women's health and lacks education on the area, is online reading the news and sees information about women's health. This easy find is an opportunity for the person to learn the information he or she wants and provide a public health message. However, there are many other mediums for SOCMRKT, such as billboards, signs, television advertisements, pamphlets, posters, and other materials with health messages. Examples of other promotional materials with health messages are pencils, water bottles, t-shirts, bags, etc., SOCMRKT is the application of commercial marketing principles aimed at influencing and improving behavior in a group (Doyle, Ward, & Oomen-Early, 2010; Goldman, 2003).

## Concepts of Population, Community, Subpopulation, Aggregate, and Stakeholders

The American Nurses Association (2013) defines population as "the total number of people living in a specific geographical area (e.g., town, city, state, region, nation, multinational region)" (p. 3).

"A *community* is a set of people in interaction, who may or may not share a sense of place or belonging, and who act intentionally for a common purpose" (for example, living in a neighborhood or sharing a health concern) (American Nurses Association, 2013, p. 3).

According to the American Nurses Association (2013) *subpopulations*, *groups*, or *aggregates* consist of people experiencing a specific health condition (e.g., disease, disabilities, pregnancy); engaging in behaviors that have the potential to negatively affect health (e.g., smoking tobacco); or sharing a common risk factor or risk exposure, or experiencing an emerging health threat or risk (e.g., victims of a disaster or a disease outbreak) (pg. 3).

A *stakeholder* is defined by the American Nurses Association (2013) as "a person or organization that has a legitimate interest in what the public health entity does" (p. 68).

## Benefits of SOCMRKT in Population Health

The most obvious benefit of SOCMRKT is the positive change it can result in, cause, or bring about (Weinreich, 2011) in a health area. Enablers and barriers to SOCMRKT in public health nursing were studied by researchers Knibbs and Leeseberg Stamler (2009). Enablers reported by public health nurses are learning about SOCMRKT in their baccalaureate nursing education, evidence-based, and the client-centered approach. Another reported enabler is the trusting relationships that public health nurses have with the community. Recently, baccalaureate nurse education has included basic social marketing knowledge. However, SOCMRKT may not have been an included content area for nurses who completed their baccalaureate nursing education prior to 2009 (Knibbs & Leeseberg Stamler, 2009). Advanced practice nurses have an opportunity to lead the way for teams in the workplace regarding social marketing to improve health outcomes.

Other benefits to organizations are publicity that SOCMRKT could bring. Trusted health messages may impact consumers to choose a specific hospital (Peck, 2014). A communication strategy and SOCMRKT policy are for organizations to be clear that there is some control and direction to the messages attached to their organization name (Ramsay, 2011). SOCMRKT is a cost-effective way to promote population health messages (Cecchini *et al.*, 2010; Huesch *et al.*, 2016; Lister *et al.*, 2015) aimed at improving health.

## Limitations of SOCMRKT in Population Health

SOCMRKT campaigns require many resources, such as human, time, and money. SOCMRKT is very time consuming to create. Barriers to SOCMRKT reported by public health nurses were heavy workloads, time constraints, and lack of role clarity for the nurse (Knibbs & Leeseberg Stamler, 2009). Knibbs and Leeseberg propose continuing education in SOCMRKT and increases in public health nurse staffing to address the concerns (2009). Additionally, monies are required to implement SOCMRKT in population health. Often, population health budgets are lacking appropriate resources to fund SOCMRKT.

The confusion about the concepts of social media and SOCMRKT is another limitation. Weinreich (2011) explains that SOCMRKT is not just the use of health messages or educational materials to communicate, but a well-intended program that uses a systematic process of SOCMRKT. This requires knowledge about the SOCMRKT process and the ability to lead and implement a SOCMRKT campaign. Weinreich (2011) cautions against the confusion of SOCMRKT and social media marketing as these two terms are not the same. Social media marketing does not use the SOCMRKT process that intentionally plans campaigns for maximal impact.

## Theoretical Foundations of SOCMRKT

SOCMRKT is based on marketing theory and theories of planned behavior change. Several theories of planned behavior change are good possible fits for SOCMRKT to improve health behaviors. Each campaign should include the theory of planned behavior change that is the most suitable. These theories can help nurses understand how to help populations improve health behaviors. A review of marketing theory, transtheoretical model, and behavioral modification are included in this section.

### Marketing Theory

Marketing principles include a systematic inclusion of managing consumer relationships with the product, costs, benefits, and how to access the product (Lefebrve, 2013). The use of marketing principles in business has a significant impact on the sales and profits of companies that target marketing toward specific consumers (Lefebvre, 2013). Marketing theory is driven by selling the product for profit because of the intervention.

## Key Differences Between Marketing and Social Marketing

According to Weinreich (2011), there are key differences between marketing and social marketing. Marketing focuses on the consumer with a motive that the consumer will make a purchase to benefit the marketer. In contrast, with social marketing, the focus is on the product (a healthy message) with a motive to increasing health to benefit the population. In population health and SOCMRKT, the product is the health message.

## Transtheoretical Model

The transtheoretical model (TTM) explains the change of behavior over time in stages (Gilbert, Sawyer, & McNeill, 2015). A brief synopsis of the stages is explained next (Diehr *et al.*, 2011; Gilbert *et al.*, 2015; Sharma, 2017). During the first stage, known as the *precontemplation* stage, the person has no intent on making a change for the next six months. In the second stage of *contemplation*, the individual understands the need for a change. Throughout the third stage, *preparation*, one plans for the change that is soon to occur. The fourth stage, or the action stage, is when a deliberate change occurs. The *maintenance* stage is the fifth stage to occur, in which the change of behavior has been sustained for about six months. The stages are linear in this description, but happen in a variety of orders and regression may occur (Sharma, 2017). Individuals move through the TTM stages at varying rates.

## Behavioral Modification

The use of SOCMRKT in public health to improve health behaviors of a group fits with behavioral modification (Hastings, Angus, & Bryant, 2011). Behavioral modification is apt for public health campaigns designed at decreasing or stopping a given behavior, such as *do not text and drive*. Likewise, behavioral modification is appropriate for increasing a behavior, such as physical activity for at least 30 minutes a day. Reinforcement (positive and negative) and punishment (positive and negative) are the main premises of behavioral modification. Ways to increase a behavior include positive reinforcement (a desirable consequence) or negative reinforcement (removal of a negative consequence). For example, to increase physical activity to at least 30 minutes per day, a positive reinforcement is to hike at a park and enjoy nature. An example of negative reinforcement is the effect of naturally lowering the person's blood pressure. Punishment to decrease or stop an unwanted behavior uses positive punishment (an undesirable consequence) or negative punishment (the loss of something that is desirable). For example, for the unwanted behavior of texting while driving, a positive punishment is a traffic ticket for texting while driving. A negative punishment is losing one's driver's license for repeated texting while driving.

### Purposes of SOCMRKT

The purpose of SOCMRKT is the focus in this section. The overall purpose of SOCMRKT is to improve the quality of health in the lives of the people in the community (Wymer, 2015). Carvalho and Mazzon (2015) recognize the impact SOCMRKT has on humans being able to reach their full potential. Carvalho and Mazzon emphasize the importance of preventing and treating illnesses in relation to promoting well-being (2015). SOCMRKT is one strategy that advanced practice nurses can think and act upstream in population health. Health promotion and disease prevention messages tailored to a specific population are inexpensive methods of delivering public health information to communities.

A great deal of healthcare dollars involves the use of money thrown downstream, which means money spent to treat health conditions that already exist. The notion of spending money upstream in population health is the idea of preventing health concerns before occurring, which has a better return on the investment (Mohan & Patrick-Mohan, 2008; Nies & McEwen, 2015). Cecchini *et al.* (2010) found that by using a multi-intervention strategy, a significant number of chronic diseases can be prevented, and this saves the cost of treating the chronic diseases. Data collection included the countries of Brazil, China, England, India, Mexico, Russia, and South Africa, to study predictive cost effectiveness. Specifically, Cecchini *et al.* (2010) reported for a cost of 80 cents per person in Russia for a SOCMRKT media campaign, one case of ischemic heart disease can be prevented for every 230 Russians. Therefore, the upstream intervention of SOCMRKT is cost effective.

One excellent point made by Mohan and Patrick-Mohan (2008) is that in order to think and act upstream in public health, skills such as partnering with the community, organizing with the community, political advocacy, interprofessional collaboration, team building, and public speaking are necessary. Specific to SOCMRKT, advanced practice nurses must be able to implement these skills to improve population health.

## Ethical Considerations with SOCMRKT

There are many ethical considerations for SOCMRKT. Over the past several decades, the use of SOCMRKT in population health has increased (Coles, 2015; Threatt, 2009). In addition, ethical issues related to SOCMRKT of health messages have drawn attention (Guttman & Salmon, 2004). From target audience selection (known as audience segmentation) to persuasive tactics, which may include guilt and fear (Guttman & Salmon, 2004) there are ethical concerns at every step of the SOCMRKT program planning and implementation.

### *Audience Segmentation*
Audience segmentation in population health SOCMRKT refers to the grouping of populations based on their current behavior patterns (Grier & Bryant, 2005). Audience segmentation is one method used to narrow the SOCMRKT project when only so many funds are available (Slater, Kelly, & Thackeray, 2006). Simply put, it costs less money to target an audience of 1,000 people as opposed to 100,000 people. Social marketers often are faced with making decisions about focusing on a narrow aggregate and often select the highest risk persons. For example, it would be great to focus on the entire population to deliver tobacco prevention messages, but this is not feasible based on money available. This creates an ethical dilemma for the social marketer in population health. The ideal course of action is to reach all persons with the health message, but fiscal limitations prohibit this action. Thus, fiscal responsibility versus delivering healthy messages to all becomes a dilemma. Social equity is a major principle of public health (Guttman & Salmon, 2004). In keeping with a utilitarian approach, the social marketer selects the target audience that can benefit the greatest number of people (Newton, J. D., Newton, F. J., Turk, & Ewing, 2013).

### *Guilt and Fear*
Should gruesome images be included in SOCMRKT populations to signal importance, reality, and capture attention? Startling and morbid images may be perceived by some audiences as gory turn-offs that are disturbing and counterproductive for the message (Guttman & Salmon,

2004). While others may view the images as important reminders intended to deliver messages about health and safety. Advanced practice nurses should review the research literature regarding the use of shock tactics in SOCMRKT for intended populations. Additionally, ethical checks with the agency's SOCMRKT policy should be included in every SOCMRKT campaign plan.

*Professional Boundaries*

Advanced practice registered nurses (APRNs) should be very careful to maintain professional boundaries. Social networking with patients or clients, as well as their family members, on programs such as Facebook or Twitter, would be inappropriate on the nurse's personal accounts. It could be perceived as a breach of confidentiality based on the communications. At the very least, it crosses the line of the professional relationship for the APRN. APRNs should know their employer's policy about socializing with patients/families.

An agency or facility may have a social networking account. Peck (2014) reported that social media strongly influences consumers when selecting a hospital. So, it is common for an agency to have a social media account. This creates the need for an agency or facility policy to make the boundaries clear to employees. APRNs may be assigned to post health messages using the software. The agency or facility should include information in the SOCMRKT policy about what is appropriate for posting and communication.

*Legitimate or Illegitimate Messages*

Another ethical area is the legitimacy of social marketing messages. Most SOCMRKT messages in population health are legitimate health messages crafted and marketed by a reputable agency or facility. However, there are some illegitimate SOCMRKT messages that are fraudulent with the intention of seeking resources, such as money from victims. APRNs should be aware of any fraudulent health schemes in their practice area so they can respond to patients and families' questions. Olivier, Burls, Fenge, and Brown (2015) published an article about mass marketing fraud in which they state vulnerable adults are often targeted populations. The authors warn against how convincing the scammers can be and that they often use social media to reach their victims. Unauthorized images, endorsements, false results, and inaccurate data are often used to persuade the victim into giving money or purchasing a product. The use of a framework to test suspicious social media for legitimacy is recommended (Bhat & Abulaish, 2013). The U.S. Health and Human Services (2013) has a resource for finding quality resources in e-Health that can also be applied to SOCMRKT to test for accurate and trustworthy information at https://www.healthit.gov/patients-families/find-quality-resources.

All healthcare agencies and facilities that use SOCMRKT should have an organizational policy that includes ethical statements on the 8 Ps of SOCMRKT in population health. The agency SOCMRKT policy will provide guidance for the agency and employees (including the APRN) to keep the SOCMRKT campaigns consistent with the organization's mission and values. Practitioners using social marketing must consider these ethical areas when planning a social marketing plan. Additionally, the social marketing plan should be consistent with the overall agency mission and values. A sample SOCMRKT policy written and adapted by the Centers for Disease Control and Prevention (2015) is found at https://www.cdc.gov/socialmedia/tools/guidelines/pdf/social-media-policy.pdf. This resource provides an example for any advance practice nurse that works at a facility that has not yet established a SOCMRKT policy.

## The Ps of Social Marketing (SOCMRKT)

Eight Ps of SOCMRKT serve as the conceptual framework. The traditional four Ps of marketing include product, price, placement, and promotion. Four additional SOCMRKT Ps include publics, partnership, policy, and purse strings (Sharma, 2017). The intended persons for SOCMRKT are the population, subpopulation, or aggregate, depending on the program and purpose. For the purposes of this section, the term population is used.

1.  The *product* is developed in program planning. Think of the product as the behavior to change in a specific population (Longest, 2015). For population health SOCMRKT, an example is to promote breastfeeding. Other examples of the product, or behavior to change, is the use of helmets while riding bikes or diabetes care.

    Firestone, Rowe, Modi, and Sievers (2017) completed a systemic review of the effectiveness of social marketing that includes 125 studies. Some studies focused on behavior change and some on health outcomes of SOCMRKT. The projects that had positive results included audience insights. The results of this systemic review support knowing the specific population and including the population specifics in the SOCMRKT plan.

2. It is also important to consider the price, which considers money, human resources, time, and effort (Doyle *et al.*, 2010). The target population surrenders something when they adopt the new behavior (Longest, 2015). Perhaps instead of drinking soda pop, drinking water is adopted for a healthier behavior. The price paid is drinking soda pop. Small, slow, steady changes may be easier prices to pay and, therefore, more successful. For example, a focused, small SOCMRKT message, such as walking for 30 minutes per day with the price being 30 minutes of time, is a much more palatable price than to change one's complete diet and add one hour of physical activity per day. It is important for advanced practice nurses to recognize and incorporate the concept of price in SOCMRKT.

3. The *place* refers to where the product is distributed. Examples are billboards, television, newspapers, schools, churches, community centers, and online (Weinreich, 2011). The place for SOCMRKT is tailor made for the targeted population. For example, when the desired population is women in the region or state, television commercials with health messages shown during television shows watched by female dominated audiences speaks to matching the place to the targeted population.

4. *Promotion* is similar to place, but promotion includes how to keep interest in the product so consumers will purchase the product (Doyle *et al.*, 2010; Weinreich, 2011). The medium for the SOCMRKT refers to the promotion. Again, the promotion is wrought to the targeted population. Some examples include health fairs, television commercials, radio advertisements, newspaper advertisements, Facebook, Twitter, billboards, press releases, posters, billboards, state fair booths, and contests. Incentives may build long-term interest in the product. For example: a Minnesota State Parks program promoted physical activity (and park use) by a year-long point game for walking, hiking, and boating at state parks to celebrate the Minnesota's State Parks and Trails 125 years' anniversary. Prizes include a 125 sticker and bragging rights (Minnesota Department of Natural Resources, 2016). The 2016 program was titled *125 Miles by Bike, Boot or Boat*, and was designed to keep interest in physical activity at Minnesota parks for the duration of one year.

5. The targeted population and their secondary population are *publics*. The primary population means the targeted population, while the secondary population refers to the friends and family of the primary population (Sharma, 2017; Weinreich, 2011). Nurses are familiar with knowing their client, and that is what publics require. To illustrate the publics, assume the primary population is adolescents. The developmental considerations are critical aspects to include when describing the publics. The communication styles and behaviors of adolescents are quite different from elderly persons. The social marketing plan that targets the adolescent population is unique for the target population. A population health nurse that uses SOCMRKT to decrease soda pop consumption in teenagers and increase water consumption, designs it with the teenagers in mind. Adults refrain from telling the teenagers that water is a healthier choice than soda pop. Instead, posters promoting water consumption and contests in high schools to sample and vote for favorite bottled and flavored waters are held. Peer teenagers lead the water sampling and voting contests in high schools. Students can vote online for their favorite bottled water. The secondary population in this example is the parents of the teenagers who receive a letter, as well as notification in the school newsletter, about the water promotion activities in high schools. The parents (secondary population) are included in the communication about the project and can provide support for the teenager at home, such as purchasing their favorite bottled water.

   Now consider that a population health nurse wants to promote water drinking in the elderly population. The approach is tailor made for the elderly primary population. Newspaper advertisements, in addition to posters and flyers at the Senior Citizen Center and local healthcare clinic, are avenues to communicate drinking extra water. Tap water and iced tap water may be the most successful message communicated to the elderly population. Having elderly vote online for their favorite bottled water may not be an effective option with this population. The secondary population is the friends and family of the elderly. Messages for this population might include checking with any elderly family member or neighbor to encourage water consumption. Informational flyers may be sent to the elderly or circulated at the Senior Citizen Center, local pharmacy, local health clinics, and their family members as well. This is an example of a major difference between SOCMRKT and social media.

6. The next P is *Partnership* with the community. Partnerships with the community, other healthcare providers, and agencies benefit success by communicating with the stakeholders (Doyle *et al.*, 2010). Additionally, sharing resources for the social marketing project is also beneficial. According to the American Nurses Association (2013), collaborating with stakeholders is desirable to improve the quality of health in populations. Earlier in this chapter, Mohan and Patrick-Mohan (2008) presented ideas related to thinking and acting upstream in public health (skills such as partnering with the community, etc.). Partnership with the community is an important aspect of SOCMRKT that is much deeper than a description of the people; it is the development of understanding and insight about the population (Lefebvre, 2013). Advanced practice nurses who develop partnerships with stakeholders will increase the likelihood of successful SOCMRKT.

7. Policy is an important element of health programs and SOCMRKT. It is best when policy and health program are consistent. Policy is the creation of an atmosphere that will continue the intended change. For example, to improve the nutritional health of public school lunches, the creation of government policies that require standards in lunches for federal subsidies exist (United States Department of Agriculture, 2016). Examples may be health policy or legislative. Consider the political climate for the intended health program. For example, marketing birth control in a high school would be controversial at best. However, marketing and providing condoms in a public university setting would probably not be as controversial. The advanced practice nurse must consider the perceptions of the population when planning a social marketing project.

8. The amount of money available for a SOCMRKT program is termed *purse strings*. Inquire about any agency monies available in the budget to fund the project. What grants are possible options to request monies? The advanced practice nurse should network with other agencies to find information about grants. Some agencies have grant officers that may be aware of leads for grant funding. Another opportunity is to consider other agencies and businesses that are stakeholders in the project and may donate monies. For example, businesses that sell breast pumps may have an interest in funding projects that promote breastfeeding. Have an idea of how

much money is wanted to request before talking to agencies and businesses, as this is a good question to anticipate.

## Examples of SOCMRKT Projects

Depicted in this section are examples of SOCMRKT projects. A variety of overall topics related to products help provide samples that may provoke ideas or how one can plan a SOCMRKT campaign. The examples may also clarify the aspects of SOCMRKT. Lilley explains that data is available about health practices of communities by zip code (2008). The data available in public healthcare point to where smokers live. This provides valuable information about where to target SOC-MRKT to improve health behaviors. SOCMRKT is an intervention to prevent tobacco use (Lilley, 2008). While Lilley (2008) promotes the use of data to target specific behaviors in populations, Diehr *et al.* (2011) narrow their work on when the most impact for tobacco prevention can net. Nonsmokers were the focus in a primary and secondary prevention project to study when to use SOCMRKT for the maximal effect for tobacco prevention (Diehr *et al.*, 2011). Selected were the segmented population and people in the precontemplation stage of the transtheoretical model. Nonsmoking life expectancy was the measure. Through studying hypothetical populations, Diehr *et al.* (2011) found the greatest impact to prevent tobacco use is by using SOCMRKT interventions to never-have-smoked populations. These results help advanced practice nurses know at what stage SOCMRKT to prevent tobacco use will have the greatest success.

In nursing, the implementation of SOCMRKT has yet to be fully realized (Knibbs & Leeseberg Stamler, 2009). Although some nurses are engaging in social marketing to improve population health outcomes, not all nurses use the SOCMRKT strategy. Many nurses are not knowledgeable about SOCMRKT and lack the skills to implement SOC-MRKT. Baccalaureate and higher education levels in nursing include the specialty of population health courses in nursing programs. Further, a role of the advanced practice nurse who precepts and mentors other nurses is to include experiences with interdisciplinary SOCMRKT interventions.

Beth Mattey, a school nurse at Mt. Pleasant High School in Wilmington, DE, teamed up with students and school officials to use social marketing to prevent tobacco use in the adolescent population (Mattey, 2003). The program was called Knights Against Tobacco and was led by fellow peers. The social marketing medium was posters, multimedia, music, and interactive games. Mattey reports a decreased attitude of tobacco use acceptance at Mt. Pleasant High School after implementation of the social marketing program (2003).

Konradi and DeBruin (2003) implemented a SOCMRKT campaign to promote the use of Sexual Assault Nurse Examination (SANE) services on a college campus. Posters were placed in residential halls and public bathrooms that college students use. The posters included information about SANE services and stressed encouraging others to use SANE services. Participants completed a survey. Participants reported an increase in seeing the SANE messages after two interventions (Konradi & DeBruin, 2003). Women reported more recognition of the SANE services poster messages than men did. Konradi and DeBruin recommend that future campaigns have a stronger focus on reaching males (2003). Strategically placed posters are a strategy to reach populations.

### Outcomes of SOCMRKT

The fundamental question, "Does SOCMRKT work with Population Health?" is the central topic in this section. When contemplating the use of social marketing, the advanced practice nurse must inquire about the effectiveness of SOCMRKT. Additionally, the advanced practice nurse should consider what variables might affect the outcomes of SOCMRKT in population health. Earlier, this chapter explores select social marketing project. Next, the outcomes of SOCMRKT are the emphasis.

*Loving Arms* is a program that is part of Women, Infant, and Children (WIC) to promote breastfeeding (Mitra, Khourty, Carothers, & Foretich, 2003). In Mississippi, SOCMRKT to increase public awareness was used in the form of a video that was shown to women early in pregnancy to promote breastfeeding. Mitra *et al.* (2003) reported the video was effective in promoting breastfeeding. In a similar social marketing program of *Loving Arms* in Iowa, the media campaign included newspaper advertisements, radio advertisements, television commercials, and outdoor billboards (Szcodronski, Dobson, Losch, & Bryant, 2002). The breastfeeding rates were higher in the hospital after birth and at 6 months in mothers in the WIC program (Szcodronski *et al.*, 2002). Additionally, the researchers reported that survey results of participants included a more favorable attitude of breastfeeding in the WIC *Loving Arms* program (Szcodronski *et al.*, 2002). The effectiveness of social marketing in these projects is positive and consistent.

Violence prevention was studied using a collaboration among the National Center for Injury Prevention and Control (NCIPC) and a research marketing communications and management firm to reframe perceptions of violence prevention and injury (Austin, Mitchko, Freeman, Kirby, & Milne, 2009). The team developed short messages to communicate to audiences. The messages were "Keeping people injury free makes communities safer," "When we prevent injuries, we help America thrive," and "We'll live longer, and be stronger, in a world without injuries" (Austin *et al.*, 2009, p. 43–44). Data was collected using focus groups and interviews with primary (the targeted population) and secondary (friends and family of the targeted population) audiences about the health messages. Participants reported favorable perceptions of the messages (Austin *et al.*, 2009). Quality made social marketing messages have both the primary and secondary audiences in mind.

A study of health outcomes from condom social marketing reported resistance from the church related to condom use (Knerr, 2011) in a review of the literature reported in 2001, 2007, and 2010. Access to condoms was improved after SOCMRKT, but more so in men than women, and more in urban dwellers than rural dwellers (Knerr, 2011). Further, similar SOCMRKT campaigns should key in on target populations to decrease the divide in gender and urban versus rural settings for greater success. A condom SOCMRKT campaign in Cameroon that targeted youth aged 15–24 years, resulted in an increased use in condoms for females and males (Meekers, Agha, & Klein, 2005). As discussed earlier in this chapter, some SOCMRKT campaigns may cause concern in secondary populations (friends and family), such as when targeting 15-year-olds with condom messages. The buy-in of the secondary population may sway the success of the project. When nurses and teams use focus groups and interviews with the stakeholders while planning a SOCMRKT campaign, these concerns will often emerge, as well as ideas for how to incorporate the secondary population's concerns in the project.

The *Whatcha doing?* SOCMRKT campaign is aimed at increasing fruit and vegetable consumption and physical activity in Nebraska adolescents at public high schools (Struthers & Wang, 2016). Data were collected over six years in the adolescent population and the outcomes were an increased amount of physical activity and fruit consumption. The amount of vegetable consumption and the campaign attitude was not statistically significant (Struthers & Wang, 2016). Elements of the *Whatcha doing?* campaign included a fun and interactive campaign. Buzz agents were teenagers (stakeholders) involved in the campaign who owned the campaign (instead of adults) (Struthers & Wang, 2016). This was a strong use of empowering partnership based on knowing the target population of adolescents.

A majority of SOCMRKT campaigns with published research have positive outcomes. There are some limitations or considerations that nurses should consider. Best practices for successful SOCMRKT campaigns are to plan according to the 8 Ps. The 8 Ps of SOCMRKT provide guidance for advanced practice nurses to develop a successful SOCMRKT campaign.

**Specific Dynamics for the Advanced Practice Nurse: Think 8 Ps**

Incorporation of the 8 Ps of SOCMRKT by advanced practice nurses when planning and implementing a social marketing program cannot be stressed enough. Ideas for how a nurse can "Think 8 Ps" are further addressed in this section in relation to the nurse specific dynamic. The nurse is at a great advantage with advanced assessment skills, education, and experience in providing cultural care. Assessment of the target population is a critical aspect of SOCMRKT. This is a strength of nurses. Talking to stakeholders in the targeted population using focus groups, interviews, telephone interviews, and surveys, provide valuable information about their knowledge levels, attitudes, values, beliefs, behaviors, and practices (Keller *et al.*, 2004). Assessment of the usual communication practices of the population is also valuable information. For example, does the population use online sources to receive their health information? Are they connected to Facebook, Twitter, and other electronic media? What are the literacy levels and preferred language of the population? The answers to these questions can help design a customized SOCMRKT plan. After a portrayal of the intended population, the APN can identify and describe the secondary population. How should the family and friends of the primary population receive communications about the SOCMRKT campaign? Consider what might help the secondary population support the primary population. Remember the human element. This is an easy step for nurses, since they have such trusting relationships with their clients. A successful SOCMRKT campaign reaches people by touching them.

Determining the product or health message is a vital step for nurses to explore with stakeholders. The health message should be narrowed and incorporate the knowledge levels, attitudes, values, beliefs, behaviors, and practices of the target population (Keller *et al.*, 2004). Start with determining goals, objectives, and then a catchy health message statement are important activities for nurses. It is wise to show a pilot group from the population the message and seek their response. This can be helpful in refining the message or knowing the intended response was heard in the pilot group.

Direct the place (where) and promotion (how) to fit the target population. For example, when the target population is young to middle-aged females, what is the best way to reach this population? For example, if they are mothers, it may be at activities related to their children. Do they read their children's school newsletter? Are they on Facebook? Where do they routinely interact in the community? What television shows do they watch? By now, the importance of knowing the population is clear and is a critical aspect to consider for the best program outcomes.

Population health nurses are skillful at finding resources. When the agency budget does not include monies for SOCMRKT projects, there are some ideas that nurses can employ. By partnering with others, this increases the number of resources available for access. Therefore, perhaps nursing does not have monies for SOCMRKT projects, but another department or agency might. APNs should network and explore these options with partners. Additionally, some employers may provide resources to implement projects that affect employee wellness, such as pay for the printing of posters or advertisement. Think about who will gain from the health message that is marketed, because this may sponsor or open some resources for use in the project. For example, if the message is to improve dental health, some dentists, dental colleges, or a dental association may provide resources for the project. Be creative and use networking skills to find resources to add to the purse strings.

Skipping any of the planning items for the SOCMRKT campaign may lessen the effectiveness of the product. Advanced practice nurses should be sure to include all 8 Ps of social marketing in population health to ensure the greatest change of success. Collaborating with stakeholders, including other health professionals, are excellent resources to help with the project.

### Nursing and Social Marketing Worksheet

The following worksheet is a great resource for starting a SOCMRKT project using the 8 Ps of SOCMRKT (Sharma, 2017; Weinreich, 2011). Nurses can use the worksheet to write out some ideas or notes as a starting point for planning a SOCMRKT project. This is especially helpful before meeting with stakeholders to discuss ideas.

*TABLE 17.1.  8 Ps of Social Marketing in Population Health.*

| 8 Ps of Social Marketing | Prompts | Ideas/Notes |
|---|---|---|
| Product | What is the intended health behavior change to be adopted by the target population? | |
| Price | What will the target population give up for the behavior change? | |
| Place | Place and promotion are closely related, but think of place as where. What place will you use to deliver the health message? Consider the internet, schools, grocery store, community center, church, park, etc. | |
| Promotion | How will you communicate the health message to the population? Consider advertisements, letters, flyers, health fairs | |
| Publics | Identify and describe the primary population and the secondary population. Consider their unique culture of communication, their values and beliefs, literacy and health literacy levels, socioeconomic status, support systems, ethnicity, developmental respects, etc. | |
| Partnerships | Make a list of the stakeholders that have interest in the project. Be sure to communicate with the stakeholders in the planning, implementation, and evaluation of social marketing. | |
| Policy | What policy supports the project you are planning? | |
| Purse strings | How will the project be funded? Is there money in the budget to use? What grant or donation could be requested? What organization/ business has an interest in the project? | |

## Conclusion

SOCMRKT is a valuable skill and tool for the advanced practice nurse to implement to improve the quality of health in populations. The purpose of SOCMRKT in population health is to deliver health messages aimed at improving the quality of health. Advanced practice nurses should use a theoretical foundation that fits the specific SOCMRKT campaign and targeted population. The 8 Ps of SOCMRKT are helpful guides to planning the SOCMRKT campaign. The advanced practice population health nurse draws upon nursing experiences with clients that include a unique understanding of the human touch and brings this to SOCMRKT campaigns.

## Tool Kit and Resources

*Social Marketing Case Study 1 Resources*
*(Resource Author, Title, Description, and Website Address)*

Centers for Disease Control and Prevention, Suicide and Self Inflicted Injury: This resource has United States (U.S.) suicide and self-inflicted injury statistics. http://www.cdc.gov/nchs/fastats/suicide.htm

Governing the States and Localities, State Suicide Rates: Suicide rates reported by states are reported at this source. http://www.governing.com/gov-data/health/state-suicide-rates-total-deaths-statistics.html

American Foundation for Suicide Prevention, Suicide Statistics: This resource reports suicide rates and facts. Data is stated by age, race/ethnicity, and suicide methods in the United States. Suicide attempts/self-injury statistics are included. https://afsp.org/about-suicide/suicide-statistics/

National Institute of Mental Health, Suicide Statistics: This resource provides suicide data in comparison to other causes of death and displays suicide data over time. http://www.nimh.nih.gov/health/statistics/suicide/index.shtml

The Ohio State University, Youth Suicide Rates in Rural Areas: This resource discusses the difference in youth suicide rates and methods in urban versus rural areas. https://news.osu.edu/news/2015/03/09/youth-suicide-rate/

American Association of Suicidology, National Suicide Statistics: This resource houses some suicide data broken down by other characteristics, such as profession and sexual orientation. http://www.suicidology.org/resources/facts-statistics

## Tool Kit—SOCMRKT Quality Improvement Resources

This section includes recommended resources about SOCMRKT. The resources are great references but also have some good examples that can stimulate ideas.

*Social Marketing Quality Improvement Resources*
American Journal of Public Health Video: The Laugh Model: Reframing and Rebranding Public Health Through Social Media: This fantastic video resource introduces the Laugh Model to reframe

and rebrand public health messages. https://www.youtube.com/
watch?v=JCuW6lY3PFw

Centers for Disease Control and Prevention: Gateway to Health Communication & SOCMRKT Practice: This is an excellent website. It
provides information about researching, planning, and evaluating
SOCMRKT. It includes research summaries, journals and reports,
nonprofit organizations and research centers, research and data tools,
and evaluation resources. http://www.cdc.gov/healthcommunication/research/

Chuck Malcomson at Hubspot Blog: Brilliant Healthcare SOCMRKT:
This website is a blog, but it describes 8 examples of excellent
healthcare SOCMRKT that might offer some ideas or stimulate some
creativity for a SOCMRKT project. http://blog.hubspot.com/marketing/brilliant-healthcare-marketing#sm.00196829z12t1dewxcd1jlgu
x13j2

Katie James: Evaluation of a SOCMRKT Campaign: This is the dissertation of Katie James published in the digital commons at the University of Nebraska. Katie studied a SOCMRKT program to prevent
foodborne illness that she called 4 Day Throw Away. She has some
great ideas in her dissertation. http://digitalcommons.unl.edu/cgi/
viewcontent.cgi?article=1032&context=nutritiondiss

Larry Hershfield and Jim MIntz: Tools of Change: This website provides resources for social marketers, including a planning guide, information about the 4 Ps, tools of change, and case studies. http://
www.toolsofchange.com/en/programs/social-marketers/

Substance Abuse and Mental Health Services Administration: Ten
Steps for Developing a Social Marketing Campaign: This resource
includes helpful steps for implementing a SOCMRKT project. http://
www.samhsa.gov/capt/tools-learning-resources/developing-social-
marketing-campaign

The Community Tool Box at the University of Kansas: Chapter 13 Implementing SOCMRKT: This is Chapter 13 of a Creative Commons
textbook that provides a rich resource of information about how to
implement SOCMRKT. http://ctb.ku.edu/en/implement-social-marketing-effort

The Community Tool Box at the University of Kansas: Chapter 2 Conducting a SOCMRKT Campaign: This is Chapter 2 of a Creative
Commons textbook that does an outstanding job explaining the ins
and outs of a SOCMRKT campaign. There are a number of Chapters,

but we choose our favorites to include in the resources. Should you be interested, check out any of the other Chapters of interest. http://ctb.ku.edu/en/table-of-contents/sustain/social-marketing/conduct-campaign/main

W. Douglas Evans (2006): How SOCMRKT in Healthcare Works at National Institutes of Health: This is an informative resource about SOCMRKT in healthcare and includes information about the SOCMRKT wheel. http://www.ncbi.nlm.nih.gov/pmc/articles/PMC1463924/

## Tool Kit Social Media Resources

This section includes social media that for use with SOCMRKT plans.

Instagram is an online social network in which you share pictures with those in your network. Available at https://www.instagram.com/

Vimeo is an online video sharing network. Available at https://vimeo.com/

Facebook is an online social network for sharing of messages, photos, and videos. Available at https://www.facebook.com/

You tube is an online video network where videos can be shared with friends, family, and the world. Available at https://www.youtube.com/

Flickr is an online photo organization and sharing media. Available at https://www.flickr.com

Babbly is an online sharing social media system where you can share content. Available at http://babbly.com/

Twitter is an online social media-sharing network. Available at https://twitter.com/

Snapchat is an online messaging that sends images. Available at https://www.snapchat.com/

Periscope is a social media that allows live video streaming. Available at https://www.periscope.tv/

Statistica includes consumer survey results. For example, the preferred social media sites for teenagers and young adults are found at http://www.statista.com/statistics/199242/social-media-and-networking-sites-used-by-us-teenagers/

The reliability of this data is unknown. Available at https://www.statista.com/

*Discussion Questions*

Are all the health messages information you read on social media accurate? How would you know if the information is credible or not? How would the average citizen know if the information is credible or not? How might inaccurate social media messages mislead people? Explain two ethical dilemmas of social marketing that includes misleading health information?

Explain the similarities and differences between SOCMRKT and social media, including two examples of each.

Compare and contrast SOCMRKT methods for the two target audiences of teenagers and the elderly. What is one source of data that can be used to know how to reach your population with social media?

You are working as an APRN in a Family Health Clinic. A colleague of yours at another agency tells you that he/she recently developed a SOCMRKT campaign to promote immunizations in infants to age 19 years. Your colleague asks you to look over the campaign plan and provide feedback. Describe the elements you will check as you evaluate the plan.

You are working as an APRN in Acute Care. One area identified for quality improvement is better handwashing among the interprofessional healthcare team. You decide to use a social marketing campaign in the workplace as an intervention. Using the 8Ps as your guide, explain how you will plan for this campaign.

Brainstorm creative ways of reaching a population of adult Deaf women with health education messages about self-breast exams and routine mammography. How might you reach this population? What would you do to find out more information about this population?

## Case Study 1

Rick, a Psychiatric Mental Health Nurse Practitioner has noted a trend in the patients/families that he is seeing in the local clinic. Since suicide is a common concern that Rick is seeing in his practice, he contacts Suzie, a colleague from school who works at the public health department, to discuss this concern in the community. The conversation stimulates further discussion between Rick and Suzie.

Together, Rick and Suzie partner to develop a SOCMRKT intervention plan. Rick and Suzie have asked you to work with them to develop a SOCMRKT intervention plan about suicide in your community.

Describe the rates of suicide in your community.

Does any specific aggregate have higher numbers of suicide (age, gender, rural, city, etc.)? (Write approximately one paragraph)

Write a one-paragraph summary of your target population or the public (the 5th P in social marketing according to Sharma, 2017).

State in one or two sentences what the product or intended health behavior outcome is for the SOCMRKT project.

1. Identify possible resources in your community related to suicide.
2. Identify the health message you want to communicate in the SOC-MRKT plan.
3. Describe the place and promotion (where and how) you will communicate the health message to the targeted population.

## Case Study 2

You are working in the local public health department as an Advanced Practice Nurse Leader. You are in charge of leading an interdisciplinary SOCMRKT campaign for the public health department. There is only enough money in the budget for one major SOCMRKT campaign in this year.

- How will you determine the topic and audience for the SOCMRKT campaign?
- State the product and the public.
- Once you determine the topic and primary and secondary population, how will you communicate with the stakeholders to develop partnerships?
- What policies relate to the product and/or publics?

## Case Study 3

Use the same product and target population used for case study one or two for this activity. Write a catchy, short message (one short sentence or less) that you will use in social marketing. Think through the values and beliefs of the population related to the product when you write the message. It might be helpful to review some previous examples of messages in this chapter. Another example to stimulate ideas is the Take Care of Your Heart and Know Your Numbers! (Mayo Clinic, 2014) campaign, which encouraged publics to have their blood pressure checked.

## Case Study 4

You are an Advanced Practice Registered Nurse in a local health promotion agency that is focused on promoting healthy lifestyles in children and families. You have been tasked with planning a SOCMRKT campaign, but have a limited budget to use for the project. Your supervisor tells you that you will need to use audience segmentation to narrow the target population. What ethical principle(s) will you use to make decisions about the target population for the project?

Describe the ethical dilemma involved.

## References

Affinito, L. & Mack, J. (2016). *Socialize your patient engagement strategy: How social media and mobile apps can boost health outcomes.* Farnham, GB: Routledge.

American Nurses Association. (2013). Scope and standards of practice: Public health nursing. (2nd ed.). Silver Spring, MD: American Nurses Association.

Austin, L., Mitchko, J., Freeman, C., Kirby, S., & Milne, J. (2009). Using framing theory to unite the field of injury and violence prevention and response: Adding power to our voices. *SOCMRKT Quarterly, 15*(sup1), 36–54. doi:10.1080/15245000902962623

Carvalho, H. C. & Mazzon, J. A. (2015). A better life is possible: The ultimate purpose of SOCMRKT. *Journal of Social Marketing, 5*(2), 169–186. doi:10.1108/JSOCM-05-2014-0029

Bhat, S. & Abulaish, M. (2013). Community-based features for identifying spammers in online social networks. Paper presented at 100–107. doi:10.1145/2492517.2492567

Cecchini, M., Sassi, F., Lauer, J. A., Lee, Y. Y., Guajardo-Barron, V., & Chisholm, D. (2010). Chronic diseases: Chronic diseases and development 3: Tackling of unhealthy diets, physical inactivity, and obesity: Health effects and cost-effectiveness. *The Lancet, 376*(9754), 1775–1784.

Centers for Disease Control and Prevention. (2015). CDC Enterprise Social Media Policy. Retrieved from https://www.cdc.gov/socialmedia/tools/guidelines/pdf/social-media-policy.pdf

Coles, L. (2015). *Marketing with social media: 10 easy steps to success for business.* Queensland, Australia: Wiley.

Diehr, P., Hannon, P., Pizacani, B., Forehand, M., Meischke, H., Curry, S., & Harris, J. (2011). SOCMRKT, stages of change, and public health smoking interventions. *Health Education & Behavior, 38*(2), 123–131. doi:10.1177/1090198110369056

Doyle, E. I., Ward, S. E., & Oomen-Early, J. (2010). *The process of community health education and promotion.* Mountain View, CA: Mayfield Publishing Company.

Eggleston, E. M. & Weitzman, E. R. (2014). Innovative uses of electronic health records and social media for public health surveillance. *Current Diabetes Reports, 14*(3), 1. doi:10.1007/s11892-013-0468-7

Eke, P. I. (2011). Using social media for research and public health surveillance. *Journal of Dental Research, 90*(9), 1045–1046. doi:10.1177/0022034511415277

Evans, W. D. (2006). How SOCMRKT works in health care. *BMJ, 332*(7551), 1207–1210. doi: 10.1136/bmj.332.7551.1207-a

Firestone, R., Rowe, C. J., Modi, S. N., & Sievers, D. (2017). The effectiveness of social marketing in global health: A systematic review. *Health Policy Plan, 32*(1), 110–124. doi: 10.1093/heapol/czw088

Fung, I. C., Tse, Z. T. H., & Fu, K. (2015). The use of social media in public health surveillance. *Western Pacific Surveillance and Response Journal: WPSAR, 6*(2), 3–6. doi:10.5365/wpsar.2015.6.1.019

Gilbert, G. G., Sawyer, R. G., & McNeill, E. B. (2015). *Health education: Creating strategies for school and community health.* (4th ed.). Burlington, MA: Jones and Bartlett Learning.

Goldman, K. D. (2003). SOCMRKT concepts. In R. J. Bensley & J. Brooking-Fisher (eds.). *Community health education methods*, (pp. 83–105). Sudbury, MA: Jones and Bartlett.

Greenwood, S., Perrin, A., & Duggan, M. (2016). Social media update 2016. *Pew Research Center.* Retrieved from http://www.pewinternet.org/2016/11/11/social-media-update-2016/

Grier, S. & Bryant, C. A. (2005). Social marketing in public health. *Annual Review of Public Health, 26*(1), 319–339. doi:10.1146/annurev.publhealth.26.021304.144610

Guttman, N. & Salmon, C. T. (2004). Guilt, fear, stigma and knowledge gaps: Ethical issues in public health communication interventions. *Bioethics, 18*(6), 531–552. doi:10.1111/j.1467-8519.2004.00415.x

Harvey, P. D. (1999). *Let every child be wanted: How SOCMRKT is revolutionizing contraceptive care around the world.* Westport, CT: Auburn House.

Hastings, G., Angus, K., & Bryant, C. A. (2011). The sage handbook of SOCMRKT. Los Angeles, CA: Sage Publications.

Haustein, S., Peters, I., Sugimoto, C. R., Thelwall, M., & Larivière, V. (2014). Tweeting biomedicine: An analysis of tweets and citations in the biomedical literature. *Journal of the Association for Information Science and Technology, 65*(4), 656–669. doi:10.1002/asi.23101

Huesch, M. D., Galstyan, A., Ong, M. K., & Doctor, J. N. (2016). Using social media, online social networks, and internet search as platforms for public health interventions: A pilot study. *Health Services Research, 51*(3), 1273–1290. doi:10.1111/1475-6773.12496

Kass-Hout, T. A. & Alhinnawi, H. (2013). Social media in public health. *British Medical Bulletin, 108*(1), 5–24. doi:10.1093/bmb/ldt028

Keller, L. O., Strohschein, S. Lia-Hoagberg, B., & Schaffer, M. A. (2004). Population-based public health interventions: practice-based and evidence-supported. Part I. *Public Health Nursing, 21*(5), 453–468. doi: 10.1111/j.0737-1209.2004.21509.x

Knerr, W. (2011). Does condom SOCMRKT improve health outcomes and increase usage and equitable access? *Reproductive Health Matters, 19*(37), 166–173. doi:10.1016/S0968-8080(11)37558-1

Knibbs, K. & Leeseberg Stamler, L. (2009). Exploring perceived enablers and barriers to SOCMRKT use in public health nursing. *SOCMRKT Quarterly, 15*(3), 100–112. doi:10.1080/15245000903151010

Konradi, A. & DeBruin, P. L. (2003). Using a social marketing approach to advertise sexual assault nurse examination (SANE) services to college students. *Journal of American College Health, 52*(1), 33–39. doi:10.1080/07448480309595721

Lefebvre, R. C. (2013). *SOCMRKT and social change: Strategies and tools for improving health, well-being, and the environment.* San Francisco, CA: Jossey-Bass.

Lilley, R. (2008). Nurses get a lead on SOCMRKT. Primary Health Care, 18(2), 12–13.

Lister, C., Royne, M., Payne, H. E., Cannon, B., Hanson, C., & Barnes, M. (2015). The laugh model: Reframing and rebranding public health through social media. *American Journal of Public Health, 105*(111), 2245–2251. doi: 10.2105/AJPH.2015.302669

Longest, B. B. (2015). *Health program management: From development through evaluation* (2nd ed.). San Francisco, CA: Jossey-Bass & Pfeiffer.

Luxton, D.D., June, J.D., & Fairall, J.M. (2012). Social media and suicide: A public health perspective. *American Journal of Public Health, 102 Suppl 2*(S2), S195–S200. doi:10.2105/AJPH.2011.300608

Mattey, E. A. (2003). Knights against tobacco: Teens lead the charge to prevent tobacco use among adolescents. *Pediatric Nursing, 29*(5), 390, 393.

Mayo Clinic. (2014). Take care of your heart and know your numbers! Retrieved from http://newsnetwork.mayoclinic.org/discussion/take-care-of-your-heart-and-know-your-numbers/

McCreanor, T., Lyons, A., Griffin, C., Goodwin, I., Moewaka Barnes, H., & Hutton, F. (2013). Youth drinking cultures, social networking and alcohol marketing: Implications for public health. *Critical Public Health, 23*(1), 110–120. doi:10.1080/09581 596.2012.748883

Meekers, D., Agha, S., & Klein, M. (2005). The impact on condom use of the "100% Jeune" SOCMRKT program in Cameroon. *Journal of Adolescent Health, 36*(6), 530–530. doi:10.1016/j.jadohealth.2004.10.012

Minnesota Department of Natural Resources. (2016). 125 miles by bike, boot, or boat. Retrieved from http://www.dnr.state.mn.us/125/125miles.html

Mitra, A. K., Khoury, A. J., Carothers, C., & Foretich, C. (2003). Evaluation of a comprehensive loving support program among state women, infants, and children (WIC) program breast-feeding coordinators. *Southern Medical Journal, 96*(2), 168–171. doi:10.1097/01.SMJ.0000053675.41623.15

Mohan, A. & Patrick-Mohan, C. (2008). Throw the money upstream: An alternative strategy to improve public health. *Nonprofit and Voluntary Sector Quarterly, 37*(1), 34S–43S. doi:10.1177/0899764007310532

Newton, J. D., Newton, F. J., Turk, T., & T. Ewing, M. (2013). Ethical evaluation of audience segmentation in social marketing. *European Journal of Marketing, 47*(9), 1421–1438. doi:10.1108/EJM-09-2011-0515

Nies, M. A., & McEwen, M. (2015). *Community/Public Health Nursing.* (6th ed.). St. Louis, MO: Elsevier.

Olivier, S., Burls, T., Fenge, L., & Brown, K. (2015). "Winning and losing": Vulnerability to mass marketing fraud. *The Journal of Adult Protection, 17*(6), 360–370. doi:10.1108/JAP-02-2015-0002

Peck, J. L. (2014). Social media in nursing education: responsible integration for meaningful use. *Journal of Nursing Education, 53*(3), 164–169. doi: 10.3928/01484834-20140219-03

Ramsay, M. (2011). Social media etiquette: A guide and checklist to the benefits and perils of social marketing. *Journal of Direct, Data and Digital Marketing Practice, 12*(4), 389.

Sharma, M. (2017). *Health education and health promotion.* (3rd ed.). Burlington, MA: Jones & Bartlett Learning.

Slater, M. D., Kelly, K. J., & Thackeray, R. (2006). Segmentation on a shoestring: Health audience segmentation in limited-budget and local social marketing interventions. *Health Promotion Practice, 7*(2), 170–173. doi:10.1177/1524839906286616

Struthers, A. & Wang, M. (2016). Buzz agents in a teen-driven SOCMRKT campaign: Positive campaign attitude leads to positive changes in health outcomes. *SOCMRKT Quarterly, 22*(3), 218–235. doi:10.1177/1524500416637052

Szcodronski, H., Dobson, B., Losch, M. E., & Bryant, C. (2002). Iowa's implementation of the WIC national breastfeeding promotion project: Loving support. Retrieved from http://www.orau.gov/cdcynergy/soc2web/Content/activeinformation/resources/SOC_WIC-Iowa_breastfeeding_report.pdf

Threatt, S. R. (2009). *Facebook and the ideal social marketplace: A study of the marketing benefits of social media practices.* (Order No. 1467532). Retrieved from ProQuest Dissertations & Theses Global. (304999249).

United States Department of Agriculture. (2016). National school lunch program. Retrieved from http://www.fns.usda.gov/nslp/national-school-lunch-program-nslp

US Health and Human Services. (2013). E-Health. Finding Quality Resources. Retrieved from https://www.healthit.gov/patients-families/find-quality-resources

Weinreich, N. K. (2011). *Hands-on social marketing: A step-by-step guide to designing change for good.* (2nd ed.). Thousand Oaks, CA: Sage Publications.

Wymer, W. W. (2015). *Innovations in SOCMRKT and public health communication: Improving the quality of life for individuals and communities.* Cham, Switzerland: Springer.

# Index